LET'S EAT RIGHT & EXERCISE

An Entertaining Senior Fitness Guide

SPYDER JOHNSON

SpyderJohnson.com

Let's Eat Right & Exercise – *An Entertaining Senior Fitness Guide*
Published by SpyderJohnson.com

Print ISBN 978-0-9899211-0-7
Ebook ISBN 978-0-9899211-5-2
Photos by David Steele (dsteelephoto.com)
Illustrations by Worldwide
Cover illustration by Victor Manuel Nieto
Cover design by Dar Albert, Wicked Smart Designs
Formatting by BB eBooks (bbebooksthailand.com)
This book is written by a 1957 geezer for geezers.

Publication Data
Johnson, Spyder
Let's eat right and exercise: an entertaining senior fitness guide /
Spyder Johnson
Fitness, senior / nutrition / weight loss / humor

"I'm growing older, but not up."

– *Jimmy Buffett*

To fellow baby boomers who have unselfishly given your time and energy for the benefit of others. You can get in shape!

"I ain't old, but I've been around a long time."

– *Delbert McClinton*

About the Author: SpyderJohnson.com offers personal trainer services and more.

About the Illustrators: Eight artists from around the world created the 57 illustrations in this book. It was a total pleasure working with and being surrounded by such talent, creativity and professionalism. I describe it as magical. We became friends during the process.

I can't give enough credit, for they added a whole new dimension to the book. I also have to give special thanks to my photographer, formatter and designer, as these are true arts. This world is full of incredible, mostly unrecognized artists. Contact me at spyderjohnson@outlook.com if you would like to use any of them for a project.

Much heartfelt thanks to Victor Manuel Nieto from Venezuela, Iulian Thomas from Romania, Moroccan from Morocco (who wishes to remain anonymous), Liri Bahar from Israel, Anouk de Vries from Finland, Ambrosius Yunias from Indonesia, Muhammad Taufiq Hidavath from Indonesia, and Angelo Quintero from Venezuela.

Contents

Introduction

Well, we've made it this far. I'm guessing if you're reading this book, you're in your so-called golden years like me. In other words, you're old. You're pretty much a geezer.

I don't know about you, but mine has been an up-and-down affair. Life is one big curveball. You ride on top for a while, then awaken one morning to find out it has all crumbled and crashed. You carry on and rebuild. Decade after decade rolls by as the torturous, teasing cycle continues.

The problem with all this is that we prioritize to survive. Certain things become important while others slide down the prioritization scale. Too many times the loser in this survival mechanism is our health. There are relationships, careers, and a thousand other things that become more important than taking care of ourselves.

Then one day, sooner or later, reality slaps you in the face. An event, diagnosis or some physical crisis alerts you to the fact that you've neglected the most important element, your physical body. You suddenly see the light.

So that day arrives. You realized you've erred with your priorities and you're now going to do something about it. You're going to make health a priority. Maybe you've experimented in the past with Snake Oil Bob's overnight weight-loss lotion. You know, he's the guy on late night television that convinces you in a weak moment to mortgage your home and purchase his miracle salve.

You do this and you're optimistic as can be. You wipe it all over your somewhat-chunky body at night with aspirations of waking up whip-thin and raring to go participate in a triathlon. Instead, you wake up with a still chunky, but oily body, and you're now broke and homeless.

The point here is that gimmicks don't work. Fitness and weight loss are multi-billion-dollar industries and that naturally brings in the sharks. You're old and wise now, so there's no need to dwell on that fact. Let the sharks swim somewhere else. There are advantages to being a geezer.

Here's what works. Here's the secret to losing that extra weight. You have to *eat right and exercise*. It's the simplest concept of them all. Watch what you put into your mouth and move your body. That's it!

What you're going to learn in this book has been repeated in hundreds of books and articles. It's basically common sense. Eat more fruits and vegetables, drink a lot of water, and make sure your protein source is lean. Get that excess weight off and *keep it off*. Anyone can lose weight, but the true winners maintain it for the long run. This book is designed just for that, developing long-term habits for life.

As far as exercise goes, get the heart beating by moving your body and eventually add a few strengthening exercises. I'm really into the flexibility component of exercise, especially at our geezed-up age. Sometimes we wake up stiff as boards. You know what I'm talking about. You're rubbing one of those geezed joints as you're reading this. We're going to reverse that and bring back some of that youthful elasticity. I'll get to the details of this later.

You'll also learn to say NO. You'll wage war on the processed foods that relentlessly conspire to take control of your body. They and their corporate masters desire to transform you into a deep-fried, salty, sugar-encrusted, clogged-heart, sedentary slug with a debit card. Don't be naïve. They're more concerned with the bottom line and purchasing a bigger house than anything else.

Many of you are active and relatively fit and simply wish to up the ante a bit. You desire to take it to the next level. That's great, this book will take you there. However, I take special pride in helping someone who is at the bottom fitness level. I've helped a couple of people who were *extremely* overweight to become fit.

The emotions I felt when transforming hopeless despair into unconditional self-worth were off the charts. To feel responsible for changing someone's life at that level generates a rewarding satisfaction that words can't describe. Are you at that lowest level of fitness? Read this book, apply it, become fit, and tell me about it. I want that high again.

Educating yourself about what you *should* do is easy. A first-grader could easily grasp these simple concepts. Even my less-than-ambitious dog Gizmo could learn it if he so desired. This stuff is incredibly easy to comprehend once you slice away the constant societal advertising bombardment that attempts to persuade you otherwise.

Be your own person and make your own choices. Do you really need a slick advertising firm to choose what you're pumping into your body? No, you don't, especially when they don't always have your best interests at heart. Use your well-earned wisdom to make your own decisions. We're old geezers and proud of it.

The objective of this book is *how* to achieve it. You will learn how to motivate yourself. It's all about desire. It's about wanting it! It requires dedication and discipline. I'm aware those two words scare the heck out of the average human being.

Dedication and discipline are not what people want to hear. They would much rather stick their head in the sand and avoid them. To even see those two words in print make most people shiver in fear. They run for the hills when they're told they have to apply dedication and discipline to a task. You're going to develop an entirely different outlook and embrace it. *Then you won't believe how easy it becomes.*

At that point you'll effortlessly and automatically station your healthy nutrition habits (this is *not* a diet!) and exercise routine under your protective dedication/discipline umbrella. Your desire and determination will be the fuel that shoots you to the top. You're going to master all these D's, dedication, discipline, desire, determination, and then you're off to the races.

You're going to be primal and raw. Primal and raw are pure animal energies, and that's who we are at our core. That youthfulness that you thought was long gone will reappear in a huge way. Sensuality will seep from your soul because you're so confident and radiant. You're hot and you know it. It'll resonate from within and everyone will see it. The eyes don't lie. You'll feel so *good* about yourself, but you'll present it in a humble manner.

You're going to fascinate everyone that inhabits your world. You'll be talked about when your friends gather at their gossipy luncheons. They'll wish they were you. You're going be the star among your peers. You're going to strut your stuff in a classy style. You'll catch others looking at you in admiration. You're all about elegance, sensuality and libido with an appetite for life. You're the catch of the day.

This isn't going to be as hard as you think. It really is as easy as eating right and exercising. You not trying to be on the cover of some magazine or become the weight-lifting champion of the universe. You're too damn old for that and you know it. What you *do* want is to become leaner, stronger and look good. Being all geezed-up doesn't mean you're done forever. There's still some treasure left in that old tank. You can still turn a head or two.

Oh yeah, vanity is a great motivator. All you pretty girls can turn back the time machine a little bit and get yourself in shape. Get out there and prance around your remaining years with that sexy little smirk that's been driving men crazy since the caveman era. And guys, you'd better get in shape too, because your pretty lady is going to have guys relentlessly chasing her 24/7 every week of the year. You can't fall behind and let the pool boy capture your prize.

Along the way we'll take a look back at the interesting life of Zarkoff Zucchini. He was the pioneer and driving force of the vegetable rights movement. He also had an eye for the pretty ladies which caused some real problems. And maybe he drank a little too much.

There's no doubt his legacy will be stained by his indiscretions, but nevertheless he'll go down in history as the most iconic vegetable ever sprouted. Every genius is flawed to a certain degree and Mr. Zucchini was no exception. He excelled in the fields of vegetable equality and STD antibiotic consumption.

So, that's it. Let's get on with it. Let's get to work. You'll have to put up with my silly zaniness which I do apologize for, but it's really out of my control. I get bored when it's all serious. If you like, simply skip over the nonsensical parts and return to the basics. There's a segment of you readers who won't care for campy frivolousness, but don't let that stop you from absorbing the good stuff. This nutrition and exercise plan will work and I'm really proud of it. Life is a party and it's more fun when you're fit. *Let's eat right and exercise!*

> *I'm a geezer,*
> *I'm so wise.*
> *I eat right,*
> *And exercise!*

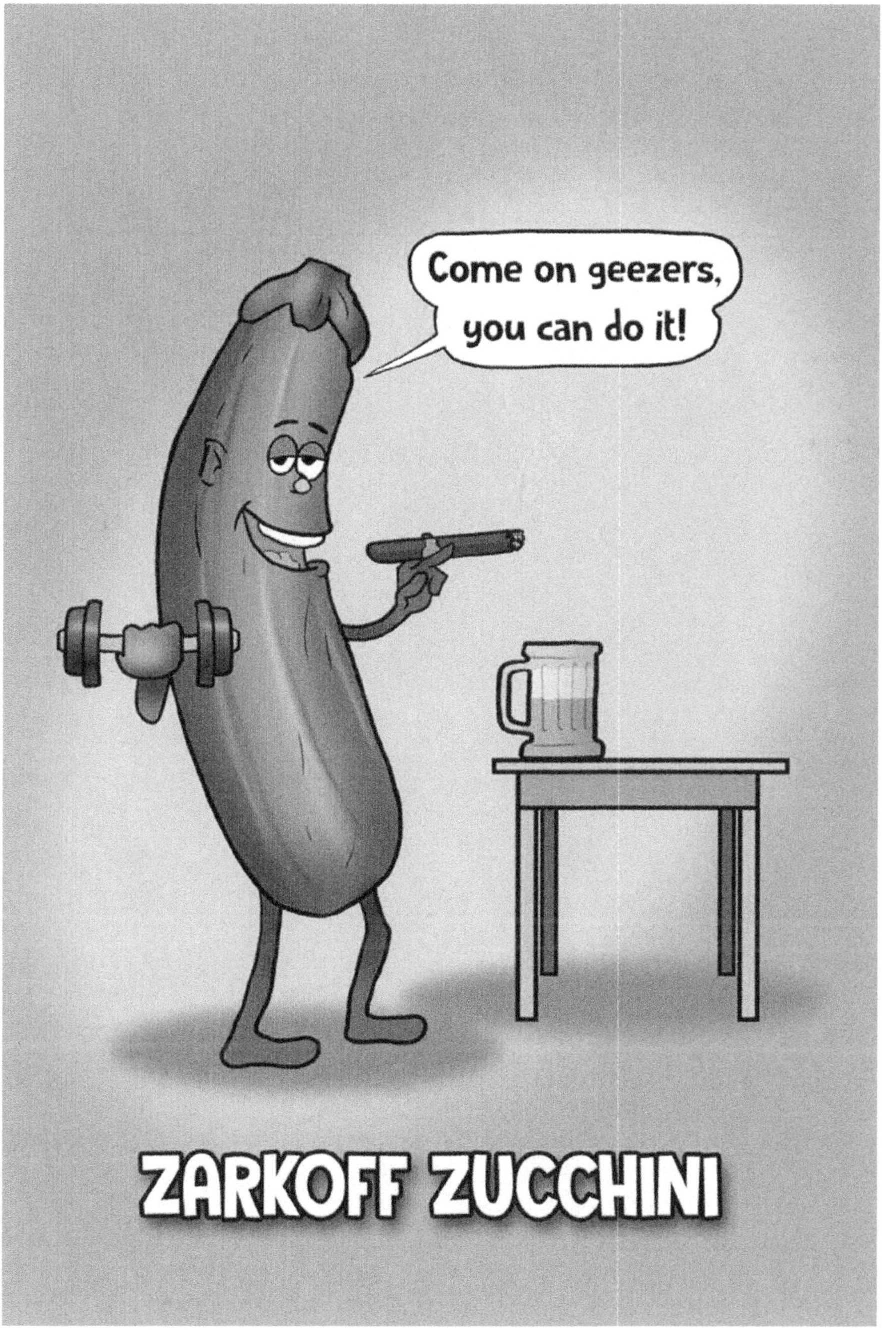
Come on geezers,
you can do it!
ZARKOFF ZUCCHINI

CHAPTER 1

You Can Do It!

"You can do anything you want to do if you want it bad enough."
Bill Russell

Top Priority

How bad do you want it? Do you *really* want to lose some weight and tone up? If you *really* don't want to become fit, then just close this book right now. Don't return it to Amazon, because I could use that dollar. Stretch out on the sofa, grab a Hollywood gossip magazine, and chew on something greasy or sweet. An old *Matlock* television rerun sounds good, or maybe something with Bill Murray in it. He's always funny.

Seriously, there is a right time and place for everything. If you're not in the right frame of mind this will never work. Not only will you fail, but you'll possibly become so discouraged that you'll completely give up on your dream of becoming fit.

Don't give up. Reanalyze your situation. Make a better plan of attack. Get yourself psychologically prepared for this. Half-hearted attempts are doomed and destined for failure. Don't be a loser. Show those doubters, and you know who they are, that you're going to blast them away with a fit body. Win at this game, and win big.

There really is no other option. If you don't take care of yourself, who will? Do you really think your grandkids are going to tear themselves away from their techy gadgets to research senior fitness? I don't think so. You can't cave in to Father Geeze, or it will be a cookies and cream future that will eventually catch up with you.

As you know, we've all got one foot in the grave already. Do we really want to just give up, dive into the grave, and let them cover us with dirt? And that fiery-oven cremation option doesn't sound too appealing either. There's much more fun to be had before the ultimate retirement. Get fit, cause some trouble, and give them something to talk about. Let's go down fighting. I'm not ready to go yet. Are you?

Life is full of choices. Every minute of every day we make decisions that affect us, some big and some small. Our lives are a result of the choices we make and we've all made some bad ones. Just ask my two ex-wives. They could have thought things through a little more before hitching to my wagon. Luckily for them they upgraded as soon as possible.

Fitness is all about priorities. Throughout my life I've prioritized different things at different stages. Little League baseball, education, money, and career were the standards, along with a few others that would have been better left alone. Today fitness and health are top priorities. Eating right and exercising are ingrained into my being. Getting to that point required some behavioral changes, some easier than others.

You'll find that when you get serious about becoming fit that you can't have it all. Sacrifices will be necessary if you want to succeed. Certain foods you'll have to kiss goodbye, at least for a while. You'll also have to figure out what's sliced away to make time for your exercise routine.

Time is one thing that won't budge for you. You're going to have to give something up in order to fit in in your exercise routine. Maybe you spend every waking moment helping the sick, the poor, the homeless, and fighting world hunger. If so, I say continue on and you're probably destined to be eternally fit in heaven.

For the rest of us sinners, it will be easier to find the time. An exercise routine could replace time otherwise spent slugging down drinks at the local bar, gossiping about who's hair is dyed when they claim otherwise, debating whether Harry and Susie have a thing going on, or shopping for that hundredth pair of shoes that won't fit into your crowded closet. There are countless areas that qualify to be eliminated. Some of them could even be deemed a complete waste of time.

Twenty or thirty minutes a day, that's all it takes. Eventually you can work yourself up to an hour, which includes stretching, a little weight work and some walking. An hour of television seems to be a logical place to start in my opinion. Is it really necessary to watch the weatherman every fifteen minutes? Did the forecast change so dramatically that grapefruit-sized hail will soon be pounding you on the head?

Is that sporting event *really* that important? Those guys change teams like they're on a merry-go-round. Put yourself and your health a little higher on the priority list. Display some of that team loyalty you have towards yourself. Tape the game if it's really that important. Get yourself fit and you'll relate to those fit athletes in a way that others can't.

Is it absolutely critical that you watch that movie again that you so loved back in 1980? How about sitcoms, reality shows, talk shows and such? The list goes on and on. Surely you can find one of these intellectual wastelands to be a sacrificial time-lamb. The point here is that most of us *can* find time for exercise.

That old movie,
Such a hit.
Turn it off,
Go get fit!

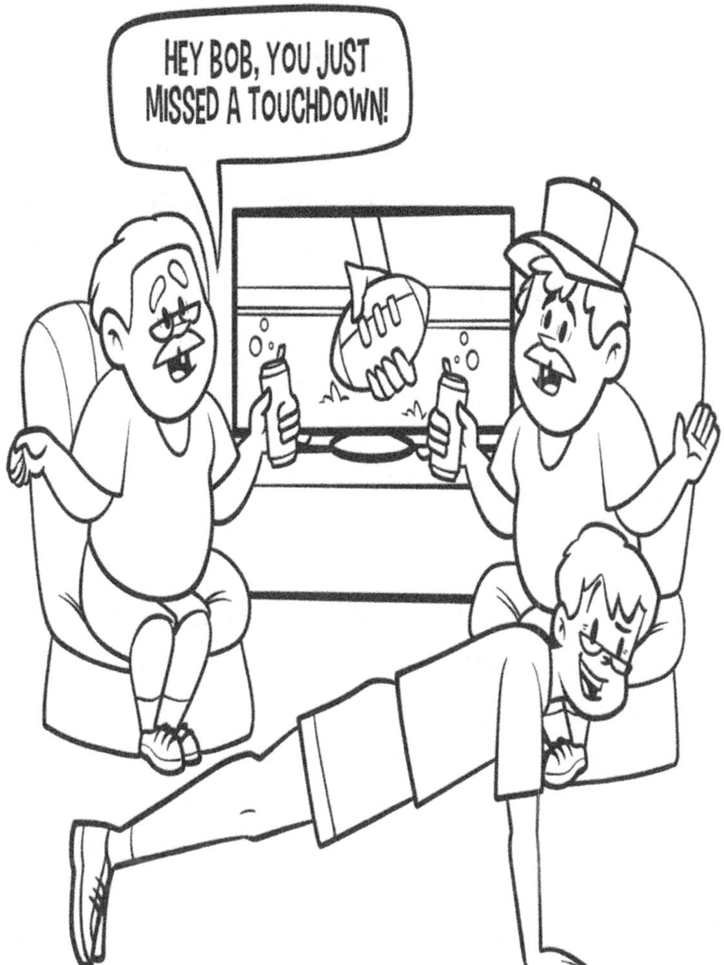
HEY BOB, YOU JUST
MISSED A TOUCHDOWN!

Top Priority II

Now comes something more difficult, changing eating habits that have been ingrained for decades. The good side of this is that once you're over the hump it becomes easier to say *no*, no to the foods that are your enemy, no to the foods that stand in your way, no to the foods that have controlled you for a lifetime.

It's all about priorities. You have to sacrifice the fatty little antagonists that tempt you every second of every day. That early morning doughnut is a good example. He just lies there like a devil in waiting.

"Umm, I'm so delicious," he says to you. You have to fight back because it's really you who has the power here. He's nothing compared to your will of steel if only you use it. It's an easy win if you're in the right frame of mind.

Now if the doughnut is female, watch out! Female doughnuts are much smarter than males. These sweet vixens sneak into your mouth and march unopposed into the stomach. Then they proceed to make themselves at home and settle into waistlines and buttocks.

The key here is to identify the female as she lies in her doughnut box. One thing to look for is freshness. She will appear fresher than the males because she was late getting to the oven. She was doing her makeup.

Now you know the dangers associated with doughnuts and other visually appealing delicacies. As always, beware of the females in every species. Some of the upcoming Zarkoff

Zucchini tales will certainly verify this fact. Many of you men will relate. A jealous female is *not what you want*. Avoid this situation at all costs. The great Zucchini learned this the hard way as you will find out.

Just remember, fitness is your new *top priority*. It's really as simple as that. Becoming lean and strong involves making sacrifices and making the right decisions. It's a 24/7 commitment that involves hundreds of little decisions every month. Before long, the choices will become automatic. Choose the right path and those little decisions add up to a big result. It's really not as hard as it sounds and it can be *fun*, especially when that mirror stares back at you with a smile. Strut your stuff, baby.

Oh, so alluring,
Oh, so sweet.
Don't you do it,
Watch what you eat!

The Mindset

When it comes to dedication and discipline, there's one thing you always need to remember. The mind rules the body, the body doesn't rule the mind. If you're in the proper frame of mind you can accomplish anything. The sheer will of a determined human being is a powerful force of unrelenting strength. The possibilities are endless as to what can be accomplished when *you really want it.*

Eating right and exercising, that's our goal. That's a very manageable endeavor when you think about it in simple terms. We're going to engage in a war, a war between our powerful mind and two clear, distinct enemies. The enemies are bad-food products and time-wasters. Bad-food products stand in the way of eating right. Time-wasters stand in the way of our one-hour exercise routine. They really don't stand a chance if a battle plan is set in your mind.

As far as eating right, the enemy enters through a tiny hole we call the mouth. Controlling words that flow from that creature may be a difficult task, but controlling what enters into it foodwise doesn't need to be.

When you think about it, the bad-food enemy doesn't stand a chance. Look at it like this, you're guarding a border into a country. The border is that minute hole where bad things try to slip into your body and commit terror events like making you fat. Don't let this happen! Guard that mouth, for it's the gateway to Heaven for fatty foods.

It's fatblob paradise once they make it through your mouth. As you're mindlessly watching Archie Bunker for the thousandth time, they're invading human cells and setting up shop inside your body. As you're laughing at Archie, they're laughing at you. Once they settle, they tell all their buddies about their wonderful new home. Doughnuts, greasy foods, fatty meats and the like are all cordially invited to join them in your stomach.

Your stomach is party-central and they're going to party like John Belushi. It's champagne, strippers of the male and female variety, various white powders, and general debauchery. It's hedonism at its finest.

Blobs enter when you're most unaware. They're working while you're preoccupied with the latest Hollywood gossip. Artery-clogging substances approved for entrance include high-fat meats, and all creamy, sweet, salty, buttery guests.

Decoders have intercepted fatblob messages in the past. Below is a typical telegram. Once this occurs the victim is in deep trouble. The unfortunate target in this particular case is named Goober. Previous blob communities built inside Goobers had been very successful. Here's the Goober-gram.

To all fatblobs: You are cordially invited to enter Goober's mouth for a free tour. Our beautiful community is set in a stunning, high cholesterol/triglyceride environment. Fabulous artery tours guarantee a twisting, turning adventure of clogged arteries like you've never seen. You'll witness challenging blockage stations where blood is at a near standstill!

Come and visit Goober soon. His mouth offers a safe and easy entrance. We're fully insured, crime-free, and have excellent schools and medical facilities. We love fat! We love Goober!

If your name is Goober, change it to prevent a blob invasion. That's enough of this silliness and I appreciate you tolerating it. Now we know how the enemy thinks and operates. The lesson here is to use your mind to control that little hole where food enters your body. Fiercely guard it as if your life depends on it, because it does. That takes care of the bad-food enemies.

Goober note: Goober was the original surname of a close friend of mine. We've joked about it for decades. The joke continues. I love all Goobers.

> You be lean,
> You be strong.
> You do right,
> Don't do wrong!

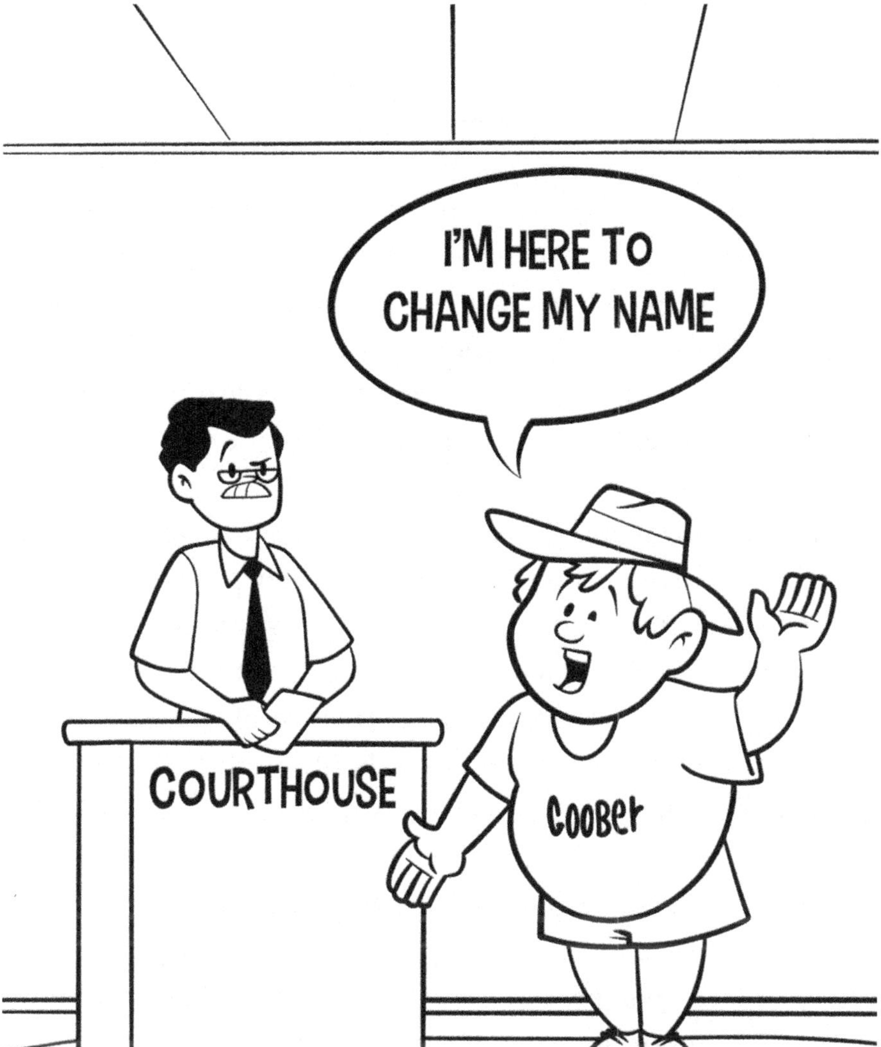
I'M HERE TO CHANGE MY NAME
COURTHOUSE
Coober

The Mindset II

Now we're going to deal with our second type of enemy. Time-wasters are by far the number one reason people don't stick to their exercise routine. Over and over, I'll hear someone say, "I don't have time for exercise."

The truth is they *do* have time for exercise. It's just that time-wasters are standing in the way. Time-wasters are semi-invisible beings that exist for one purpose, to manipulate humans into wasting time. You'll find them hanging around places where sluggish energy resides. Their primary haunt is television territory, but they lurk in the shadows anywhere there's an opportunity to steal your precious time.

These time thieves have no scruples at all. They're worse than a common criminal who steals little old ladies' purses. They're diabolically programed to take your most valuable resource, *your time,* and convert it into intellectual and physical droppings. Squandering time is their game.

These weasels hold their power only because you *give* them power. Somewhere in the past you have declared something important enough to claim an hour of your time every day. What actually happened was one of these little connivers *convinced* you it was important.

Take a hard look at your daily schedule. By daily, I mean every second, from the time you wake until the time you close your eyes and begin your Freudian dreaming. Surely there's *something* during all those waking moments that can be sliced away and converted to a more productive activity.

I'll regress once more to the principal time-waster habitat, a television viewing area. How many hours do you spend watching TV? Is each of those hours vital to your survival? Can you ruthlessly tear out an hour and replace it with exercise? Can you reclaim what's rightfully yours from those devilish schemers?

I'll bet you can create an hour right there. If not, let's move on. Maybe you're not a television person. Review your schedule, every valuable second of it, and pick and choose and grind away at it. If you want it bad enough, you'll scrape together sixty minutes of relative wasteland that you'll turn into your exercise time. Once you get into the habit of exercising, you'll realize its value. Evict that time-waster out of your life.

If you're still having difficulty finding your exercise time, then it's time to delve into the creative realm. Use that part of your brain that solves problems, creates solutions, and helps you wiggle your way out of precarious situations with little white lies that you apologize to God for later.

You know you can do it. Your mind is a powerful tool in your quest to become fit and transform your body. Unleash that creativity and find time to squeeze in that workout. You'll soon be addicted and you'll never look back. *Let's eat right and exercise!*

> *If you want it,*
> *You will find.*
> *You can do it,*
> *You'll find time!*

Have Fun

Having fun is an art. There was no one better at it than Zarkoff Zucchini. He was the king of all things fun. Let's delve a little into his background, as he lived quite the exciting life. His STD history alone verifies this. He was living proof that any vegetable could make a difference in the world and have fun doing it. That's why his legend lives on today.

Zarkoff Zucchini was born of Czech heritage. The zucchini patch where he was conceived doubled as a high-end brothel for prominent, wealthy vegetables. The rich felt very comfortable frequenting this establishment as discretion was placed at a premium. Zarkoff was a result of the union between the madam of the brothel and the director of the International Vegetable Association. Zarkoff possessed quite the family pedigree.

Zarkoff's parents were both quite the characters. Their relationship was a discreet one. Both were vibrant, spirited individuals, zucchinis of sophistication, wealth and taste. Hence the creation of such an iconic force like Zarkoff Zucchini. Newborn Zarkoff bounced out of the womb all wrapped in a layer of rich, dark, soil. He started out life as a dirty bastard.

Zarkoff was a rowdy youth and engaged in nefarious behavior. After several incidents he was sent away to Bad Veggie Penal Institute. This proved to be a decisive period for the mischievous lad. A year in prison persuaded young Zarkoff to pursue better options. Greatness lay ahead for him.

Upon release from prison, Zarkoff enrolled at prestigious Oxford Garden University. He graduated with honors a year ahead of schedule despite being named drinker/partier-of-the-year for three straight years. He learned early on that having fun was a pursuit where he excelled. He was especially popular with the pretty coeds on campus.

Upon graduation Zarkoff worked as an administrator for Veggie Lives Matter, a vegetable rights organization that offered assistance to abused produce. Zarkoff immediately found his place and took off like a rising star. He helped many victims, most of them pretty females. He would take them on weekend jaunts to "further his investigative curiosities" into their particular cases and gather more information.

Zarkoff became proficient in legal parlance and soon he was testifying in abuse cases as an expert witness. He quickly discovered that he had an aptitude for persuading jurors. Zarkoff's natural charm, good looks, and his practical manner of disclosing the facts won over many hearts.

Zarkoff Zucchini hit the stratosphere of his profession when he took the stand in his own defense. The young zucchini had taken a pretty eggplant to dinner and all was going well. They were into their third bottle of wine and his leggy date was becoming amorous. The evening promised to be an exciting and sensual one.

Then it happened. A waiter came over and snatched Zarkoff up with a spatula. He raced inside the kitchen and placed the shocked zucchini upon a plate alongside a hamburger. What followed was mental and emotional abuse in the most severe manner, as the courts would later agree. Because vegetable discrimination is so dear to my heart, I will reference the court case that followed three months later.

It was a highly anticipated event. This landmark Supreme Court civil rights case pitted Ground Beef against Zucchini. The plaintiff, Zucchini, claimed he was moved to a dirty side dish after Ground Beef invaded his space.

Oral arguments were heard on June 17, which happened to be National Vegetable Day. This created compassion from the court and they sided with Zucchini. The result was a ruling that discrimination had occurred against the young squash. Zucchini was awarded his own dinner plate, silverware, and stud privileges in a local produce market.

The scope of the landmark decision electrified the veggie world. The vegetable community erupted in celebration. Parties ensued and there were many veggie hangovers the next day.

Zarkoff Zucchini went on to become an international celebrity. He authored several books and starred in an adult vegetable film. He opened up several strip clubs. He started a celebrity tequila.

However, not all was peaches and cream for Zucchini. He found it hard to handle fame and fortune, especially when it came to pretty girls. He could never say no to a pretty face, and relationship after relationship crumbled as the result of his numerous affairs.

Jealousy issues eventually defeated him. He married and divorced due to his constant womanizing and masterly adroitness at contracting and spreading STDs. He died an early death at the hands of his girlfriend Yellow Squash after she caught him in bed with a pretty cucumber.

The resulting media coverage was sensational. Zucchinis became popular in restaurants worldwide in honor of the fallen hero. The veggie community owes much to the randy youth that was Zarkoff Zucchini. He will never be forgotten.

This heartwarming and heartbreaking tale brings us full circle to our subject at hand. To be lean and strong, you have to *have fun* doing it. To lose weight and become fit, you have to *have fun* doing it. Zarkoff Zucchini's method of having fun is not advisable unless you love relationship drama and constant doses of antibiotics, but we can still learn from him. We can make things fun via other methods. Let's discuss some of these.

Poor ole Zark,
Had too much fun.
Now he's dead,
Now he's done.

BISTRO

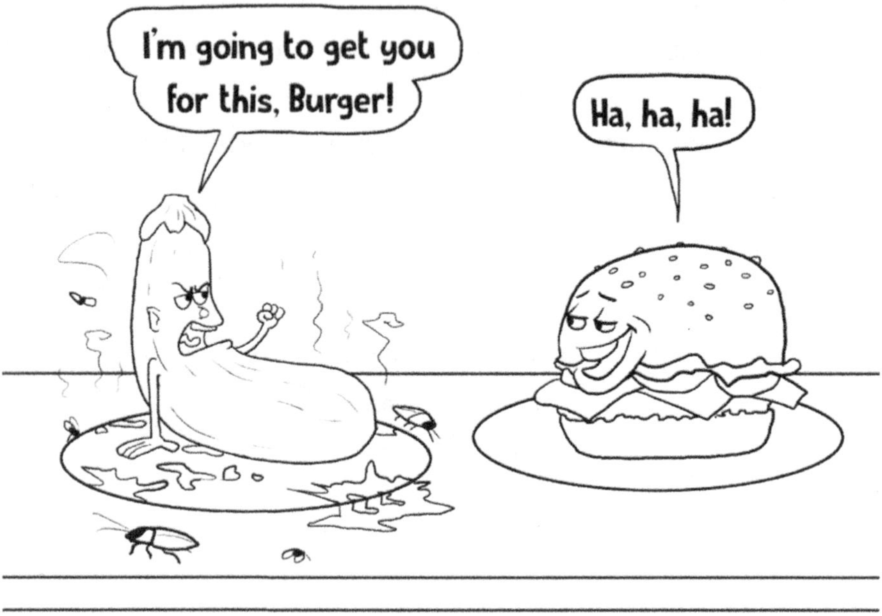

Have Fun II

One of the first steps towards having fun is to simplify and minimize. Slice away all that stands in the way. Clutter is a major enemy and formidable opponent in your battle to become fit. It's not only physical objects that oppose you, it's also clutter of the mind and emotions. If you have a thousand little daily obligations to attend to it affects what's really important. All of us have a certain amount of daily energy. When it's used on trivial pursuits it's gone forever.

Do you really need three houses and all the mental, emotional and physical exertion that go along with them? Do you really need loads of material objects that you think better your life, but instead hinder you on a daily basis? Do you really need to plan every second of your day doing things that mean nothing in the big picture?

Step back for a moment and look at yourself. Are there things in life that you're doing because you're worried what others might think if you didn't do them? Are there things in your life that you possess because Joe and Sally across the street possess them? Isn't life hard enough with just what's thrown against us by the universe?

Every day some unexpected event or obstacle appears that requires attention, some larger than others. Bank your emergency energy just as you would prepare for the future financially. Use your valuable mental, emotional and physical energy on what counts. And what counts more than your health?

Minimalism is relative. Get tough on yourself and slice away the clutter. Decide what you really need and what's draining your energy. Get rid of it, sell it at a yard sale, or give it away. And that's just the physical stuff. Deal with the time clutter and take some time for yourself. Be ruthless and deal with any emotional baggage that weighs you down day after day, week after week, year after year. Look *within* instead of running from place to place in a vain effort to appear normal and successful.

Be yourself, as you are a unique individual. If people want to declare you as strange, so be it. Embrace your true nature and let it run free. Years ago, I accepted my so-called weirdness and I've never regretted it. So what if I eat differently at the neighborhood cookout, live without all the latest gadgets, and possess minimal furniture and possessions? So what if I walk around in circles all over the neighborhood wearing a big floppy hat that shields me from the sun and admittingly looks ridiculous?

In a thousand years, will anyone be running around the planet saying Spyder Johnson sure was one big weirdo? No, I'll be dead, they'll be dead, and the world may or may not still be around. Live it your way and make health and fitness a priority. It's you who is the decider, not societal molders and shapers. Focus on what's important. Cut away the clutter, be yourself and get the last laugh.

Gotta be real,

Gotta be true.

Gotta be yourself,

Gotta be You!

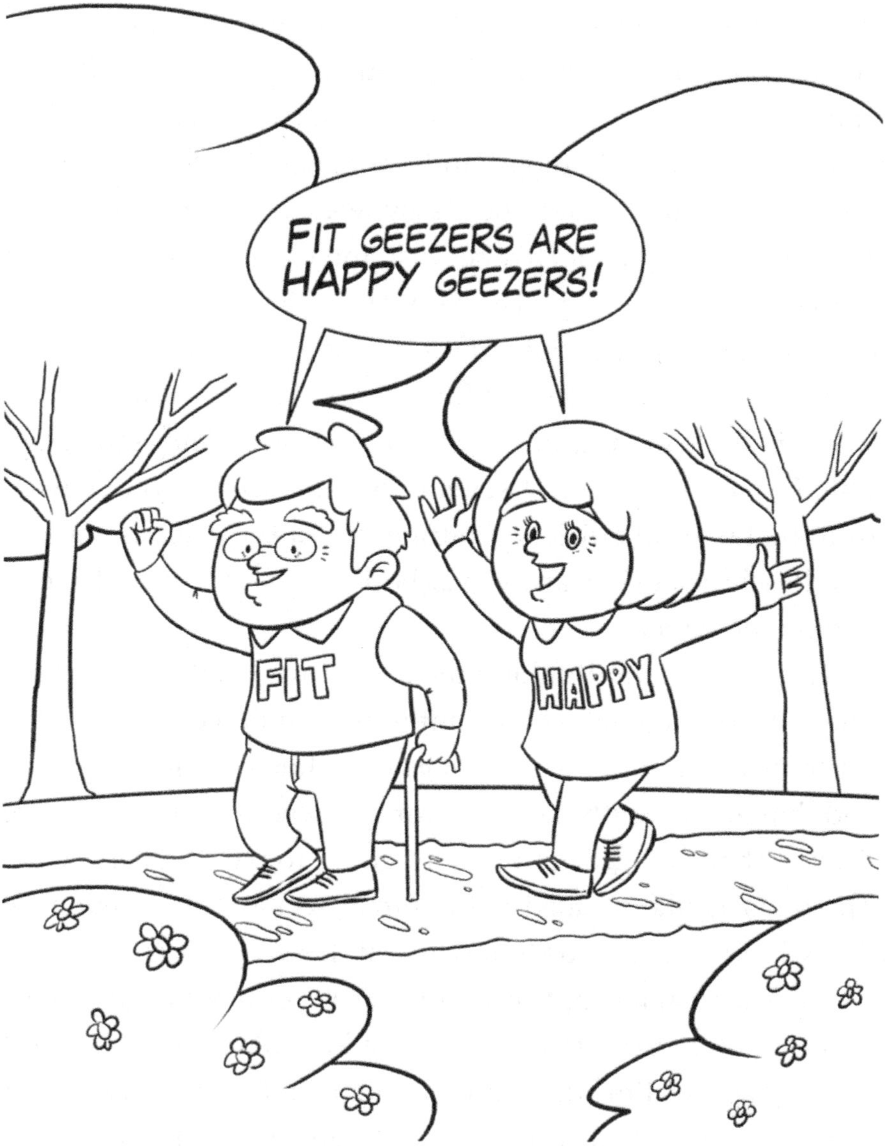
FIT GEEZERS ARE HAPPY GEEZERS!
FIT
HAPPY

Have Fun III

It's an overweight world and becoming more so every day. Have you ever wondered how humanity, and the United States in particular, ever slipped to such obesity levels? A combination of technology and processed foods seem to be the main suspects, but the "easy way out" mentality also appears to be a factor. It's because the easiest way is usually the least physical way. The body was designed to be used, otherwise it slowly disintegrates.

Our bodies are naturally fine-tuned machines that normally operate lean and mean, taking in fuel and efficiently utilizing it. Over the last several decades we've gotten away from that natural efficiency. Sitting in front of a computer and mindlessly snacking away has become the norm and we're paying the price.

It's time to stop thinking the easiest way is the best way. I guess it's human nature to want to be pampered, whether the server is another human or a sort of technology. Kicking back and having everything done for us seems to be what we desire. That's all great, but we're going to pay the price later. The body is like a caged wild animal seeking the freedom of the wilderness. It needs to move or it dies.

Let's look at a simple example of the "easy way out." Have you ever seen cars circling a parking lot looking for the closest parking space? I'm sure many of them have a valid reason for doing so. The handicapped, elderly and the sick are among the many who need to be as close as possible to their destination.

It's the others that humor me as I observe them circling the parking lot like vultures. After ten minutes of navigating tight corners and straining their necks, they'll finally be rewarded as someone pulls away from a prime spot. They'll gleefully wait, oblivious to the traffic jam they've created behind them.

When they finally pull into that spot, they're smiling from ear to ear. Then I watch as a fit, healthy person exits the car and proceeds to their destination. The look of joy on their face amazes me. Really? True happiness can be found from saving twenty steps in a parking lot? As for me, that wouldn't do the trick. All the stress involved in winning that coveted prize just wouldn't be worth it.

I'm parking in the back of the lot where I don't have to fight for it. My heart doesn't need the wear and tear of stressful parking lot warfare. Call me a loser if you want, but I'll go ahead and walk those extra steps to avoid that mess. It's not a competition to me. I guess those people feel victorious with their temporary ownership of a prime parking spot. They're probably inside buying champagne to celebrate the occasion.

I can't help but expand on the world of parking lot politics. I actually saw this with my own eyes. Two cars approached a prime parking spot in front of a gym. The rest of the parking lot was practically empty, but apparently this particular space was extremely valuable.

One slipped in ahead of the other and claimed his prize, causing much anger from the loser. The enraged loser got out of his car and approached the victor in a threatening manner. I actually thought these two adults would engage in violent confrontation.

And here's the amusing thing. They're two fit men going into a gym to work out and they're fighting over taking ten extra steps to the entrance. Wouldn't the ten extra steps just add to their fitness level? Does getting emotionally upset to near coronary-failure levels contribute to their well-being? Is it possible their priorities might be misplaced? Is it really worth it?

That's just one glaring example of the "easy way out" mentality. Much of the "easy way out" focus seems to be on avoiding walking and moving. Try to change your mindset when it comes to moving your body. Look at it as an opportunity rather than a challenge.

Walk to that diner around the block instead of driving. Take the stairs instead of the elevator. Add thirty minutes to your workout by exercising in your home and eliminating the roundtrip drive to the gym. Anything and everything should be considered.

Anytime you have a choice, consider an option that involves moving your body. It's the way we were meant to be. Cage your body into a technological prison and it will resist. It wasn't meant to be waited on hand and foot. It wants to treat you right, but you have to treat it right as well. Free it up and let it run wild. It matters not that you're sixty or seventy years of age. As a matter of fact, that's when you need movement more than ever. The easy way isn't always the best way.

> *Move your body,*
> *And you'll see.*
> *You'll look good,*
> *Fit you'll be!*

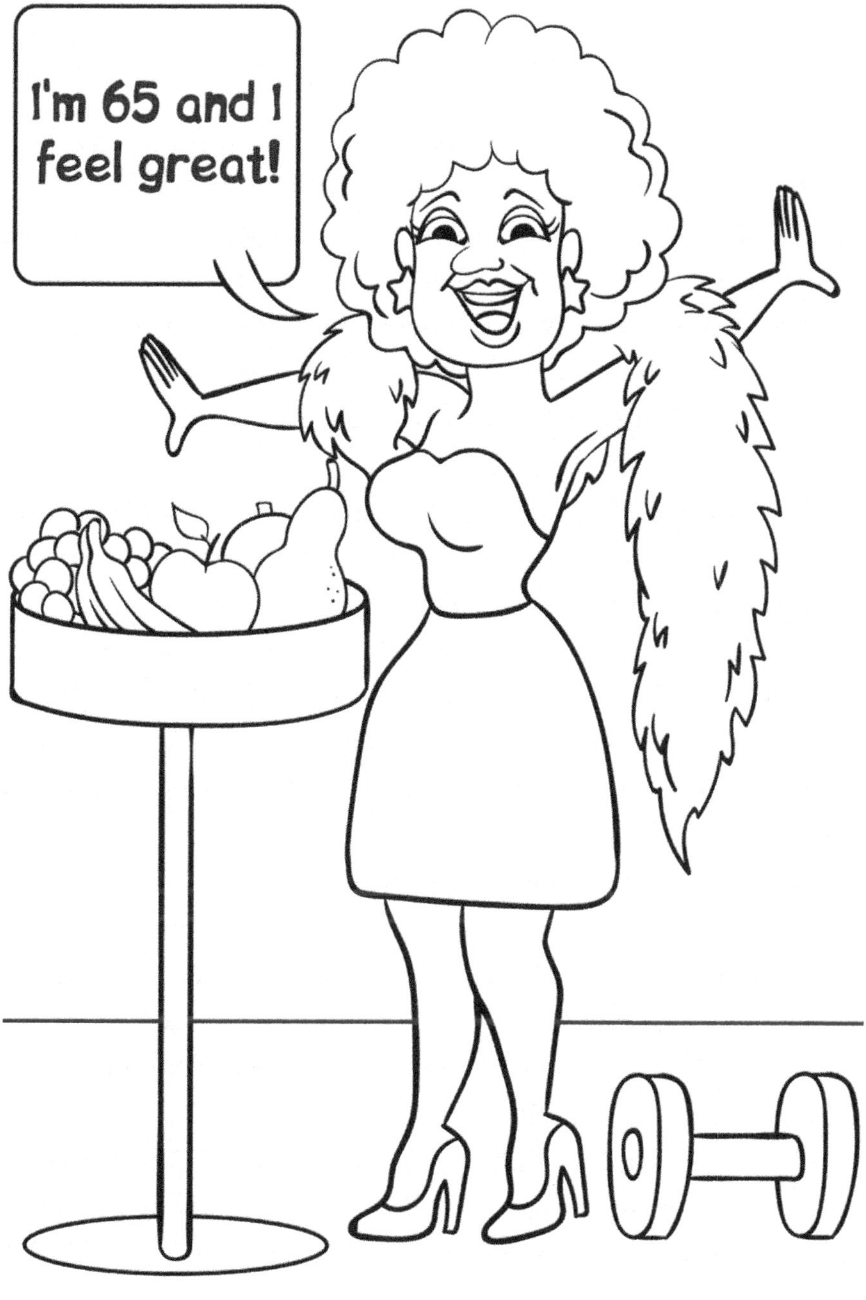
I'm 65 and I
feel great!

Have Fun IV

It is of the utmost importance that you have fun in life. A big smile just paves the way for a smooth ride ahead. Zarkoff Zucchini was the quintessential fun-lover, the master of balancing work and fun. He never let a day go by without enjoying himself. Sometimes he enjoyed a tad too much and it came back to haunt him. The following story illustrates one of these fun-gone-wrong events.

"Yes, please, I'll have another of each," said Zarkoff. The pretty scallion waitress smiled and nodded in acceptance. She picked up his empty glasses and trotted back to the bar.

Zarkoff plopped his feet into the water as he stared at the deep blue sea in front of him. His lounge chair was placed surfside. The gentle waves rolled over his legs. He took a long puff from his Luis Concepcion, the world's finest Cuban cigar. The mid-morning sun was warming his body and the weather was perfect. The rum, tequila, beer and all the bikini-clad girls were just what he needed. Oh, how he loved Mexico.

Zarkoff had two full days of enjoyment ahead of him before he was to speak at the International Vegetable Awareness conference. He would be receiving an award for all his efforts toward vegetable equality.

"Here you go, Mr. Zucchini," a voice called out. It was the pretty scallion waitress, loaded up for his fresh round of drinks. "Here's your triple rum on the rocks, your double shot of tequila, and your liter of beer. Enjoy, Mr. Zucchini." She smiled and walked away.

Zarkoff quickly downed his tequila and took a big gulp of his beer. The day was getting brighter by the moment. All he needed now was a little female companionship and it would be perfect. Then his day took a turn like no other.

"Hi Zarkoff, do you remember me?" a voice called from behind. Zarkoff turned and saw a most disturbing sight. It was Tottie the Hottie Tomatillo, a stripper acquaintance of his. Joining her was her mother and grandmother. This would be trouble indeed.

"So you lie to me, you lie to my mother, and you lie to my grandmother," said Tottie. Her face was flushed with anger. "You're going to pay the price now, you slimy weasel!"

Zarkoff was trapped and he knew it. He had hoped he would never run into Tottie again. The last night they were together he had been especially drunk. He had promised her that she could travel the world with him and be his one and only girlfriend. That's when things got quite complicated. His philandering ways caught up with him.

Zarkoff realized he had previously dated her mother *and* her grandmother on previous visits to Mexico. He had not been truthful to them either. They too thought they would be his one and only. Oh, how he wished he could take back those awful lies. He would do anything to go back and do things the right way. Now he had three hot-blooded tomatillos out for blood.

Zarkoff never saw the first blow coming. The baseball bat smashed into his ribs, fracturing several of them. Tottie's grandmother reared back and took another swing. This time she nailed the other side. Zarkoff heard the bones shatter as the girls laughed.

"How does that feel, Mr. Romeo, liar pig!" screamed Tottie. "You're in big trouble now."

Tottie walked into water and slapped her hands on the surface. "Come and get him, Jezzy. Bring all your friends. He's all yours!" Tottie then leaned over in front of Zarkoff. He was doubled over in pain. She laughed in his face.

"I just called in my pet jellyfish. Jezzy and all her ocean friends are going to zap you with cheater juice. You really screwed up this time, you worthless scumbag zucchini."

Zarkoff was helpless. The pain in his shattered ribs was horrific. Tottie and her mother dragged him into deeper water. Then he felt the first sting. "Ohh!" he cried out.

"Good girl Jezzy!" shouted Tottie. "You and your friends sting that scoundrel!"

Then it was one sting after another. At least fifty jellyfish were stinging every part of his body. Zarkoff had never felt worse pain in his life, and he had seen some harsh times. Maybe this was the end. Maybe he was going to meet his maker. Or maybe he was going straight to Hell for all his misdoings. Just when he thought things couldn't get worse, they did.

"You get him, Sally!" cried Tottie. "Be a good shark and eat that degenerate sleazeball!"

Sally the shark was happy to do it. Her shark husband was a liar and cheater and she felt compassion for Hottie. She crunched down on Zarkoff's arm and tore it off. "Yum," she said as she swallowed it down. One of his legs was next. "Umm good," said Sally. Zarkoff was preparing for death.

"It ain't over yet," declared Tottie. "Sherry Stingray's gonna fill you with cheater poison. How's that gonna feel, you deviate skirt-chaser!"

Zarkoff felt the barbed stinger enter his back and extend into his chest. The toxic venom rushed directly into his heart, bursting it. Sherry pulled out her stinger and swam away laughing. She was no fan of cheaters either.

At that moment Zarkoff felt himself being pulled back to shore. A lifeguard had heard the commotion and rescued him. Some beachgoers helped subdue the angry tomatillos. Medics were immediately called in. As Zarkoff fell out of consciousness, he heard one remark that it was doubtful he would survive. Another commented this was the worst cheater revenge he had ever witnessed.

Zarkoff's eyes closed, but not before he saw Jezzy Jellyfish a few feet away in the sand. She was laughing hysterically, overcome with joy, waving her tentacles at Zarkoff. She blew him a kiss as he passed out.

Zarkoff awoke from his coma eight months later. Doctors told him of his heart transplant and new pig heart. All of his ribs had been removed and replaced with chicken wire. He now was the happy owner of two prosthetic limbs. He had permanent brain damage from the massive amount of venom injected into him.

Zarkoff didn't care to hear it. He was Zarkoff Zucchini and he was out to have fun. He got out his little black book and began calling girlfriends. He was way behind in the fun department and was determined to catch up.

While it's critical that you have fun as you chase your fitness goals, it is *not* advisable to carry things as far as Zarkoff.

When fun turns into stress you've gone too far. When extreme violence occurs, you've definitely crossed the line. When love of fun constantly places you in ICU, you absolutely should seek mental health counseling.

Zarkoff likes girls,
And he drinks.
Zarkoff acts,
Before he thinks!

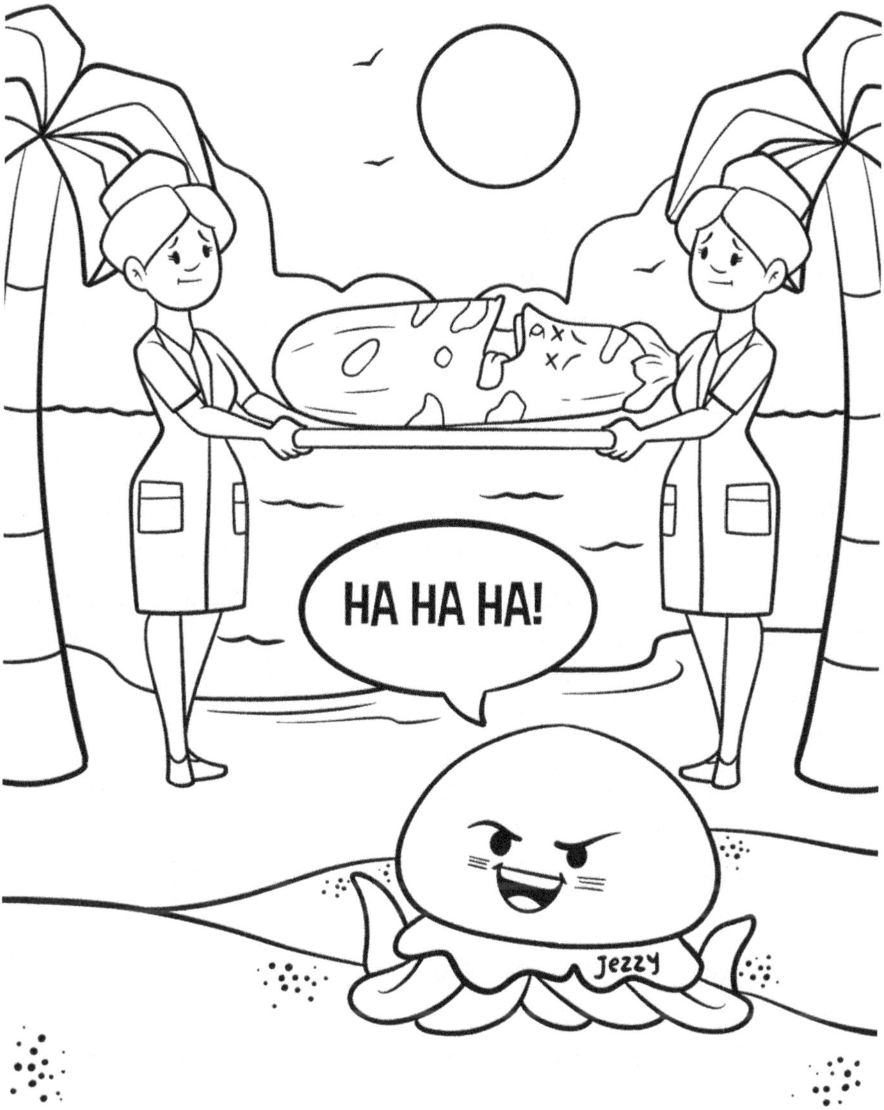
HA HA HA!
Jezzy

Have Fun V

Let's get back to the real world, if there is such a thing. There is nothing more important than a sense of humor. You have to be able to laugh at situations that inevitably will be imposed upon you in your quest to become fit. Most importantly you have to be able to laugh at yourself!

When you think about it, this whole exercise thing is a relatively recent aspect of human history. For the first million years or so, early man wouldn't dare think of expending valuable energy unnecessarily. Humanity was too busy trying to survive. Hunting wild game and roaming the countryside gathering nuts and berries provided more than enough exercise.

Then they had cavewomen awaiting them back at the cave. Early cavewoman was a very sensual creature and expected her man to display copious amounts of kinetic energy. Cave babies were necessary to propagate future cave society.

Somehow, we have evolved from these fit, muscular, well-toned beings into television butterballs. Long gone are the days of yesteryear when we ran around showing off chiseled bodies beneath tiny loincloths. Now twenty buffalo hides couldn't cover many of us. All that aerobic exercise pushing the TV remote doesn't seem to be doing the trick.

You can see the need to laugh. When you sit back and analyze human behavior, we really are sort of a clownish species. That makes it easy to find humor in nearly everything we do. You don't have to look very far.

Birds, animals, insects, they all seem to use common sense as they wander through life doing whatever it is they do. We humans bounce around from gimmicky fad to gimmicky fad in our struggle to impress other humans who are doing the same. Who needs a sitcom when you have free entertainment watching humanity aimlessly wander the corridors of Planet Folly? This is especially true in the weight-loss and fitness arena.

Utterly ridiculous would be an accurate description of some of the weight-loss methods proposed by the scammers who prey on the desperate. Let's turn the table on these vultures and laugh back at them. Refuse to buy into their pipe dream fairy tales. Make them get a real job instead of tricking good-hearted people into handing over hard-earned money in exchange for a glitzy packaged illusion. I hope they come back in another life as a floor mat.

The bottom line here is to keep a healthy sense of humor as you work to achieve your goals. Battle through the challenges and obstacles that stand in your way and laugh in their face. Make a joke of it on the outside as you relentlessly chase it from the inside. It makes the dedication/discipline pill so much easier to swallow.

Having fun fits right in with maintaining a sense of humor. Think about it for a moment. When you're having fun, the world just seems to be in sync with your energy. Life is a breeze when you're laughing, at least for that moment. Time and space blend into your essence and the world becomes problem-free. Now who doesn't want that!

Laugh and joke,
Wear a smile.
We're only here,
For a little while.

Have Fun VI

Now think about when you're not having fun. Pretend you're doing something you absolutely can't stand to do. How about this scenario? You're driving a large truck laden with dangerous explosives. One bump too many and the truck and you will be blown to smithereens. That next pothole could be your last.

But wait, the situation is worse. You're trying to get to La Paz, Bolivia from the town of Coroico. You're driving a 43-mile stretch of road called Yungas Road, better known as "Death Road." The reason for this is it claims 300 lives per year. This high mountain road features hairpin curves, heavy rain and fog, unpredictable landslides, and cliffs that drop 2,000 feet. The road is single lane, muddy, and there are no guardrails to prevent you from going over the edge.

Imagine you're on this incredibly dangerous road. You're on pins and needles from worrying about those explosives that are bouncing around in the cargo area. The blinding rain and thick fog make it nearly impossible to see the road. You're struggling to just see three feet ahead of you. A landslide occurs in front of you and giant boulders begin crashing into the truck. It's getting difficult to maintain control. Conditions couldn't be worse.

Those are reasons enough to be a little on edge, right? I doubt you would consider that fun. There are other issues that make matters worse. The truck is old and dilapidated and the brakes are prone to failure. They're currently on fire and smoking heavily as you're navigating the most dangerous curve on the highway. Your tires are completely bald and are apt to blow at any moment. You're a nervous wreck.

Just when you think matters couldn't get worse, they do. A shot rings out and a large-caliber bullet shatters your shoulder. Then a second shot enters your thigh. It's true what you had heard. There are snipers stationed on the highway who target truck drivers. The situation is getting out of control. A third bullet goes through your ear.

Suddenly you feel a sharp pain in your one good leg. You look down and see an angry Bolivian lancehead snake latched onto your ankle. This extremely poisonous snake is not happy that you invaded his space. The dilapidated truck is his home. He is repeatedly biting you and distributing his deadly venom. You are about to lose consciousness as venom spreads through your body.

Just then your co-driver awakens from a drunken stupor he was trying to sleep off. He's been drinking a lot due to some personal issues at home. He grabs a long knife and begins stabbing you in the back of the neck. He thinks you resemble his neighbor whom he just caught sleeping with his wife.

Is this situation fun? I think not. This is about as bad as it gets in my opinion. The odds of surviving this trip are slim and getting slimmer by the moment. Being shot, stabbed, and bitten by a snake while driving the world's most dangerous road in a deathtrap of a vehicle carrying explosives is not my idea of fun. It is indeed a precarious situation.

Let's turn this situation around. Now imagine you're on a sandy beach, cool drink in hand, a handsome man or beautiful girl is waiting on you hand and foot. You get a text informing you that your long-lost Aunt Jesse just passed and left you ten million dollars. She now resides in Heaven, so she upgraded. Now, this is what I would definitely consider *fun*.

Let's compare the two situations. On one hand we're about to die a horrendous death on a mountain road, something we hate. On the other hand, we're living like rich royalty, something we love. One is fun and other is not fun. So now we all know the value of having fun.

Now comes the tricky part. You have to deceive your mind into having fun. Imagine doing a crunch or a pushup, walking a mile, or lifting a dumbbell. I have to admit that sometimes these don't seem like the most fun things in the world. But lucky for you, you're now going to compare it to driving that truck. You can apply the truck-horror principle to your diet regime also. It will make that salad taste a whole lot better. It's all in the mind.

Once you compare the two, exercising and eating right becomes easier to imagine as fun. You now realize it could be worse, *much* worse. The point here is to *make it fun*. It really is all in your head. You honestly don't have a choice because you *have to* get fit and healthy. You *have to* eat right and exercise. It's all about attitude and the way you approach everything. Legendary fun-lover Zarkoff Zucchini would certainly approve. Have fun!

> *Make it fun,*
> *Fun in the mind,*
> *You'll get fit,*
> *You will find!*

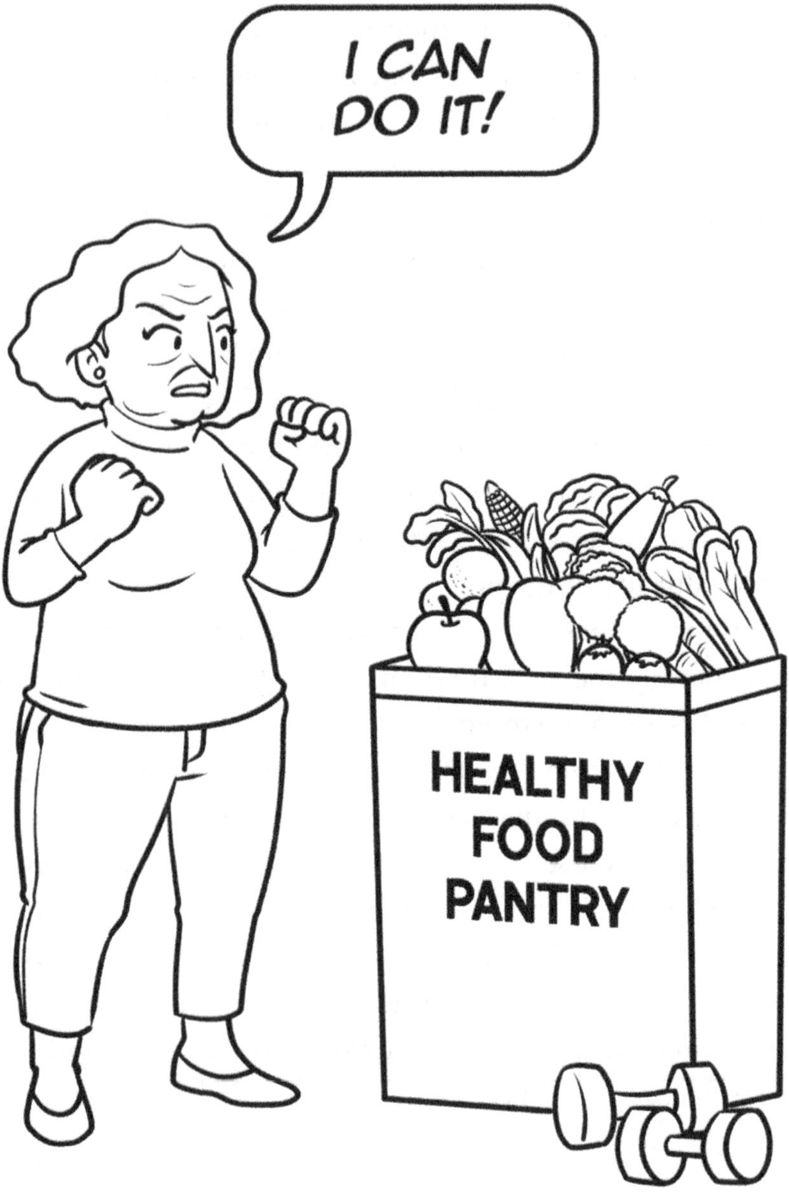

BELIEVE IN YOURSELF

CHAPTER 2

You Can Do It II

"The starting point of all achievement is desire."
Alvin Walker

Think Long-Term

Now this is a really serious subject. It is extremely critical that you take a long-term view of your fitness program. You didn't get out of shape in one week and you're not going to get back into shape in one week.

As a matter of fact, and get prepared for this horrifying bit of information, it will take a year. You heard it right, *a year!* You must exhibit patience. You have to get psychologically prepared to deal with this. If you don't, you're doomed for failure.

The reasons for this are numerous. Once again, it's all about how you look at it. Getting fit is a marathon, not a sprint. Your sprinting days are long gone, but with all that wisdom you've acquired you're very capable of winning a marathon. Leave the quick-fix mentality to the young kids who have so much to learn. We've all been in their shoes. They'll learn the hard way the same as we did.

The number one reason why we have to go slow, in case you've missed it, is we've aged. We're certified geezers. Our bodies react slower, our metabolic rate is reduced, and our joints are more susceptible to injuries. Those are just a few reasons to ease into it smoothly and soulfully. There are dozens more.

One year from now, that's the attitude you have to maintain. You can't be jumping on those scales five times a day checking your weight. Don't worry, if you do as you should, the weight will come off. Grind it out and stick to your routine. Be patient, let the system fall into place, and success will be yours. You'll become leaner and stronger and your confidence will be sky high.

Another reason there is no need to hurry is the nature of time as we age. Most of us agree that the older we get the faster the years seem to speed by. There's something about being geezed-up that makes the clock tick faster. On one hand that seems to be not so good, however in this case it works to our advantage.

Try this simple example. Think about exactly a year ago today, where you were, what you were doing, and the circumstances surrounding you at that time. Doesn't it seem like almost yesterday?

Now imagine you and your new body that you'll possess if you put a year of discipline and dedication into it. You'll look back in one year at this particular moment and realize it was really nothing timewise. As slow as some moments drag on, the year still passes like the snap of a finger.

It's a lot like writing this book. If I didn't think of it as a one-year project it would have intimidated me. On a great day I would produce maybe one percent of my final product. It just crept along incrementally. That made it so easy to give up and say why bother, but I didn't and you're now reading it.

Just as I had to look at the finish line while writing, you'll have to keep your eye on your final goal. One day will go by, a week will pass, then it's a month, then two, four, six months. Then you bear down and barrel through it and before you know it you've made it. A year of hard work, dedication and discipline finally paid off. It was just another year in the big scheme of things. *But it won't be just another year.*

It will be one of the most successful years of your life. You'll be so proud of yourself and what you accomplished. Your healthy habits will be ingrained into your being. Your mindset will be that of a winner. You'll feel confident and sexy and ready to conquer the world.

Pick the exact day that you're going to start this program. Take a picture of yourself, date it, and put it away. Pull it out after one year and jump for joy because you did it. You accomplished your goal and you did it all on your own. Go out and celebrate because you earned it. You're a fit geezer.

> Don't you worry,
> Have no fear.
> You'll be fit,
> In One Year!

Never Give Up

This topic needs to be discussed early on because it's of utmost importance. It is likely many of you will occasionally stumble in your journey towards being fit. It's completely normal. I know I did when I started many years ago. It can be very disheartening to slip and fall off track.

Before we proceed further into this important subject, I would like to relate an example of falling down and picking yourself back up. It involves our late hero, the one and only Zarkoff Zucchini. His persistence exhibited no boundaries in his determination to conquer the demons that led him into sinful temptation.

Over and over, he kept failing within romantic relationships. Saying no to sexy fruits and vegetables was extremely difficult for the concupiscent youth. He couldn't stop himself. His desires ran rampant.

Zarkoff had been seeing her for over a month. Carla Cabbage had knocked him off his feet the moment they met at the Cabbage Patch Brewery. She had sparkling blue eyes, blonde hair and a striking smile. Her smooth-leafed, firm-headed body sent his libido racing skyward. As far as Zarkoff was concerned, she would be his one and only forever.

One evening Zarkoff stopped off at Olive's Bar and Grill, an after-work hangout for the locals. One drink certainly wouldn't hurt before he headed over to Carla's place. It might even spark him up a little romantically. He ordered his customary Bloody Mary with three extra shots, a double shot of tequila, and a liter of beer. After downing his drinks, another round suddenly appeared in front of him.

"It's on the lovely lady standing behind you," pronounced the bartender. Zarkoff turned to see the most beautiful cauliflower he had ever seen. She was absolutely stunning with her white fleshy head and sparkling eyes. Wow!

"Mr. Zucchini!" she exclaimed. "I admire your work and I've always wanted to meet you, so I bought you a drink."

Zarkoff was flabbergasted and astonished at his good fortune. How lucky he was to have this gorgeous veggie approach him. She looked as if she could be a fashion model. He stumbled before he replied.

"Well…umm…thank you. I am proud of my work. What is your name?"

"I'm Candy Cauliflower. I'm so happy to meet you in person. I've seen you on TV and always thought you were so handsome."

That was it. The compliment sent Zarkoff over the edge and his lusty demons came roaring back. The two of them drank and danced into the evening. Zarkoff completely forgot about his girlfriend waiting for him. The two of them were becoming amorous on the sofa when Zarkoff felt the first blow to the head.

The whiskey bottle shattered his skull, causing major brain trauma. "You cheating, dirty pig! My girlfriend saw you here and called me. You're in trouble now!"

It was Carla and she had gone completely mad. Zarkoff ducked as she took a swing at him with a vodka bottle. She barely missed and that only enraged her more. Carla jumped over the bar and retrieved a large knife. Then she expertly leaped back over, red flames exiting her eyes.

"I'm gonna get you, you piece of slimeball trash," Carla shouted. "I'm gonna slice you up like a Thanksgiving turkey."

She took a sidearm slice at him and the blade ripped across Zarkoff's throat. Zarkoff was nearly decapitated. He watched helplessly as Carla continued her violent tirade upon the rest of his body.

Carla next vicious slice severed his arm. It fell onto the floor. Yet another cut directly into his femoral artery. Blood spewed out like a faucet.

A burly patron subdued Carla as she plunged the dagger into Zarkoff's new pig heart. Carla was hauled away screaming obscenities. Zarkoff was rushed to a nearby hospital where he fell into a coma. Doctors reconnected his head. They performed transplants, brain surgeries, and other medical procedures as he slept.

Zarkoff survived this brutal attack and eventually healed. To his credit, he apologized and tried to win back Carla's affections. Over and over, he begged her to take him back. It was all in vain however, as Carla rejected all of his advances.

The moral of this story is to keep trying if you fail. It didn't do Zarkoff any good, but don't let that stop you when it comes to fitness. Zarkoff is a hopeless case. Your situation is different and not filled with such intense drama. Starting over is much easier when it's applied to eating right and exercising. Let's delve into this.

Don't be Zarkoff,
Always be true.
Stay with one girl,
Never TWO!

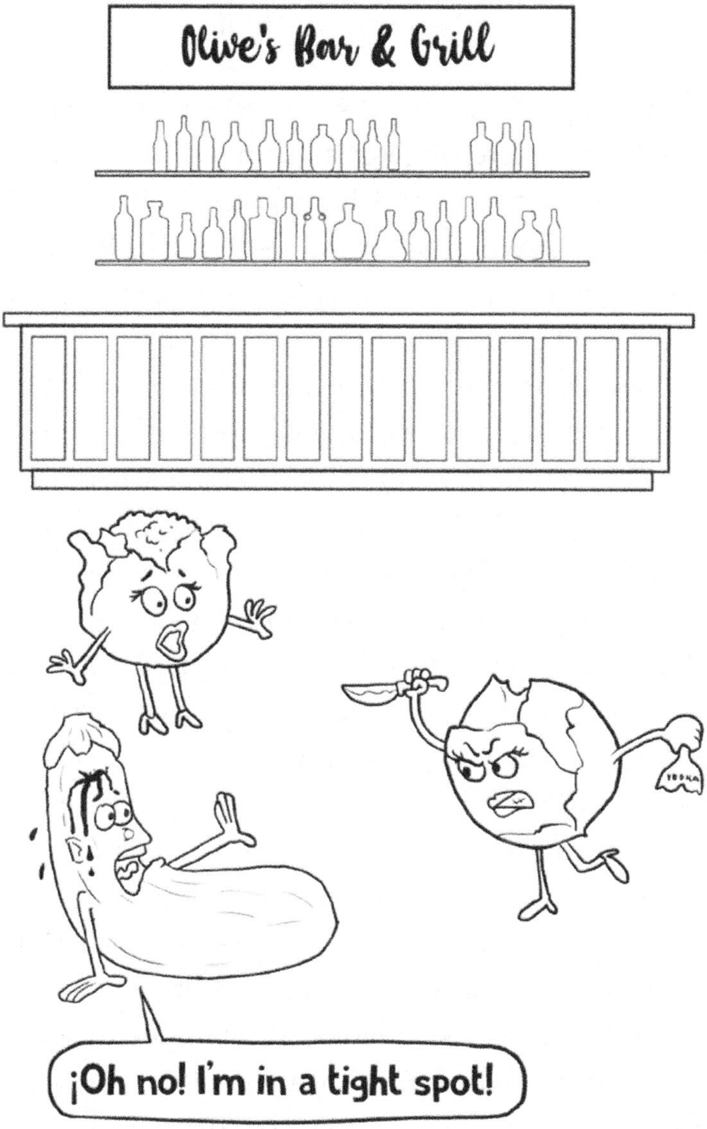
Olive's Bar & Grill
¡Oh no! I'm in a tight spot!

Never Give Up II

You're cruising along and it's all falling into place. You're eating right and exercising just as planned. Then it happens. It can occur unexpectedly and hit you like a brick in the face. You can be proceeding along so well and suddenly you fall off a cliff. Your expertly laid plans destruct and you stop eating right and exercising.

This can occur due to many reasons. So many times, it is emotional in nature. Death, divorce, problems with children and grandchildren, there are countless scenarios that can and do affect your emotional state. Emotions are a fragile area that affect every aspect of your life.

Maybe you just wake up one morning and you're feeling a little depressed. Sometimes it can be as simple as a rainy day, or even a bad hair day. Whatever the reason, whenever you slip and miss a day you must continue onward. You can't fall apart at this point.

While we can never escape these situations unscathed, we can deal with them in a constructive manner. It's like the old saying "It's not what happens to you, it's how you handle it." We're wise enough now to understand life is a roller coaster of emotions. The true survivors are the ones that who come through the other side with a positive outlook. Be one of those individuals and stay focused on your goals.

Let's imagine you're moving right along in your fitness program. You're exercising for a half-hour every day and eating the right foods in the proper proportions. You're as happy as Zarkoff in a house of ill repute. Suddenly a call comes in from your daughter. Your grandson has been injured in a car accident. There's not a lot of situations worse than this.

It's completely normal that exercising is off the agenda and has slipped down the priority scale. Maybe you miss a day, then another and another. You're eating unhealthy foods as the crisis continues. You simply don't care about your exercise and healthy diet. All that concerns you is your grandson's well-being.

At some point the situation is at least partially resolved in one manner or another. Then you step back and realize everything you've worked for is potentially slipping away. This is a critical decision point and separates the winners from the losers. You've resumed the unhealthy eating habits that plagued you for decades. You've completely given up on your exercise routine.

You have to look at it this way. I've put X number of weeks or months into this and I haven't lost that. The only thing I've lost has been the time when I was consumed by a genuine crisis. *You have to pick up where you left off!*

A warrior mentality has to take over. Pick up the pieces and carry on like a true survivor. Look at the top performers in any arena, athletes for example. Although they may possess extreme talent in what they excel in, it's usually something else that separates them from their peers. It's that pure will to win, that drive that comes from deep inside.

Use whatever motivation possible to stand up and fight. Adversity is the name of the game in life and we're never going to avoid it. I remember how a famous race car driver once dealt with adverse conditions. It was one of the most prestigious races of the season. The race track was wet, bumpy, and extremely treacherous. All the other drivers were whining and complaining before the race about how difficult the track was.

They interviewed this particular driver. He smiled as he told the interviewer he liked a difficult track. Everyone was in the same boat, so to speak. He explained that it was an advantage to him because he didn't care what the conditions were. It was a level playing field in that respect. The other drivers were psychologically weakened and were now his prey. He was out to win the race.

He did win that race and you can win yours too. Challenges can and will occur and you accept them and even embrace them. It's all in the mind. The mind controls the body, the body doesn't control the mind. Get back on that horse and ride off into the sunset just like those ole cowboy movies. Be the hero of your own desires and make it happen. Do it for yourself and do it with purpose. Let nothing stand in your way. It starts with you and ends with you. Do you want it? Go get it!

It's not easy,
Getting fit.
Stay with it,
Never quit!

Women & Men

Women and men are different, just in case you didn't know. I happen to have been born into the weaker gender. We men blaze through life thinking we're the stronger of the two sexes. Nothing could be further from the truth.

I do realize that the human race in general is a pretty screwed-up species, but women appear to have it more together than their male counterparts. Women are the controllers even though it can be clandestinely so. Look at everything that happens and trace it back to where it originated. You'll find a woman at the source. Then glance in the periphery and you'll see their male subjects wagging their tails in blissful obedience.

Women definitely rule the planet. Women have the goods that transcend materiality, that *something* that men will never possess. Eons will continue to pass and we'll never come close to attaining your unreachable status.

There you have it in all its simplicity. You women kick back, perched up there enjoying your lofty status, watching us men scurry around trying to appease you. We're putting on our tough protector act, erroneously thinking we're running the big show. Our defective rationale is quite comical when you think about it.

It's all a delusional defect that has plagued men since creation itself. I guess we should blame it all on that apple. You know, the one we were told not to eat, but was so irresistibly tempting that we had to have a bite. Humanity lost all rationality at that point with no hope of ever recovering. It sure makes it interesting though.

You ladies operate like magicians as we men inhabit our illusionary world. I guess we serve some sort of purpose or you wouldn't keep us around. Entertainment and amusement seem to be our mainstay. I for one am thrilled to serve you goddesses. What a dull world it would be without you. Zarkoff Zucchini would certainly agree with that.

I know what lies beyond the curtain, for behind that silky veil lies a true work of art, a beautiful pastiche of all that is real and wonderful, a flawless masterpiece of creation. We men will forever be in awe of you.

There you are in all your glory, like the queens you are, smiling down at the amusing theater beneath you. Males are no more than puffed-up puppets, operating on a subconscious level, genetically driven to appease our masters.

You may wonder what all this female ingratiating and flattery has to do with fitness. In actuality nothing, but it's true nevertheless, and more men need to realize how lucky we are to have you. All this, however, does bring me to my major point. For all the differences between men and women, when it comes to exercise and healthy eating, we're very similar.

Although the marketing gurus would like you to believe otherwise, women and men require *basically* the same nutritional needs. A healthy, balanced diet will suffice for both sexes. It really is that simple.

Don't fall for the shiny dream they dangle in front of you. This packaged powder or that gender-specific specialized nutritional bar is always the magical answer. Eat their particular product and fat will miraculously melt away, or so they say. After two servings you're transformed into a magnet for the opposite sex. You're wise and you know otherwise.

The same goes for the exercise plan. Those bozos pushing their infomercials want you to believe that because you're a woman you're doomed for disaster unless you purchase their gimmicky device. The last one I saw was the funniest ever. They claimed that sitting in their special chair thirty minutes a day would turn you into a lean, toned, head-turning stunner. I've got serious doubts about that one.

Human beings seem to enjoy complicating things. Sometimes overthinking can lead to decisions that push you further from your desired goal. Don't worry yourself to death about being too feminine or too masculine in your approach toward acquiring a healthy body. Our needs are similar. Just get out there and stick to the basics whether you're male or female. You'll make it. It's more about those two words that you'll grow to love, dedication and discipline.

Men seem to have it worse in the beat-yourself-up department. For some reason we feel we have to prove our machismo and it becomes self-defeating. This seems to be the mentality of some men and I've witnessed it. It must be some primal defect we have that infinitely tortures us. To be a real man requires a manly approach, or so our Hollywood indoctrination has led us to believe.

Here's a real example. I know a guy who literally thought he could reverse forty years of unhealthy living in one week. In his delusional state he believed that if he drank twelve protein shakes and power-lifted several hundred pounds of weight, he would get fit immediately.

I don't have to tell you how that one turned out. On day two after his premiere ferocious workout he was visiting a doctor. Muscle tears, ruptured tendons and torn ligaments were the horrendous diagnosis. It would be months before he could lift anything heavier than a coffee cup. Predictably he gave up fitness forever and resigned himself to a life of watching fit people play sports on television instead.

In summation of this gender discussion, it all boils down to applying common sense. Go with your natural instincts and don't let the image-molders fool you. The beautiful girl that's selling that glitzy exercise device is getting paid to trick you. That perfect male specimen that's pushing his version of utopia is also on the payroll.

If you still fall for it, you're on your own. Just make sure you know the expiration date on your credit card and remember that little number on the back. They'll need that to finalize their snow job and transfer your money over to their bank.

Women are lovely,
Women have smarts.
Women have brains,
And Beautiful Hearts.

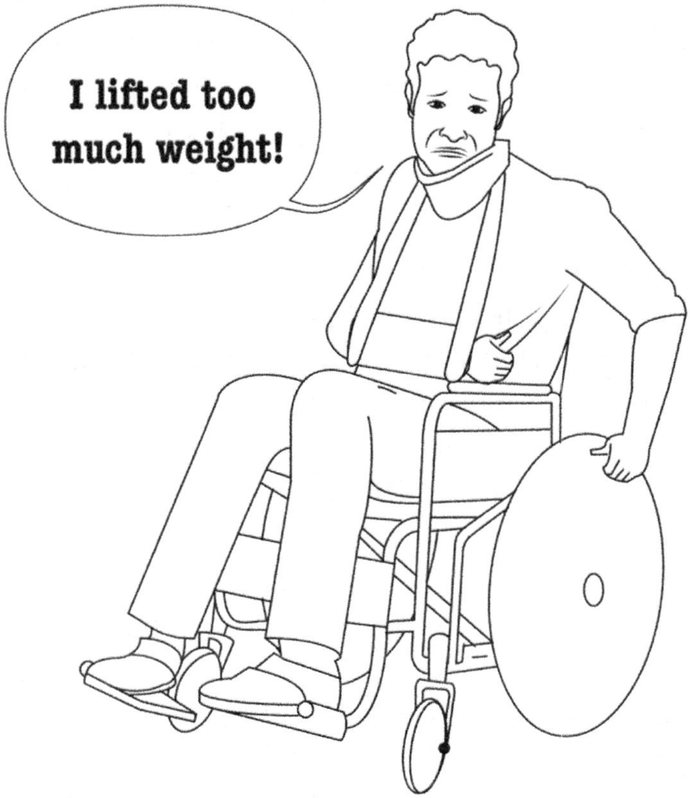
I lifted too
much weight!

Women & Men II

Relations between women and men can be complicated. I don't have to tell you this because you're a wise and aware geezer. Quite the tales we could all put together. We've learned from each experience. Zarkoff, however, was a whole different animal. He never seemed to learn. He certainly expressed a deep, genuine appreciation for women. It's just that it backfired on him sometimes. Here is a case that perfectly illustrates this point.

Zarkoff looked out at the magnificent beauty of nature. The Grand Canyon was spectacularly breathtaking. It was hundreds of miles long, miles wide, and a mile in depth. Every inch of it was a glorious treat to the senses.

Zarkoff turned to his girlfriend and smiled. Times were good and things were looking up. Relations with Barbie Broccoli had been rocky due to his numerous indiscretions, but they had finally turned the corner on all that. Maybe he would finally find some peace in a relationship. They had talked about this trip for months. Now they were finally seeing the Grand Canyon.

"Well, hello, Zarkie," a voice called from behind. "Are you enjoying your new girlfriend?" Zarkoff's body instantly went limp. There was only one person who called him Zarkie. This wasn't going to be good.

The voice belonged to Maggie Maize, better known as Maggie the Madam. She was one tough piece of corn. Maggie was the most famous brothel owner in Nevada. She had a reputation for taking no crap from anyone. No one pushed Maggie the Madam around, especially a man.

Maggie directed her attention to Barbie first. "Honey, baby," she said. "You're one pretty piece of broccoli and you can sure do better than this slimeball louse zucchini. That rotter just gave my best working girl an STD last week. Now she's out of commission for two weeks and I'm losing money. By the way, pretty broccoli, have you been checked for an STD? He probably gave it to you also!"

"Last week!" shrieked Barbie. "Zarkoff, you degenerate swine, you lowlife vermin, you wretched miscreant scoundrel! You told me you were being faithful, and the whole time you're out chasing hookers! And then you come back to me and give me who knows what! I'll show you, you faithless lying jerk!"

Barbie picked up the biggest rock she could find and sent it flying. It was a perfect shot to the side of Zarkoff's head. Zarkoff fell to the ground and from that moment on everything seemed like a dream. For sure he had brain damage again. He drifted in and out of consciousness as the two girls took turns kicking him and pounding him with rocks.

"Zarkie," said Maggie, "you're going for a one-mile ride. Barbie and I are going to throw you into the Grand Canyon!"

Maggie effortlessly dragged Zarkoff to the edge of the canyon. "Take a look down there, Zarkie! That's a long way and there are a lot of sharp rocks. This will teach you to dirty up my girls. Enjoy the ride because it will be your last. Goodbye, Zarkie!"

Barbie got in one last ferocious kick to Zarkoff's groin area. Maggie then gave a final push that sent Zarkoff plummeting into the canyon. "See you later, sleazeball lout!" she cried out.

Zarkoff fell several hundred feet, bounced off a pile of boulders, and went flying back into the air. A quarter-mile later he landed again, this time on a patch of jagged, sharp rocks. One of them pierced his abdomen. Another shredded his aorta. He bounced back up. This time he flew for half a mile before crashing face-first upon a giant boulder. It was three hours before the helicopter lifted out his limp body.

Zarkoff was pronounced dead four times on the way to the hospital. Each time they managed to resuscitate him. Zarkoff was rushed into emergency surgery. Doctors were not optimistic.

It was touch and go for nine months. Another heart transplant was performed. Most of his intestines were removed. Brain surgeries were necessary. Amazingly he survived. After he awoke from his coma, Zarkoff looked in the mirror. It was not a pretty sight. Those two girls had certainly gotten angry.

Zarkoff endured forty reconstructive face surgeries in an attempt to regain his handsomeness. Eventually he looked somewhat like the old Zarkoff. Now he could go back to doing what he did best, chasing women, and of course, paying the price for it.

As usual, there's a moral within this story. Women and men are similar in many ways, but there are differences. Treat women right or you may pay like Zarkoff. Behind each sweet smile lies a Maggie the Madam just waiting to show her colors.

Zarkoff likes women,
He likes them all.
Too many women,
Made Zarkoff fall.

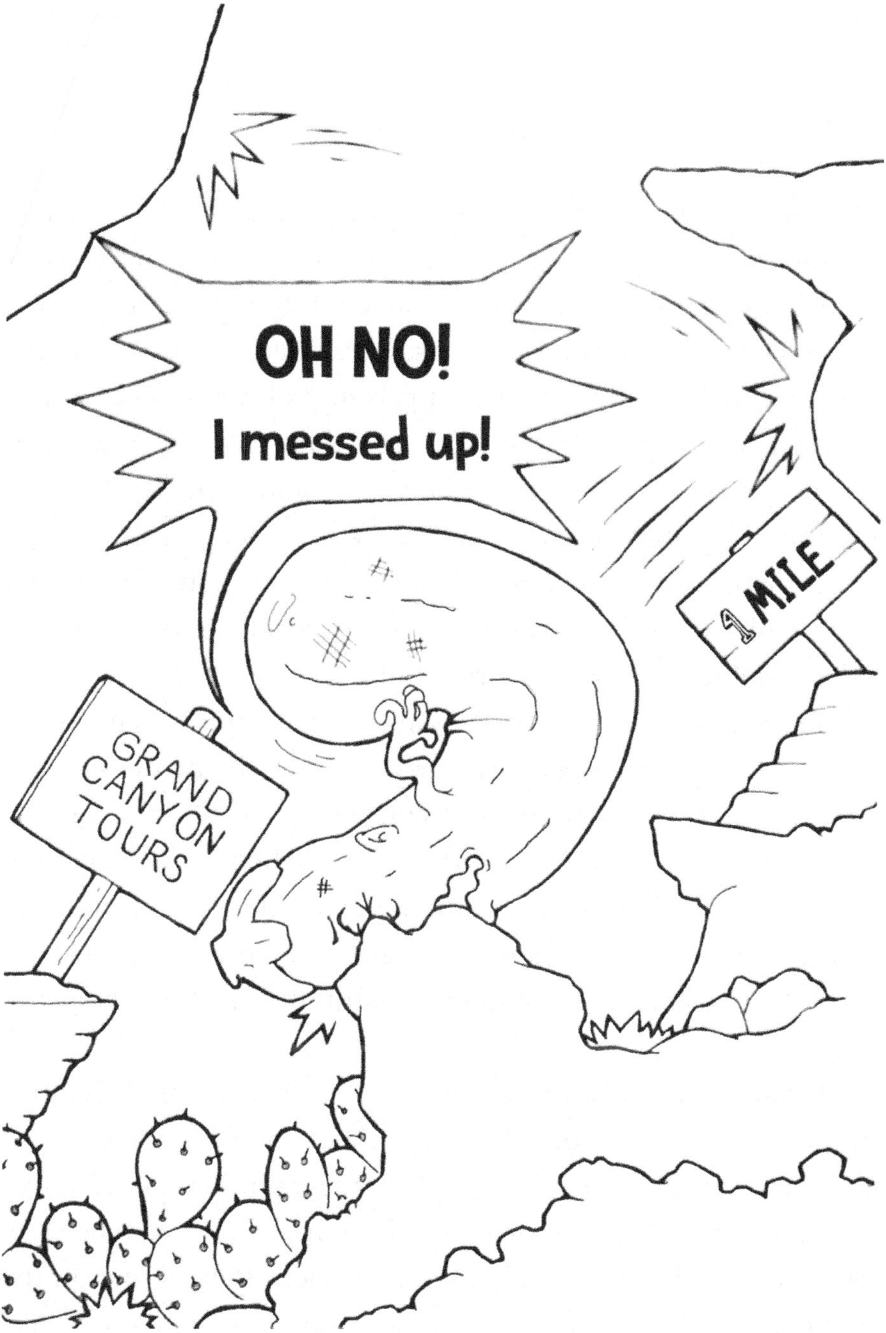
OH NO!
I messed up!
GRAND CANYON TOURS
1 MILE

Competition

Competition is a natural part of life. It exists, at least to a certain degree, in all circles of friends, family and work associates. It may be a polite and civil competition, but it's there. It doesn't stop just because you're a geezer. A geezed-up competitor is a formidable opponent to be reckoned with.

Even in the most subdued of us there lies a competitive streak ready to pounce and show its colors. Let this be you. Decide today that you are going to be in better physical shape than *everyone* in your circle. Maybe they've gotten you beat financially or in some other area of importance. If so, let this be the fuel that flames the fire within.

There is something about being fit that captures the attention of your peers, especially when they see the process in real time right before their eyes. I compare it to winning in the monetary materialistic world. That's where many people decide to display their competitive spirit. There's nothing wrong with that, but here's something I've noticed. Money and things attract a lot of attention, but being fit is a *universal* desire.

When you really think about it, what good are frivolous possessions if you don't have your health? Go ask someone who has loads of those things that question. Maybe they live in the oversized house or drive the fanciest car. Maybe they purchase all the latest gadgets the moment they arrive on the scene. Maybe they travel to all the trendy be-seen-at spots and come back sporting a tan to prove it.

I'm happy they have that disposable income that allows them to own these things and do those things. But the moment they lose their health that stuff loses its appeal. Most would trade it *all* for a healthy body. They would do practically anything to wake up every morning and *feel good* again. All those shiny objects would be swapped in a moment in exchange for a strong healthy body.

I don't know your position in the other human competition fields. Maybe you've already got all that stuff and the prestige that goes with it. If so, that's wonderful. Just realize that one day it may slip down the importance scale. I hope you won't look back and regret focusing on money instead of fitness and health. Eating right and exercising are great accomplishments. They make you shine from the inside.

Humans have a need for acceptance and like to feel important. We have a tendency to want to show off when we've attained success. Money and all the things it can buy is the most obvious method of doing this.

That may be true and great, but you know what? Being fit and healthy is so damn *primal*. It's raw and it's real and it's sexual. It's been driving humans since creation. It's desire and lust and animalistic. It transcends the day-to-day and penetrates the eternal. It's an energy that burns through the pretentious and cuts deep into the real. It's swagger and confidence and in-your-face. It's humans at their most exposed, when everything else is stripped away and the truth is the only thing standing. It's who we are and what we are at our core.

Our bodies are our first possession and we should never let them slide down the priority scale. It's a living body and the only one we have, at least in this lifetime. We're born into it and we should treat it with respect. We should be held responsible for it and take care of it. To disregard it and chase after the ostentatious is a dangerous affair.

The body is your friend and you want to keep it that way, because it never loses. When you're not attentive to it, it fights back and always wins. Sooner or later, you'll pay attention to it and regret you didn't earlier. Learn it, find out what it wants, and keep it happy. It will be a very smooth ride after that.

Getting fit,
That's your quest.
You can do it,
Be the best!

Competition II

Let's go back to the competition part of all this. You want to show others, maybe someone in particular, that you can be better than them at *something*. That *something* could be a lean, strong, and healthy body. Don't dig yourself into a hole by telling them you're *going* to do it. *Just do it.*

Read this book and every other book you can find on attaining a fit and healthy body. Pick and choose your plan of attack. Then go for it without pomp and ceremony. It's going to be a process, but here's the nice thing about that.

You want to *win*. That's what this is all about. To win in the fitness arena takes time. You need to be slow, steady and methodical. However, the day will come when they first notice a difference in your appearance. It may be weight loss or simply that glow that appears when things are going in the right direction.

At this point they're playing catchup with you. Never give advice unless they ask. Help them, but tempt and tease them by leaking the secrets little by little. After all, you're out to win. Ultimately, you're the big winner when you can help others see the light as you did.

For the time being though, you've got to keep a little distance between you and the competition. Time is your friend. You've got the jump on them, so keep grinding out your daily routine. Persevere, be persistent and keep going. The payoff is ahead. By the time they realize what you've accomplished, they'll be so far behind they'll never catch up. That's when you reveal all your secrets. Once they've seen your little miracle with their own eyes, they're yours to guide.

Keep at it. Three more months will go by and you'll become more fit. They'll notice. Another six months passes and you're even more fit. Maybe they're a little envious and jealous, but you're putting on your humble, unassuming act. Believe me, that's the classy way to win.

A year goes by and you're feeling like the queen or king you are. You're so far ahead they don't have a chance to overtake you. You won at a universal game. You're good at something and that something is a lean, strong, fit body that others crave. Be proud of yourself and smile. *You're a winner!*

You're so proud,
You don't quit.
You're so proud,
That you're FIT!

Doctor Visits

We're at an age where physicians and medical visits are part of our lives. Most of the time they're absolutely necessary and even vital for survival. That being said, you should always be alert and monitor yourself. Under no circumstances do you want to be diagnosed with Doctor Attention Syndrome.

I call it Agnes Syndrome after my late aunt, as she was struck with this horrible affliction. Aunt Agnes, God bless her soul, was a wonderful and kind lady. She baked homemade oatmeal cookies that were the hit of the neighborhood. And she never told my parents when she caught me cutting class as a teenager.

I think the root of my beloved Aunt Agnes' problems was more psychological than physical. She loved doctors and medicine so much that I think she became addicted to the attention. She would always return from a doctor visit looking so happy. Wearing a big smile, she would gleefully tell us how sick she was.

Agnes Syndrome is such that it lures you in incrementally. It usually creeps in after a series of traumatic events in the victim's life. Researchers have noted that when a person is faced with major trauma, such as a broken nail, they become highly susceptible to Agnes Syndrome. If they are unlucky enough to be hit with another devastating crisis, like detecting a slight tear in their favorite blouse, the situation could potentially explode.

That's exactly how my Aunt Agnes' situation unfolded. When she was hit with a third traumatic event, an ant was discovered in her outdoor storage room, she completely fell apart. She immediately raced to the doctor complaining of a variety of ailments, most of them deadly in nature. The combination of the broken nail, torn blouse and sighting an ant completely did her in. From that moment she was a lost cause with no hope.

My dear aunt survived twenty years of Agnes Syndrome before she finally passed. In those two decades she made hundreds of visits to doctors and received medication by the truckload. How she tricked the doctors I'll never know.

I have to admit the Aunt Agnes story is slightly exaggerated, but there's a lot of truth in it. You may know someone similar, or even display some of those same characteristics yourself. I think it really is a widespread problem.

Not for a moment am I undermining the value of doctors and the medical profession. They are incredible, caring and dedicated professionals who have invested years into education and training. They are deserving of praise and they should be held in the highest regard. They help people.

I personally know a well-known physician who has seen it all in his forty years of service. He's a respected author and possesses great wisdom. We briefly discussed this issue several years ago. What he told me was fascinating. He'll remain unnamed because of the whistle blower nature of it all.

He informed me that "Agnes Syndrome" was very real, and it was truly psychologically based. He went on to say certain people crave the attention they receive when they have medical issues, imagined or not.

The root of it all is a deep need for something that's missing in their life. They direct that energy into a sympathy-seeking path that usually ends up in a doctor's office. Then they have their excuse for the underlying emotional issue that's beneath it all.

He gave numerous examples. There were cases where illnesses were imagined or even faked, and others where a parent would consistently bring in their children claiming they was sick. In reality they were actually seeking attention for themselves.

This notable physician shared another interesting story. It somewhat explains the dependence, some could call it addiction, that so many people have to their medication. It all lies in the bigtime marketing of pharmaceuticals. It's not as neat and clean as you might think.

He especially delved into details of one particular drug that now invades so many with addiction. This drug was marketed with precision at medical conferences and events worldwide. Hospital administrators, top physicians and high-level decision-makers were tempted with great financial incentives. The result is our current sad situation.

That's enough of that. The lesson should be that the quick fix isn't always the best remedy. Covering up the pain, whether it's physical or emotional, isn't always the answer. Treating the symptom and not the cause is a runaway train that will eventually crash. It's not an easy task, but it's a necessary one. Running out for a penicillin shot every time you have a cold isn't the answer. If you've had relations with Zarkoff, you probably should get a dose of penicillin.

The medical profession is overall ethical and full of the best human beings on the planet. Make sure you're doing what you're doing for the right reasons. Common sense must be applied. One way to avoid some of this mess is to *eat right and exercise!*

Doctors are great, Doctors are wise. They say eat right, And exercise!

Yes, This Is Common Knowledge

You may have noticed that not one word has yet been written about the specifics of my fitness plan. You know why? It's because it's so damn easy to comprehend compared to the motivational end of this. Your head has to be in the right place and is far more important than the x's and o's of the plan. The educational process of eating right and exercising is an incredibly easy concept to grasp.

What you'll read further along in this book has been written in countless other books and articles. Many of you may read it and think, I know that already, tell me something I don't know. And you will be right.

Success in this field has more to do with desire than intelligence. How bad do you want it? I know a brilliant individual that actually works in the medical field who is eighty pounds overweight. I know another childhood friend who barely had adequate grades to graduate high school. He lost sixty pounds by eating sensibly and exercising regularly.

My childhood friend didn't possess a higher learning capacity than my overweight acquaintance. His success wasn't due to comprehending the intricacies of some complicated fitness regime. *That's because it's not complicated in any way.* It's very simple.

You will encounter every negative force that exists in your quest to become fit. Try to keep it your personal journey and keep others out of it. They will only complicate it. You will find that even though they may be in horrible physical shape, they are self-declared experts in the fields of exercise and nutrition.

There are always people who think they're know-it-alls and feel compelled by a higher power to share their gifts with you. It is useless to argue with them and a complete waste of time. Politely agree with them and continue doing your own thing. They're just trying to take something simple and turn it into a NASA rocket project. The most important component in this is *you*. Once you're committed, the rest of it simply falls into place.

That's what I hope to do with this book. I want to touch a nerve somewhere and fire up your desire to be physically fit. Everything else will just fall into place. You'll never stop learning about various things that will guide you, but the basic concepts will never change. Never stray far from the source, the root of it all, *eating right and exercising*.

I know this, I know that. I know it all, So why am I fat?

GYM

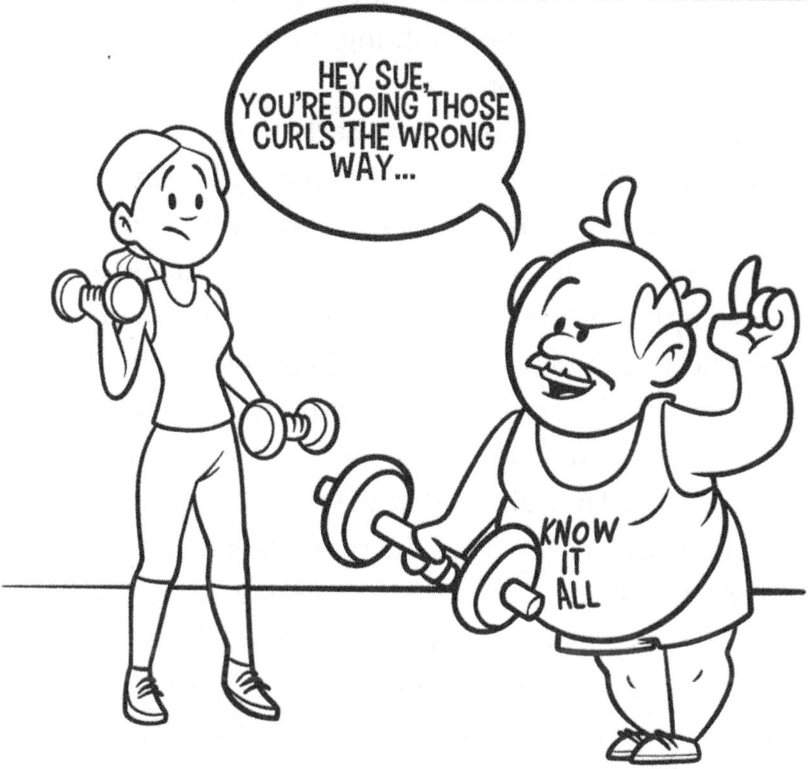

Yes, This Is Common knowledge II

Follow the script of that great visionary, Zarkoff Zucchini. He may have had flaws, but he was no average squash. He knew it was about the basics and nothing more. His simplicity was pure genius. What an icon.

As a matter of fact, there's a Zarkoff Zucchini story that illustrates how the obvious is so often overlooked. It's just as that old saying goes, sometimes you can't see the forest for the trees. Common sense can be overridden by some innate desire to overcomplicate matters. That's exactly what happened to our lovable, but somewhat disturbed Zarkoff.

Early in the days of his newfound fame, Zarkoff Zucchini found himself enjoying the company of several women simultaneously. They all lived in the same small town.

Monday was reserved for the pretty Chantel Carrot, Tuesday was for Lecia Lettuce, Wednesday was for Margie Mushroom, sexy Opal Onion claimed Thursday, Lydia Lentil was the lucky recipient for Friday, Saturday was reserved for sensual Stormy Soybean, and Sunday was Toni Tomato's day. Young Zarkoff was a busy veggie indeed and quite the juggler.

The trouble started one Friday evening. It ended disastrously for our little libido-driven veggie activist. Who knew two lovely beans could stir up so much trouble? Here's what happened.

Zarkoff was playing it safe. There had been a couple of occasions where two of his girlfriends had been dangerously close to each other. Information sharing between any two of them would not end well. This time he was taking no chances. Tonight's locale would be the zoo located in the adjoining county.

Lydia Lentil has always expressed her love for animals. The zoo would be a perfect place for her. There was no chance any of his other girlfriends would be anywhere near the place. He could finally relax without worrying about drama manufacturing spontaneously. Lydia Lentil would certainly respond with amatory rewards. She could be a wildcat when she was in the mood. Zarkoff felt really good. This celebrity life wasn't bad at all!

"Look at the little baby kangaroo," exclaimed Lydia. "He's so adorable."

Zarkoff watched as the young marsupial followed closely behind his mother. "Yes, kangaroos are such interesting animals," he said. "Hey look, there are some lions over there." He pointed straight ahead at three lions playing together.

"Oh, let's go see them!" exclaimed Lydia. "I've never seen a lion before. I'll meet you there. I need to visit the restroom for a moment."

Zarkoff walked over for a better view. He stood directly in front of the caged area.

"Don't get too close," a voice called out. "They're extremely irritable just before feeding time. They're really hungry right now."

Zarkoff turned to see a zoo employee. He had a large of bucket containing enormous slabs of raw meat. "Watch when I feed them," he said. "They'll devour this like it's their last meal on earth. I've never seen them so hungry before.

Zarkoff hoped Lydia could witness this. What was taking her so long anyway? She should be back by now. This was something that would really interest her.

Suddenly a hand appeared from behind and grabbed his left arm. Another hand snatched his right arm. In a second his hands were cuffed together with real handcuffs. What the heck was going on! Was this some kind of a joke?

He turned to see two familiar faces just before a shovel slammed him in the face. It sent him flying to the ground. It was Lydia and she had company! It was Stormy Soybean! Stormy didn't earn her nickname by accident. She was indeed a fiery storm when incited. Zarkoff had really screwed up this time. Big time!

This was what he had tried to avoid at all costs, two girlfriends interacting. No doubt Lydia and Stormy had met at the ladies' room and shared information. That was the fuel behind all this anger.

Zarkoff wiped the blood from his eyes. In horror he watched as fiery-eyed Stormy plunged a steely pitchfork into his abdomen. Lydia's shovel again slammed the back of his head. The powerful blow left him immobile. Once again, he was sure he had brain damage. Now he lay there defenseless against the two enraged-with-jealousy beans.

"How does your head feel now, you two-timing, lying, dirty, tiny wee-weed, piece-of-trash zucchini?" cried Stormy. "You gave me gonorrhea and you were going to give it to Lydia tonight. We've wrapped you in raw meat and feeding you to those hungry lions. Are you ready to be chewed upon by a bunch of ravenous wild animals? Huh, are you, you good-for-nothing, rotten vegetable?"

Zarkoff glanced down and nearly went into shock. The girls had somehow covered his entire body with large pieces of meat that the ravenous lions so craved. Now they planned on feeding him to the lions! He was in a tight spot!

The girls dragged Zarkoff to the front of the cage. Lydia had somehow acquired the key from the attendant and was preparing to open the door. In a matter of seconds he would be a goner, nothing more than minced meat for hungry lions.

Suddenly a claw pierced through the cage and ripped into Zarkoff's thigh. Blood spurted from his femoral artery. The lions were now in full fury. A huge claw slashed into his abdomen. It tore open the flesh and Zarkoff's innards rolled out. The lions quickly devoured them. Another claw ripped away a sizable piece of his chest. A lion quickly gobbled it down. "Umm good," he said to the others.

This was his last moment on earth. Zarkoff was sure of it. Why did he have to womanize? Why did he need so many girlfriends? Why, oh, why, must he die for it?

Just as a last claw tore into his pelvic area, he felt himself being pulled from the cage. Two local policemen had witnessed the commotion and subdued the girls. They dragged him away from the ravenous lions. This idiot would likely die, but at least he wouldn't be torn to shreds by hungry beasts. Zarkoff slipped out of consciousness knowing this was the end.

Zarkoff spent the next year in a coma. Doctors struggled to save him. He awakened to find himself horribly mutilated. He was told he would survive, but likely remain very ugly. He would be disfigured, but cosmetic surgeries would help. The lions had made a mess of his body. His wee was especially mangled. For sure, the girls would have been pleased to learn this.

The moral of this story as it relates to fitness is this. Never overlook the obvious and use common sense. Zarkoff should have known dating seven women simultaneously would backfire. He would eventually get caught. And he did.

In our case, common sense dictates what it takes to become fit. Anyone of our age knows that gimmickry doesn't work. Geezers have seen it all. It's the simple combination of eating right and exercising that produces results. *Don't be a Zarkoff and screw up!* Don't be delusional about fitness.

You may already know how to become physically fit. If that's the case, then close this book and get on with it. Go do it. Gain some credibility by sculpting a body that speaks for itself. Prove your knowledge through your desire. Find that desire. *Let's eat right and exercise!*

Zarkoff played,
Every day.
He got caught,
He did pay!

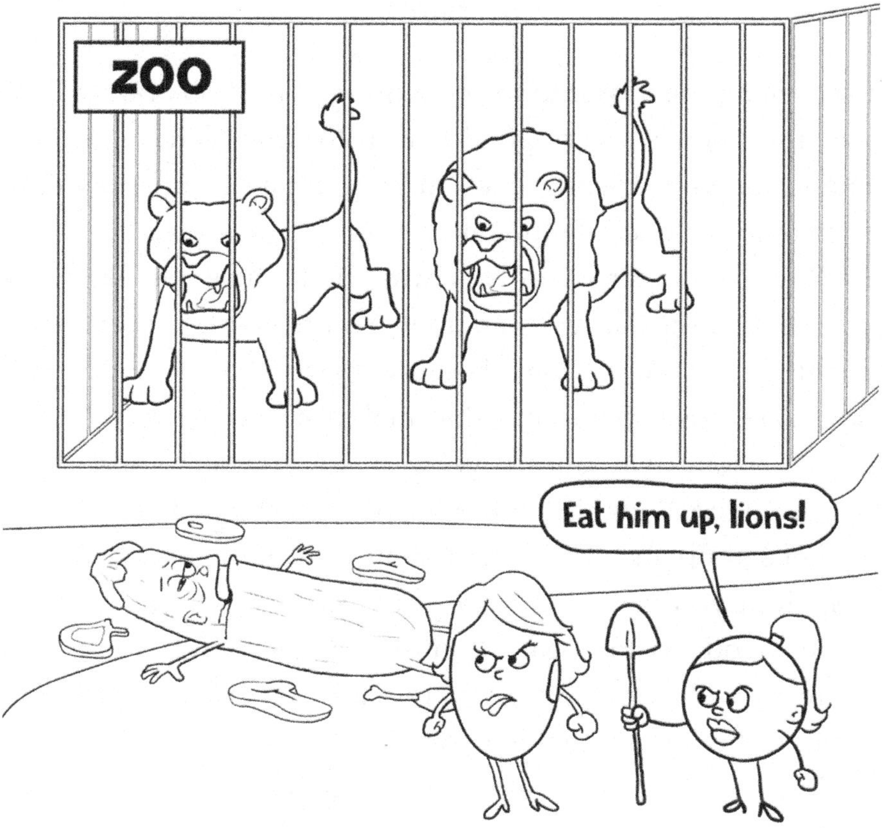
ZOO
Eat him up, lions!

Be Humble

I'm placing this closer to the beginning of the book rather than the end. There's a very good reason for this. You don't want to alienate your friends, even though it may be unknowingly and completely unintentional.

You're going to win this war, that much we know. If you've read this far, you can do it. You're going to become fit, healthy, lean and strong because that's the mentality you have. You visualize it and that makes it become reality. The end is a long way ahead, yet you see yourself, hands held overhead, breaking through the tape at the finish line.

Let's jump ahead a year, or simply several months. You've done it or you're well on your way towards doing it. You can smell blood, so to speak. You're feeling fit and strong and beaming with confidence. You're ready to explode inside and want to shout it out to the world.

Your success is an emotional experience. In most cases there were doubters, those around you who didn't think you could do it, didn't want you to do it, or both. At this point it is tempting to antagonize them with a little I-told-you-so scolding. It's human nature to want to showcase accomplishments. However, don't let that desire override your senses and create future issues in your personal relationships. Don't let emotions rule your logic.

Be very proud of what you're done, but never rub it in people's faces. Never bring up the subject of fitness around them. That would be about as tacky as a wealthy person who constantly steers conversations towards wealth and all the things it can buy. Others less fortunate will naturally take offense to such snobbery. In your case your body is your wealth. You've claimed the prize that everyone wants and it's staring them in the face. There's no need to shout it out.

Let them bring it up. Don't worry, eventually it will come up in conversation. Maybe you'll order something healthy in a restaurant and someone will comment about it. Maybe you'll receive a comment about your weight loss. However it comes up, accept it as a compliment and move on. At this point they may inquire further as to how you did it, how you succeeded in such a universal field.

Here you're at a crossroads as to how to handle the situation. You don't want to come across as a know-it-all and shove it in their face. Come out of it looking like the classy act that you are. In an unassuming way, tell them it was something you wanted to do for yourself. It was a personal goal that you set and you're grateful that you've had a degree of success. Tell them it really wasn't such a big deal.

Be humble and matter-of-fact about it. Tell them it was something you really wanted and you pursued it. Explain to them that it was hard work, but anyone can do it if they really want it. Downplay your strengths even though it may be difficult. Tell them you're just fortunate that it seems to be working out for you.

Deep inside you'll want to pronounce that it required determination and discipline of an unworldly nature. You'll feel like pounding your chest and proclaiming you're Wonder Woman or Superman. Bite your tongue, go the other route, and play the role of Common Sue or Joe Average. Save the ego theatrics for when you get back home. Then you can stand in front of the mirror and dance around like an idiot expressing your joy. For now, be a class act.

There will come a moment when someone genuinely wants to know how you did it. They'll sincerely ask for details on the methods behind your success. You may see the same fire in their eyes that you had many months before. This is when you break it down and tell them everything they want to know. They'll learn just how difficult the undertaking was for you.

They'll find out your accomplishment required dedication and discipline. They'll realize the task you've executed so successfully wasn't an easy undertaking. It required determination, an inner confidence, and a true belief in yourself. They'll admire you for what you've done and how you gracefully handled your success.

Be grateful to those individuals who doubted you, for they stoked the fire that was your success. There's always one or two that secretly wanted you to fail. They wanted to keep you down in their cellar of misery and despair. They've earned a newfound respect for you even though they may never say it or show it. Your actions and not your words proved who and what you are.

You reached for the stars and took a ride. You rode a fiery comet into the heavens and took a tour. The cosmic gods decorated you in stellar brilliance and sent you back for all the world to see. You came back a superstar, beaming with confidence, radiant energy pouring from your soul, an exhibition of calmness and coolness that speaks for itself. You did it and no one can take it away from you. You own yourself. Let others do your showcasing for you, as your actions speak loud and clear. Enjoy the view at the top for it's beautiful.

You don't quit,
You don't lag.
Now you're fit,
Don't you brag!

CHAPTER 3

Good Foods

"It is health that is real wealth and not pieces of gold and silver."
Mahatma Gandhi

Food Evolution

Up to this point we've dealt with our mental preparation, the most difficult and important aspect of becoming fit. Now it starts getting easier. We're going to get into the nuts and bolts of the overall plan. As I mentioned earlier, it's really not complicated at all. Just relax your brain and don't overthink the situation. Think back to those days of yesteryear before life became a digitally technical experience. We're simplifying, not complicating.

This chapter will explore our healthy foods. Natural and unprocessed are the key words here. In a world where everything has been altered, it's easy to forget where it all began. Food started out pure and natural before humans took it and played with it. What dummies we can be.

Let's take a potato for example. Long ago a potato was a potato, living its life so happy, growing up in peace and happiness. It would thrive in its earthly domain until it was ready to serve up mankind with a delicious, nourishing treat. Such a contented veggie it was, just kicking back and enjoying life underground, enjoying its daily routine, attending potato happy hours, and awaiting its time to surface.

When that glorious moment arrived, he popped his head out into the brilliant sun for the first time. Life had been wonderful underground, courting all the pretty female potatoes, playing potato tennis every afternoon, and enjoying all the other great potato amenities. Now the time had come to serve its purpose in life, being eaten and enjoyed by a human. It was really not a big deal, because as every potato knew, they would later be reincarnated as another potato, possibly even a coveted sweet potato.

It was more than willing to serve up early man with a healthy, tasty article of nutrition. It was mostly a baked and roasted, relatively low calorie, high fiber affair. It was the way nature intended for the potato to end its cycle of life. The potato was very willing to sacrifice its life to serve mankind's survival requirements. It was an honor. It could possibly even be listed on the Potato Memorial Hero Monument located deep underground in central Ireland.

Such was the natural cycle of the potato until approximately 1550. At least that's the date listed in the *Potato Almanac Underground History of Edible Tubers*, the highly regarded, reputable publication of upper-crust potato society.

Then everything suddenly changed. Some deranged man, reputedly under the influence of hallucinogens, had the bright idea of *improving* potato cooking methods. He found the greasiest pig fat he could find, added some possum lard, and just for good measure he threw a bucket of saturated trans fats into the mix.

Then he proceeded to cut a hapless potato up into thin slices and showing no compassion at all, laughed as he fiendishly placed the terrified solanum tuberosum into the boiling concoction of lardy intoxicants.

At this point all the other potatoes were petrified as they watched their compatriot scream in agony. As the greasy solution consumed him, they shivered in horror, knowing their turn was coming soon. In what would be known as the Great Potato Massacre of 1550, the level of brutality was beyond description.

One by one the innocent potatoes were sliced beyond recognition, thrown into the boiling mixture, and burned to a crisp. Even the women and children weren't spared. It would go down as one of the most sadistic attacks ever in potato history, a savage, bloodthirsty attack of the most callous nature.

And the torture didn't stop there. Adding to the barbary was the addition of massive amounts of salt, sugar and deadly preservatives. The hapless potatoes would be bagged, put on a shelf, and placed for sale as a snack. The once healthy, vibrant potato was now gone forever, just a footnote in Potato Almanac history. It had been reduced to a thin wasteland of nothingness that possessed no nutritional value whatsoever. Its self-esteem was now a pittance of shame. Its only goals were to make people fat, clog arteries, and attend tailgate parties. It would be commonly known as a potato chip.

So it was that the potato ended its dynasty as a healthy, happy superfood. That's just one example of the horrendous brutality humans imposed upon the vegetarian race. And it's not just vegetables that have received such heinous treatment at the hands of wicked humans. Fruits also were severely mistreated, a fact well documented by the Fruit Racial Injustice Center.

That's the world we now live in, haunted by a shameful past. While we may never bring back the innocents who were sacrificed at the hands of our evil predecessors, we can remember and honor them. The best way to honor these brave carbohydrates is to refuse to purchase or consume the processed version of their once glorious self. They've been humiliated enough already.

Don't fall for the glitzy packaging that catches your eye at the supermarket and subliminally influences you to purchase them. Walk over to the produce area and visit what remains of a once powerful potato dynasty. We cannot let history repeat itself. Remember the brave potatoes that suffered, sacrificed and gave their lives. We can never forget.

Now let's continue onward with the good foods that remain and so loyally serve us. We'll begin with the most basic ingredient of them all. Try going a week without water and see how you feel. You'll probably be pretty thirsty.

Natural foods,
They're so real.
I like the way,
They make me feel.

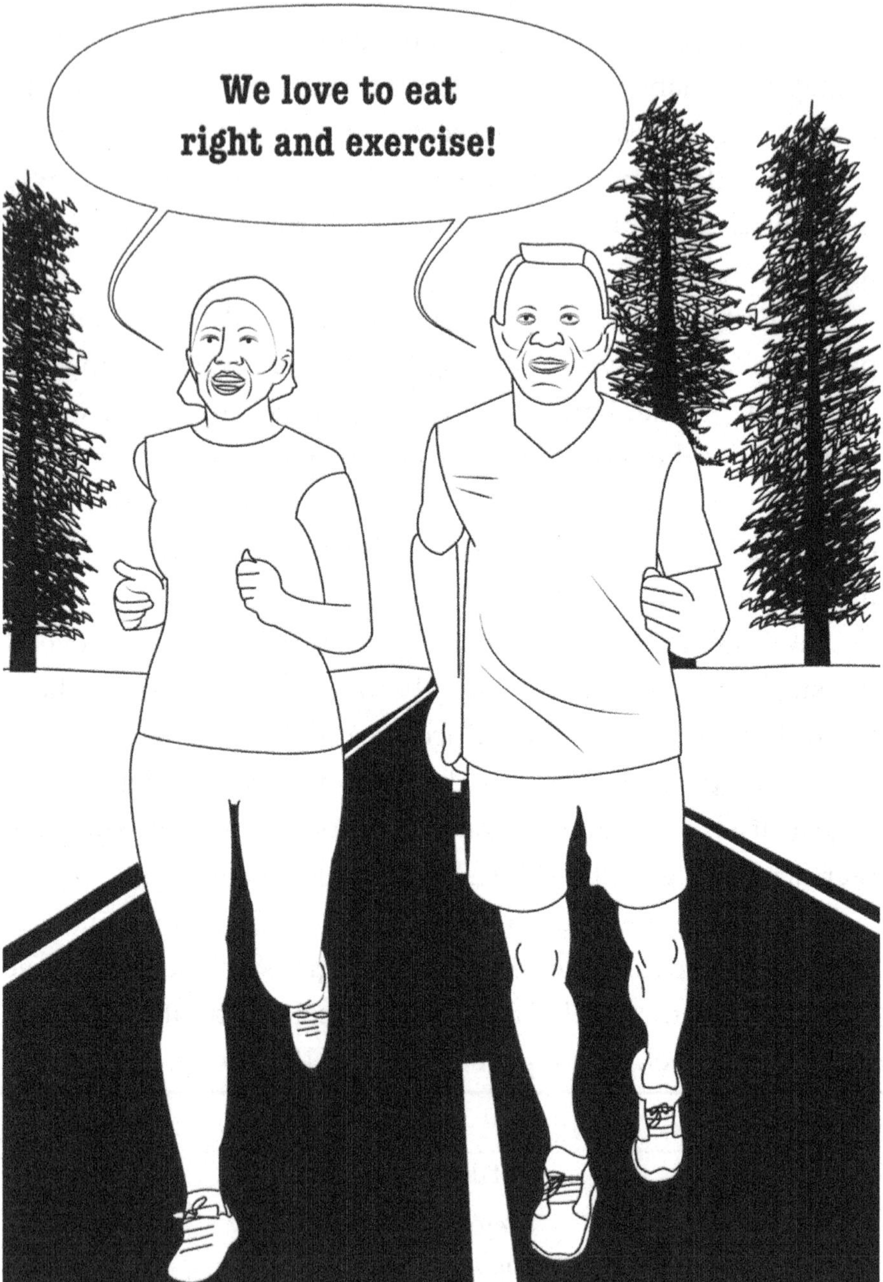
We love to eat
right and exercise!

Water

Water is the most important substance you can put into your body. Estimates vary somewhat, but roughly sixty percent of your body is water. The brain and heart contain an even higher percentage. These statistics alone should prove the value of water. Go without water for several days and you'll be on the backside of those daisies growing in your back yard. You'll be dead.

Try to get used to drinking water all day long. Start your morning with a glass of water as your body has gone all night without fuel. Continue drinking it off and on throughout the day whether you're thirsty or not.

Start becoming aware of even the tiniest feelings of thirst, for they are a signal from your body. It's telling you what it needs. Treat it right and give it what it's asking for. Push it too far and it will fight back with a vengeance. When the body gets angry with the way it's being treated it will quickly show you who's the boss. It will shut you down and you can forget working or playing or whatever it is that consumes your time. You'll be sidelined until it decides you've been punished enough.

Learn your individual needs. Optimally you should never get thirsty, or at least overwhelmingly thirsty. Keep that body lubricated and happy. A quick glass of water several times a day should do the trick, more so if you're engaging in physical activity.

Don't think that because you're in a cool environment you won't need water. Maybe you're not expending as much as you would in hot and humid conditions, but it needs replenishing just the same. A little extra water does nothing but flush out those poisons that want to homestead our bodies. Get rid of those little rascals and pee them out. Send them back to wherever they came from.

Make a habit of carrying a water bottle *everywhere* you go. Refill it constantly throughout the day. Never let yourself get caught in places without access to drinking water. Rely on your trusty water bottle to rescue you. Room temperature water is a more natural choice than cold water, so there's no need to add ice. You can drink more and drink quicker when it's slightly warmer. Fill up your tank and keep it filled.

One huge advantage of drinking loads of water is that it reduces hunger. You'll find you're not nearly as hungry as you would be if you weren't consuming water. It makes sense when you think about it. The body feels fuller when it's full of water. There's less room in there for that doughnut that's calling from the break room. You know, it's the one in the middle of the box with all that colorful sugary stuff on top. It desperately wants to escape and get cozy in someone's intestines.

Anyone who thinks they can permanently lose weight by starving their body of water is delusional. That makes as much sense as cutting off a leg to lose a quick twenty pounds. Never starve yourself of water, unless you are medically advised to do so. There are certain conditions that call for it.

Soft drinks and sugary beverages are the main enemies of water. Sure, they possess water, but they're sabotaged by other ingredients. The marketing guys figured out long ago how to trick us. Humans become easy prey once they've sipped upon that heavily marketed corn-syrupy temptation.

"Oh, it tastes so good and Cindy Celebrity is drinking it on TV," you may say. You are wrong.

Apply some common sense and don't let them run all over you. It's a war between you and the tempters. The high-paid boys back at the corporate testing laboratory have worked hard to create the perfect beverage that delights our sensory desires. Fight back and make the right choice. Choose water, that natural healthy substance that was intended for us. Say no to their doctored-up version.

There's one last thing about water. Make sure it's not poisoned by other means as well. Our industrial society has provided much for us, but there's a tradeoff. Chemicals and waste creep into our natural water systems and hide, awaiting an invasion into our bodies. They're invisible, tasteless and very dangerous.

You'll never know what hit you until it's too late. A couple of years of drinking that stuff can send you down misery lane. It's a breeding ground for cancer and tumors and nothing good can come from it. Make sure your water is not poisonous. Get it tested and make sure you trust the testers.

There you have it. Let water be your primary weapon of choice in your battle to become fit. Keep it by your side like an old cowboy and his six-shooter. Order water in restaurants instead of the pricey-concoction option. Drink it all day long. Make water your friend. Add a little lemon or lime to change it up if you like. You can't live without it. WATER.

You drink water,
Yes, you do.
It's so good,
Good for you!

Fresh Fruit & Veggies

Fruit and vegetables are key ingredients in your quest to become fit. It is especially important for us geezers. Our geezed-up systems have slower metabolisms than the youngsters. We do, however, have the wisdom and the power to do the right thing. Sometimes we may slip because we're human.

Zucchinis can make wrong choices too, as the following tale demonstrates. Of course, it involves our lovable, but seriously flawed Zarkoff. He had a difficult time escaping his lusty demons.

It was a bright, sunshiny autumn afternoon. Farmer Jones had just left after calling it an early day. Tomorrow would be a busy harvest. Most of the vegetables were at their peak and ready to be picked. A few had already been picked. The others would join them tomorrow.

Zarkoff entered the farm grounds. He had arranged an afternoon date with a saucy, red tomato that had just been picked. Her name was Tooters. They had met a couple of weeks ago when she was still on the vine. Tooters was red hot and rearing to go, Zarkoff's type all the way. Zarkoff was excited and hurriedly made his way to their rendezvous location.

Zarkoff had a steady girlfriend that he really liked. Her name was Tanya and she was also a tomato. Zarkoff had sworn to himself he would never cheat on her, but this pretty little tomato was just too tempting. What the heck, his girlfriend would never find out, so why not have a little fun?

Zarkoff saw their meetup spot in the distance. Tooters would be waiting in all her sensual glory. He couldn't wait!

It was a little patch of soil that was just perfect for romance. They would be underneath a big oak tree and the view was fantastic. Zarkoff had no doubt his little honey would be all hot and ready when he arrived. Tooters was a real firecracker. He was moments away from fun time.

As Zarkoff rounded the corner into the clearing he saw her. Wow, she looked fantastic! And what was that behind the oak tree? Was that another tomato? Wow! She must have brought a friend. He knew Tooters had a little wild streak, but this was too good to be true. Two pretty tomatoes, all for him! Zarkoff's heart raced as he neared her.

"I've got a little surprise for you," said Tooters. She flashed a wicked smile that promised all kinds of fun.

"Yes, I see," replied Zarkoff. "I can tell there's another tomato behind the tree. I bet she's as pretty as you are. I can't wait to meet her!"

"Oh honey!" exclaimed Tooters. "You have *no idea* how excited she is to see you! We're going to make this a day you'll never forget."

Zarkoff could hardly contain himself. What did he do to deserve this? He must be the luckiest man in the universe. Two lovely tomatoes both wanted him. Zarkoff's ego was riding sky high.

"Lie on that blanket and close your eyes," said Tooters in a soft sensuous voice. "You're going to get the treat of your life. My friend and I will make sure of that!"

Zarkoff laid down and closed his eyes. He pictured in his mind what carnal delights would be before him when he opened them. This must be what Heaven is like, or at least as close as you can get in this world. Pure bliss and joy, that's what this was.

"Okay, anytime you're ready," said Tooters. "Open your eyes, baby."

Zarkoff slowly opened his eyes in anticipation of the pleasures that awaited. It was definitely two beautiful tomatoes. There was Tooters in all her glory. Umm, she looked so sexy. And the other one was ...the other one was...Oh, no...the other one was his girlfriend! *His girlfriend!*

Zarkoff was in big trouble and he knew it. These two tomatoes had tricked him good. There was no way he could lie his way out of this one. Tooters and his girlfriend Tanya were in cahoots together. This was not going to end well. Zarkoff was in another tight spot.

"So, you're a cheater!" exclaimed Tooters. "Well, let me tell you something. I don't like cheaters!" Tooters reared back and gave him a stiff kick to the head that made Zarkoff see stars. Out of the corner of his eye he saw Tanya reach down and pick something up. Oh, my, it was a pitchfork! Two of them!

The first pitchfork pierced his wrist and dug into the ground. The second did the same to his other wrist. The pain was excruciating. He was now bleeding profusely and pinned to the ground by these maniacal, demonic, tomatoes-gone-mad.

"How does that feel, lover boy!" shouted Tanya. "Is this what you wanted? Is this what you wanted two women to do to you? Are you ready to take a ride, you scummy cheater?"

Zarkoff looked over at Tooters. To his horror she was approaching him and she was driving a tractor! This definitely wasn't a good sign.

"Hook him up, Tanya," ordered Tooters. "I'm gonna drag him through those thorn bushes."

Zarkoff secretly hoped he would pass out from all the blood loss, but it wasn't to be. Tanya pulled out a huge chain and wrapped it tight around Zarkoff's midsection. She attached the chain to back of the tractor. She pulled the pitchforks from Zarkoff's wrists.

Tooters revved up the tractor engine. Black fumes shot from the exhaust and into Zarkoff's lungs. He could barely breath. Tooters then headed for the thorn bushes just feet away. Zarkoff felt himself being dragged over a pile of jagged rocks. He wished he could die now and be done with it. Ever so slowly, Tooters dragged Zarkoff through the first bush.

"Oh! Oh! Oh!" shouted Zarkoff. It was the most agonizing pain he had ever experienced. Hundreds of razor-sharp thorns pierced his body as he slowly passed through bush after bush. For a full minute countless long, sharp thorns ate away at his ravaged body. He must have looked like a porcupine. The pain was beyond description.

Zarkoff finally emerged from the other side. All he could think about was how regretful he was for cheating. If he could escape this with his life, he would never cheat again. Why did he have to love so many women? Why did he always find trouble with love? It sure wasn't worth all this.

"I'm turning around, lover boy." Tooters declared. "You're going for another ride through those thorn bushes!"

This was it. Zarkoff knew he would never survive another round of torture from those unforgiving bushes and their long, sharp thorns. This was the end and he knew it. Zarkoff started praying for salvation. Better late than never.

"Give me back my tractor!" he heard a voice call out. It was Farmer Jones. He had heard the commotion and came out to investigate. The girls scattered and ran off into the distance. "Good luck, you porcupine!" they shouted in unison. They laughed as they sped away.

Farmer Jones immediately called in veggie rescue. Zarkoff was airlifted to the nearest hospital. They placed him in the ICU section reserved for chronic cheaters. Security was tight so as to keep out revengeful mates.

Zarkoff feel into yet another coma. He awoke in the hospital six months later. His body was permanently scarred for life. Some of the thorns were in so deep they would remain in his body. They would eternally serve as a painful reminder of the costs of cheating.

Zarkoff promised his new carrot girlfriend, his physical therapist, that he would never cheat again. That didn't last very long. The pretty carrot caught him with a sexy sweet potato and quickly marked him off. She abandoned him, declaring him a hopeless case. Zarkoff had lost again.

Zarkoff cried,
Zarkoff whined.
Zarkoff was,
A porcupine!

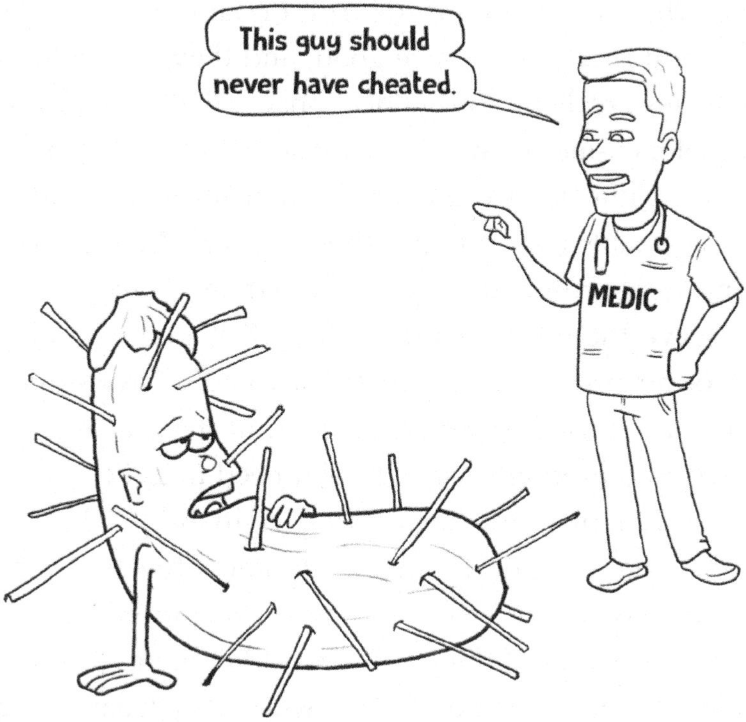
This guy should never have cheated.
MEDIC

Fresh Fruit & Veggies II

It is a fruitcake world that we live in. That alone is reason enough to eat fruit. That being said, there are many valid reasons why we should include fruit in our daily diet. They're colorful and pretty, they taste good, and they're very healthy. They're an excellent low-calorie snack that can provide a quick fuel pick-me-up, making fruit such a great choice.

In the battle to become fit, fresh fruit, along with their cousin vegetables, are the frontline soldiers. Make a habit of carrying some fruit and veggies with you everywhere you go. Never leave the house without them. If it's only an apple, a carrot, or a couple of bananas, at least you'll have something to stifle those early hunger pangs that can strike at any time.

It is very tempting to say, "I don't need to carry any snacks with me, I'm planning on coming right back." But things happen in the real world. You should know this being the old geezer that you are. We geezers have been around a long time and have seen a lot of things. The world operates as it pleases whether we like it or not. Those who are prepared are the ones that survive.

How many times have you been stuck somewhere with little or no food options? I'm sure there have been many. This is when you can completely fall off the healthy food train. The body needs fuel. There's no getting around that fact. If you can reach in that trusty cooler by your side and pull out a piece of fresh fruit or a veggie stick, then you're a survivor.

You won't be forced to go into Bubba's Grease Pit that's directly across the street. Leave that place to the waddlers. You know how much a waddler loves waddling in and out of those types of places. I could easily get used to being a waddler. Seriously though, many of us do waddle to a certain extent, but we can fix that with a few months of healthy eating and regular exercise.

If you have your little fruit/veggie container handy, you're all set. You can sit back in your vehicle or under a shade tree and relax. That boost of energy will supply you until you're back in the safety of your well-stocked home. You won't be forced to choose Bubba's Waddler Special. Today's selection is triple deep-fried fatback on a bed of salted lard, covered in a rich possum gravy. I know it sounds mouth-wateringly tempting, but stick with the fruit.

The great thing about fruit is how convenient it can be. It really is the ultimate fast food. Together with some veggie sticks they're world-class hunger-stoppers. All you're really trying to do is buy yourself some time until you're back in control of the situation. You can keep them chilled or just carry them around at room temperature.

Fresh fruit and veggies are saviors when it comes to surviving the daily grind of your battle. It really is a war with constant attacks from the enemy at all times. Processed foods are behind every corner just waiting to ambush you. You can never let your guard down.

Another great thing about the fruit/veggie snack package is that they're all healthy. Virtually all fruit and vegetables are packed with nutrition, so there's no need to research each one. They're low-calorie in comparison with almost any processed option. Bubba's muffins probably contain enough butter, fat and sugar to fuel a body for a decade.

Mix your fruit and veggie snacks on a daily basis. This will ensure that you'll receive a wide range of vitamins and minerals. Go ahead and learn all you want about fruit and veggies and the vitamins and minerals they contain. As for me, I don't worry about it. I'm confident they're all healthy and good for my body. I just rotate them around at random and it seems to work just fine. Don't be afraid to try new selections of these nutrition warriors. It might become a favorite fruit or vegetable.

Here's one last advantage of the fruit/veggie plan of attack. If you've been in the fast-food habit, you know how much money you can spend. It can add up quickly. Fruit and veggies are less expensive. You can take that extra money and start saving for a surprise gift for your girl. Make her happy and your world becomes a more pleasant place to reside. Fresh fruit and veggies, never leave home without them!

> *You wanna be pretty,*
> *You wanna be cute.*
> *Eat your veggies,*
> *Eat your fruit!*

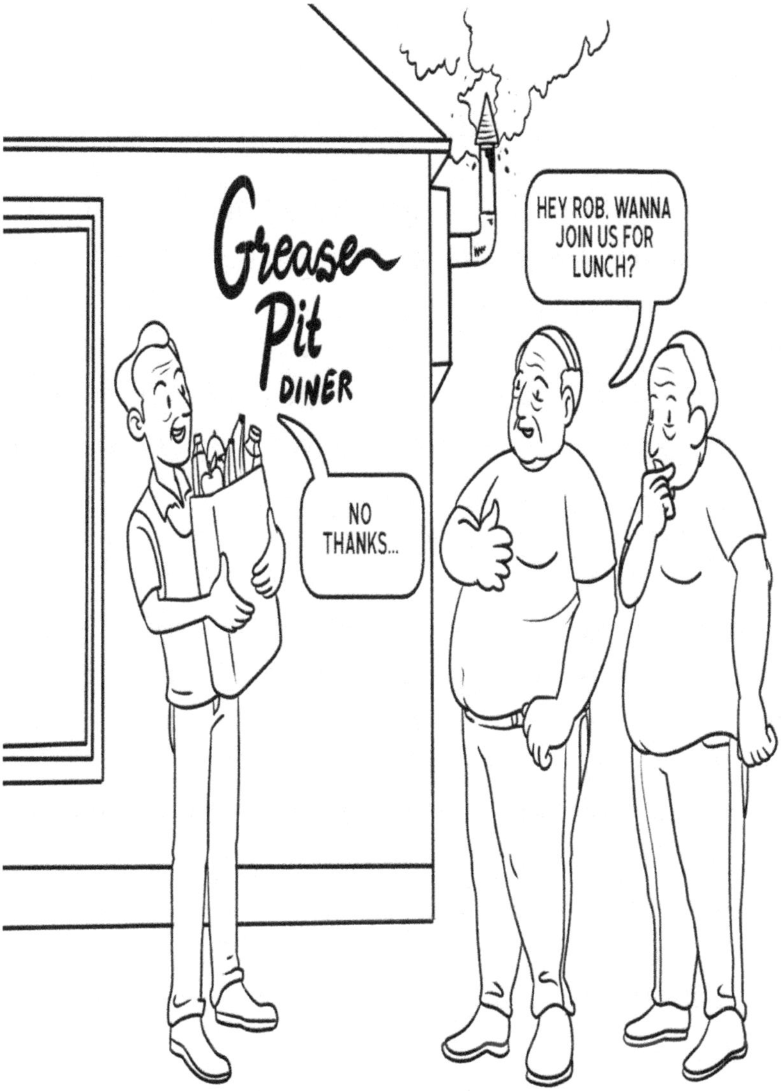
Grease Pit DINER
HEY ROB. WANNA JOIN US FOR LUNCH?
NO THANKS...

Oatmeal & Cereals

Your daily diet is a balancing act. It's all about timing and strategic planning. The body runs most efficiently when it's provided with carbohydrates, protein, and a touch of fat. The fruit and vegetables are great, but you'll need more. A complex carbohydrate is necessary to push you through the day and give you that boost of raw energy. We'll get to the protein sources in a later segment.

Many of you start your morning with a bowl of cereal. That's great, but make sure it's a healthy one. After much experimentation my choice is steel cut oatmeal. Overall, oatmeal is by far my number one choice, and the steel cut is my preferred version. Oatmeal puts most other cereals in the Cereal Hall of Shame.

Imagine your body after it has spent several hours without nutrition. It has been sleeping and hasn't fueled since dinner. All that lusty Freudian dreaming has it rearing to go and ready to be fed. You know what it needs, and it's not Sugar Smackers. Morning is a critical time and proper decisions are in order.

The worst thing you can do at this point is to saturate yourself with processed sugar. That's exactly what many people do, loading their system with an unnatural agent. Too much sugar has been proven to be related to a range of health problems, including diabetes, dementia, and of course obesity. That's right, you'll become a fatty.

Do you want to become a fatty? Most of us prefer the thinner option and the way to get there is natural and unprocessed. That's why oatmeal, especially the steel cut selection, is an excellent choice when it comes to morning fueling. It is high in fiber, minimally processed, and possesses exceptional nutritional value.

If there ever was an esculent substance it would be oatmeal. I congratulate myself on using the word *esculent,* as I had no idea what it meant until I looked it up. It helps to use weird words when you're trying to impress others with your writing. They'll temporarily think you're smart.

Some people skip breakfast entirely, thinking it's a way to lose weight. They're making a serious mistake. I've found that when you fill your body with healthy nutrition early in the day, your cravings for the bad stuff are dramatically reduced. That creamy pastry is less appealing when your stomach is full of oatmeal.

Eat to avoid eating, if that makes any sense to you. Outsmart yourself. It all becomes a psychological game that you're playing with your mind. Try to make a habit of filling up early on the healthy stuff, and you'll win the bigger battle. Trick yourself into success.

The reason many people choose those nutrition-wasteland cereals is due to taste. Those little taste bud-appeasing chunks of carbohydrates are designed for one thing, making money for their producers. How do you think those executive guys can afford their grand mansions with their fine automobiles parked by their exquisitely landscaped lawns? That's right, our sugar-saturated intestines are paying the mansion mortgage. It's all commercially driven in nature. Sweet stuff sells.

I admit that untouched oatmeal is quite the bland tasting dish. How can we get around that issue? It's really quite simple. Add some fruit, maybe some honey, or a generous pour of cinnamon. There are many ways to make it taste better. Put those old, decrepit brain cells to work and get creative. If my weathered, ancient, lackadaisical medulla can write this book, then you can certainly find a way to make oatmeal taste good. Find something healthy and tasty and doctor it up to your liking. You know you can do it.

Fatty bacon and chunks of butter are no way to start the day. Processed sugar isn't any better. Go the natural route and opt for oatmeal, or at least something that contains fewer harmful ingredients. Our bodies are our true homes and we need to keep them clean and tidy. We'll leave home soon enough, so let's not go prematurely. We're old, but we're not done yet. We have to continue living so we can annoy others as long as possible.

If you think a sugary, processed cereal is bad for geezers like us, can you imagine what it must be doing to a young child? Their bodies are in the midst of maturing and their brains are developing and they're supposed to breakfast on sugar! If you know someone who's feeding their child a substance that's fifty percent sugar, politely encourage them to change to a healthier choice. Now that would be a good deed.

The final word on cereal is to go as natural as possible. Once again, I'll delve deep into ancient caveman history. Did Carl Caveman rely on a bowl of sugar for energy to go hunt rabbits? Did Carla Cavewoman get her sexy physique by spooning sugar into her lovely self? The answer is no. We humans have been manipulated into thinking a certain way. It doesn't have to be that way. Think for yourself and make the right decisions. Your body will love it.

Oats and fruit,
That's the way.
A perfect way,
To start your day!

Complex Carbs

You've had your oatmeal lesson. It is an excellent example of a complex carbohydrate. Other examples include beans, rice, whole-wheat bread, quinoa, barley, and potatoes. There are many others, but these are the most common.

What we're not going to get into here is the science behind all this. We're going to leave that to the scholarly segment that has orgasms every time they share their knowledge. At least that PhD degree is good for something. Amino acids, fatty acids, disaccharides, monosaccharides, blah, blah, blah, we don't have time for that. We're going to get down to the practical part and get on with the program.

What we care about is information that we can convert to a healthy, sexy body. We want to take it and run with it. You want to win, that's why you're reading this book. You want to take the most basic information, apply discipline, determination and dedication, and amaze someone. Let others impress the crowd with their knowledge at the dinner table. Let them quote long medical terms as they spoon a mountain of butter on their baked potato. You'll cover yours with a low-calorie topping and keep quiet.

Don't worry, it won't be long before they'll be asking you how you did it. People will want what you have and want to know how you did it. You'll be the hero. People like to overcomplicate things, but you know the secret. Keep it simple and just go for it. People want results, not some boring display of medical-nutritional knowledge. Be the star of the show and shine for all to see.

The first hurdle we need to overcome is the mental block many have placed around complex carbohydrates. "Starchy foods," some will sneer when the subject is discussed. "Oh, I don't eat bad starchy stuff," they'll spout as they gobble down a chunk of pure animal fat.

The truth is really quite simple. Complex carbohydrates take longer to break down, therefore they energize the body over a longer period of time than simple carbohydrates. Yes, they *may* contain more calories than simple carbohydrates, but try going without them and you'll get burned in the long run. They play their role in the jigsaw puzzle of health and fitness that we're piecing together here.

Lesson one is over and the verdict is we need complex carbohydrates. Now we're going to learn how to make them a lean and healthy weapon in our fitness arsenal. Once again, it's extremely simple. Prepare them in a low-calorie manner and don't destroy everything by smothering them with a fatty item. Don't self-destruct.

The biggest mistake by far concerns the toppings. Out of habit many people cover their pasta, potato or whatever with a heart-clogging concoction that will soon convert to a roll of blubber. Instead of a tasty, lean selection, they choose to apply a topping that would provide enough calories to feed a stable of race horses.

Butter, sour cream, gravies, the list goes on and on. Stay away from these and find something lean and mean to spice up the flavor. Here we go again, delve into that creativity and design a solution that works for you. Add some spice, a healthy sauce, or anything that's low-calorie and high in flavor.

Worcestershire, low-sodium soy sauce, hot sauce, there are tons of options here. Learn to read those labels and see exactly what you're pumping into your body. As you know, I'm not a fan of sugar, but a *little* sweetness here goes a long way. It sure beats that pure-fat route that tempts us so.

I really think it's an automatic reaction for many to ruin their food with the fatty stuff. "Grandma did it, mom did it, so I'll do it," they'll say as they reach for that big chunk of butter to splash down upon the hapless potato. He's worked so hard to provide nutritional value and now he's being attacked by a big glob of fat. Please, don't do it to him. He's endured much hardship in his life and deserves better.

Cook your complex carbohydrates in a healthy manner. Stop the tunnel vision of having to do things as they've always been done. Twelve generations of bad decision making needs to end with you. I know your beloved Aunt Bessie added six pounds of butter to that famous casserole of hers. Everyone loved it, but that's probably why your cousin Grover died of a heart attack at an early age.

You know, he was the family member that raved the most about Bessie's casserole as he reached for his third helping. God bless cuz Grover, but he could have been saved. He could have won a Nobel Prize for accomplishing something remarkable had he been given a chance. Instead, he gave his life for butter.

Since you're a creative genius, it should be no problem to innovate upon recipes. You're no sheep plodding along aimlessly letting others rule you. You're in control of your own destiny. You have the power to turn a fatty dish into a lean treat and still taste good.

Think for yourself, experiment, and find out what works for you. Don't worry what others may think. Let them sneer silently as you pioneer your way into fitness. Let them sink into the fat bowl and wallow around in ignorance as you steer your way towards success.

Complex carbohydrates are great. They're energizers, high in fiber, and naturally nutritious. Keep them as unprocessed as possible and don't kill them with fat. Fit them in with fruit, vegetables and lean protein as part of your overall plan. It's as simple as can be, just do it. Be you.

> A little fat,
> Just a bit.
> That's the way,
> To get fit!

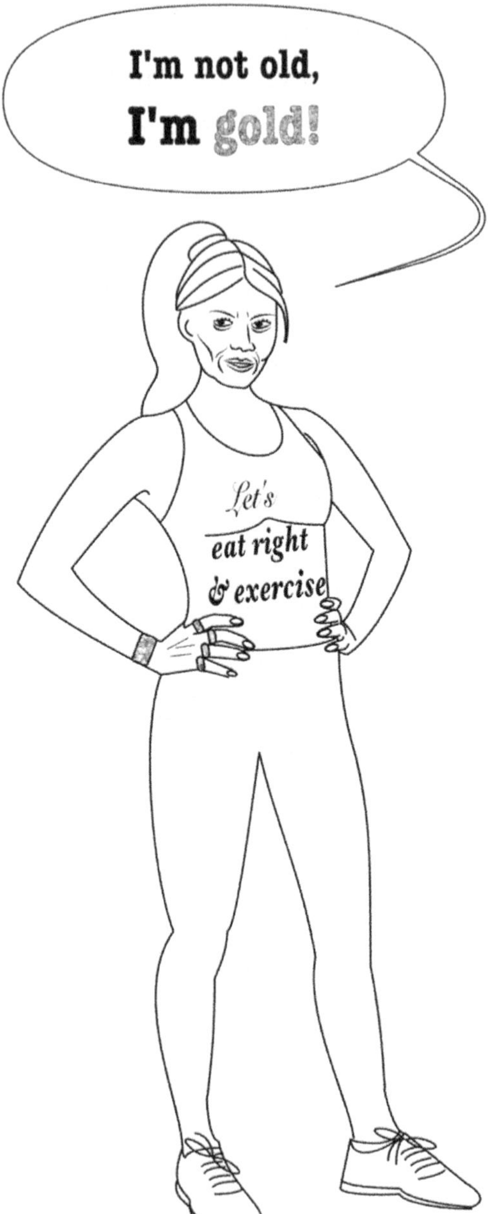
I'm not old,
I'm gold!
Let's
eat right
& exercise

Prepared Veggies

Vegetables are incredibly important in your quest to become fit. They are low in calories and packed with nutrition. I've noticed they don't get the respect they deserve. It's amazing how many people disregard them completely. They were born as vegetables and are proud to be vegetables. They shouldn't be judged simply because they're a leafy green, a pea, or a lentil. Racism is a terrible thing. Thank you, Zarkoff Zucchini! You are the spark behind the fire of equal rights.

Enough is enough. It's time to make a stand for these undervalued treasures. Vegetables have been pushed around for too long. We all need to band together and stamp out senseless acts of discrimination against these wonderful plants.

To think that a ribeye steak is superior to a cabbage simply because of ethnicity is ludicrous. All foods are created equal and should have equal rights. Segregation is still an issue as vegetables are being pushed over to the corner of the dinner plate. They have as much right to the center of the plate as meats, pasta and other more prominent sources of sustenance.

They have inalienable rights granted by the creator and we should never forget it. Prejudice against vegetables of color is especially prominent. Beets, pumpkins, rhubarbs, and many others experience this discrimination on a daily basis.

Salads, steamed vegetables, vegetable soups, all of them have been exploited long enough. They've been subjected to meat pushing them around their entire existence. This systemic oppression towards vegetables by meat cannot persist. *End Vegetable racism!*

Hopefully this emotional tirade against the horrible mistreatment of vegetables influenced you in a positive manner. It's time to put our newfound belief system into action. It's time to eat more vegetables and show those meats who really wields the power behind the veil.

Not long into the future steamed veggies, veggie soups and salads will rise and take their rightful place in carbohydrate society. We're going to learn how to treat vegetables like the royalty they truly are. We'll start with steamed vegetables.

Steamed vegetables are excellent. All you need is a pot, a steamer insert, and some fresh veggies. Treat each vegetable with equal respect so there is no internal discord among them. The steaming process can be done in less than ten minutes from start to finish.

Remember, since veggies are great raw, you shouldn't worry that they may be slightly undercooked. Also know that you don't need every vegetable each time you steam. Mix and match and rotate your selections every time you shop. You'll receive an amazing array of vitamins and minerals this way.

Steamed vegetables are great any time of day. You can make an entire lunch or dinner out of them. Eat as much as you want and fill up on them. As long as you're getting your daily protein and a few complex carbohydrates you'll be fine.

GEEZER ALERT!

I Know It's NAPPIE TIME For You GEEZER, But Continue On!

Mix and match different colored vegetables in your steamed selections. It's amazing how the different colors complement each other and add to the dining experience. Enjoy the different textures of the veggies. Some are crunchy and some even have a meaty texture. Innovate and try everything. There may be a favorite-in-waiting for you.

Okay, so you've got your veggies in a bowl and you're ready to dig in. You're going to add a little flavor to them. This is a critical decision that should not be taken lightly. What you top your veggies with determines the calorie content. Of course, the veggies are fine just the way they are, but most people like a little added flavor.

Stay away from the creamy stuff, butter, heavy oils, and anything fatty. If in doubt, read the labels or do a quick internet search of the item. A little salt or sweetness is okay as long as you don't overdo it. Most of you desire to lose weight, so don't ruin your dreams with a nightmarish topping.

Healthy sauces and toppings include my two favorites, lemon and lime juice. You can purchase the juice, or even better, squeeze it yourself. You'll never find anything to beat these two royal flavorings. They're totally natural and you can use as much as you want. Pour it on if you like. They're guaranteed to zest it up bigtime.

Other healthy options include a spicy pepper sauce, Worcestershire sauce, a low-sodium soy sauce, crushed red pepper, or anything that's low in calories. There are also loads of sauces in the Asian section of supermarkets. Take a hint from the Asians. They're pros at staying thin.

It's really unlimited as to what you can add to your steamed vegetables. Change it up daily and you'll never get bored. Don't be a conditioned recipe-head. Make your own sauce by mixing two or more, or simply create something unique. The key is to keep this stuff low-fat. The lower in fat, the more you can use. Then you can fill up and that piece of after-dinner cake won't be quite so tempting. If you do have any racist tendencies, display them against cake. Sorry, cake, you're being discriminated against and I apologize.

If you happen to be barbecuing, try grilling some vegetables. They've turned into a major favorite for me. I even purchased a tiny grill so I can efficiently cook them without a lot of expense or time. Hook up to a large propane tank and it will supply you for months. Most barbecue sauces are a little on the sweet side, but they sure are tasty. Take care with your sauces!

You can also bake veggies, or even microwave them in a crunch. I'm not a fan of microwaving, but if you're in a time crunch it will suffice. Microwaving to me seems like torture and those innocent veggies have already endured so much in their struggle for equality. Let's cook and prepare them in a humane way if possible.

The bottom line on veggies is to get used to a wide variety, cooked a healthy way, and topped with only healthy stuff. They're natural, nutritious and incredibly low in calories. Don't destroy them with salt, fat, butter and such. They've suffered enough already, having endured a long history of racial strife. Let's never forget where they came from and *never, ever* let history repeat itself.

Eat your veggies,

Every day.

If you don't,

You will pay!

Prepared Vegetables II

Due to their importance and their background of repression, veggies are being rewarded with another section. In this section we'll be addressing issues like soups and salads and how they fit in with the overall unjust treatment of these superfoods. No one should be judged because they are a different ethnicity, gender, religion, or food group.

You can't help but think about Zarkoff Zucchini anytime vegetable rights are discussed. There is no one more deserving of recognition in this field. Without Zucchini's tireless work and dedication, the vegetable community would still be stuck on dirty side dishes while burgers reap all the praise. Burgers are so undeserving of acclamation, especially the way they have mistreated minorities throughout history. Screw those mean ole burgers and their dictatorial ways.

Zarkoff Zucchini once famously dueled a burger. It became known as the Zucchini Inappropriate Advance Duel. Zarkoff became a page in European history because of it. It wasn't his proudest moment.

It all started innocently enough. It was a beautiful spring morning in Barcelona, Spain. Zarkoff was enjoying a pre-brunch cocktail at a local outdoor café. As he ordered another triple margarita, his fifth of the morning, along with another liter of beer, he caught an image out of the corner of his eye. He turned his head for a better look.

Wow! Never had he seen a more beautiful asparagus! She was having brunch with a male piece of meat. It appeared to be a medium-well burger. What was she doing with a lowly burger? She could certainly do better than that! How about a healthy, strong, handsome veggie instead! He had to go over and tell her how beautiful she was.

An opportunity quickly arrived as Burger stood and strolled towards the restroom. At this point Zarkoff lost all control of his senses. All rationale had been erased by lust and alcohol. He rose from his seat and approached the object of his affections.

"Hola, Ms. Esparragos, eres hermosa," Zarkoff stated in his most suave demeanor. "Do you speak English?"

"Yes, I do speak English," replied the pretty asparagus with a look of surprise. "Thank you for the compliment, and I do appreciate that you think I'm beautiful, but I have to let you know I have a boyfriend. As a matter of fact, he's my fiancé, and he'll be back in just a minute."

Zarkoff was now really feeling the early morning alcohol. The result was his thinking was being done with the wrong head. There was no way he was letting this pretty little veggie get away.

"Do you really want *a burger* to father your children?" he pronounced. "Wouldn't a healthy zucchini be a much better choice?" Zarkoff turned up his drink and drained it in one gulp.

The little asparagus was in shock. She couldn't believe this well-dressed, classy-in-appearance, gentleman zucchini was saying these outrageous things. "Sir, I repeat, I'm taken, and my fiancé is a very jealous type. Please leave now before he comes back."

Zarkoff looked over to his waiter and signaled for another drink. "Honey girl," he said, "Burgers make lousy lovers and you're done with him from this minute on. Come over to my table and have a drink."

"Hey!" a voice called out. "Are you harassing my fiancée?"

Zarkoff turned his head to see Burger and Burger wasn't happy. Zarkoff was now running on idealism and alcohol. All reasoning was gone. Now was the time to let it loose. He was tired of restraining his true feelings. To say he disliked meats was an understatement. Relations with burgers were particularly strained after the famous court ruling that went in his favor.

There was no love lost between Zucchini and Burger. Now it was all coming to a head. The mix of longtime loathing for red meats, the fact that a pretty vegetable chose a burger for a mate, and an overindulgence of alcohol had pushed Zarkoff over the edge.

"Yes, I am harassing your fianceé!" Zarkoff defiantly replied. "What are you going to do about it, you scum-of-the-earth burger? All you do is clog arteries and make people fat. Get the heck out of here and leave this pretty asparagus for us veggies! Run your merry way out the door back to the meat processing plant where you belong. You're a disgrace to the entire planet, you intestinal vermin, you slouchy lover, you bottom-dwelling piece of poisonous, low-life, dreg-of-society rubbish. Get out of here now!"

Utter dismay and shock enveloped Burger! Red juice seeped from his pores. He was one angry piece of meat. The other diners watched in disbelief. They couldn't help but hear the drunken outburst coming from this unassuming little zucchini.

"I challenge you to a duel!" cried out Burger. "How dare you insult me and my fianceé!" He walked behind the counter and brought out two massive serrated-blade kitchen cleavers. He threw one at Zarkoff, which he somehow caught in his drunken state.

Burger wasted no time. His first jab expertly nailed Zarkoff's eye socket. Out popped an eyeball. It rolled onto the floor. The second slash clipped his ear and it flew into a bowl of soup. His third slice hacked off Zarkoff's nose. It splashed down in a nearby patron's wine glass.

Zarkoff was completely unfazed in his oblivious stupor. He stuck out his tongue in a mocking manner as if to taunt Burger. A quick slice from Burger's cleaver sent it flying into a nearby salad.

Zarkoff remained defiant. He stuck up his middle finger as a derogatory gesture, which turned out to be a bad idea. The finger was quickly disposed of and fell into the lap of an adjoining diner.

Zarkoff wasn't done with his amputee-producing tirade. He stuck up his other middle finger and it went flying into the street. A bird quickly gobbled it up. Even though blood was gushing from numerous outlets of his body, nothing seemed to faze Zarkoff. He continued his verbal attack. The words weren't so clear without use of his tongue, but they were discernable.

"You can't kill me," he cried. "You're a pathetic loser who could never satisfy a pretty vegetable like this asparagus here.

She wants me! *Me!* Do you hear me, you sack-of-crap no-good burger garbage!"

Burger took aim at Zarkoff's jugular vein. This time he meant business. This swing would finish off the pesky vegetable that had invaded his life. Just as he reared back to end Zarkoff's existence forever, he was tackled from behind.

Someone had called the police and they quickly brought the duel to a close. Burger was subdued until his anger subsided. Zarkoff was rushed to the local hospital and taken to intensive care. He fell into his customary coma.

The entire event had been filmed by a teen with her phone. She watched it unfold from the beginning and recorded it all. It immediately went viral on every social media outlet. Zarkoff had a lot of explaining to do if he was to wiggle out of this one.

Zarkoff spent the better part of the year in his coma. He awakened and was horrified to find all his features had been chopped off. He endured numerous surgeries in an attempt to regain his handsomeness again. His international embarrassment led him into an alcohol rehabilitation program where he stopped drinking for two weeks. Upon his release, he headed to the local bar for a drink and a chat with a pretty cucumber bartender.

The moral of this sequence of events that nearly ended the life of our careless hero is this. Be passionate about vegetable rights. Zarkoff Zucchini may have defended his fellow vegetables in an improper manner, but he certainly didn't lack for passion. No piece of meat would ever stand in his way. You readers always remember this, and try to insult meats at every opportunity, but do so in a more polite manner. Avoid violence if at all possible.

This heartwarming tale of unwavering passion and love for all things vegetable brings us full circle to the importance of vegetable recognition. Let's proceed onward in memory of our visionary leader, the one, the only, the legendary Zarkoff Zucchini.

Liquor and women,
Make Zarkoff spin.
Liquor and women,
Did him in!

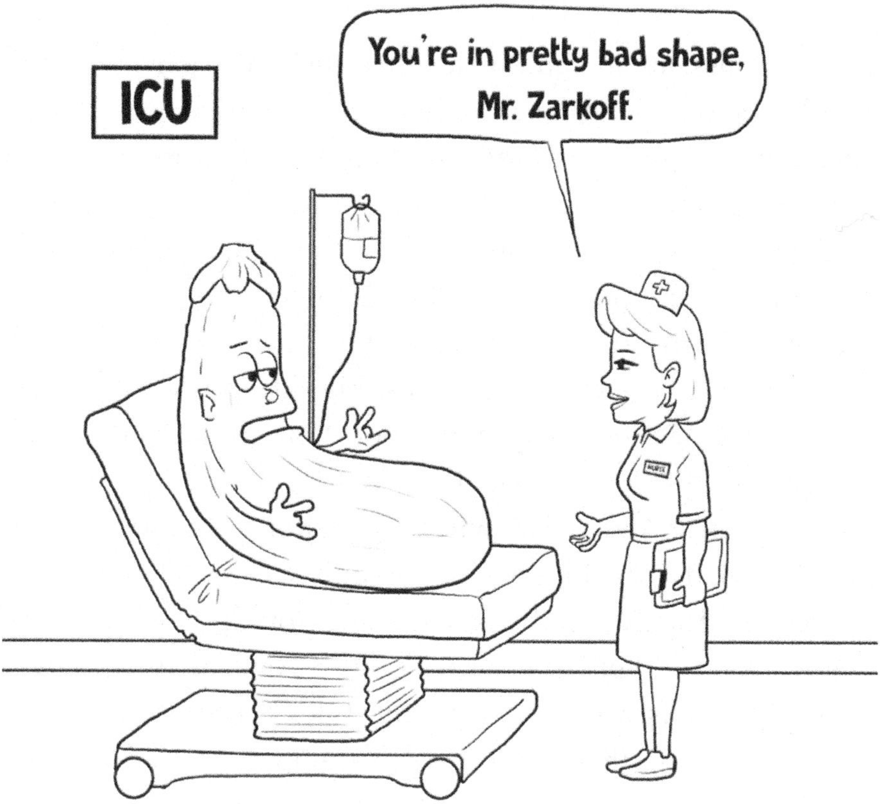
ICU
You're in pretty bad shape, Mr. Zarkoff.

Prepared Vegetables III

Let's discuss an incredibly healthy dish, the garden salad. Salads should be a major weapon in your nutrition arsenal. Salads in general are a fantastic choice, but beware of certain potential pitfalls.

The primary issue with salads is the added contents that sometimes hide under the healthy lettuce and spinach. They are often high-calorie items that you don't need or want. These include cheese, ham, bacon bits, deep-fried croutons, and a host of other fatty gangsters. You name it, there are countless ways to ruin a salad.

It's as if an evil salad witch is deviously sabotaging our healthy salad. This hideous hag is ugly as can be and wants you as unattractive as she is. Fattening you up is her primary desire. Don't let her have her way. Keep your salads healthy.

Make salads a part of your lifestyle. *Wash the ingredients thoroughly.* Keep them fresh by consuming them shortly after preparing them. Make sure vegetables are the star of the show. Include the standard items such as lettuce, cabbage, carrots, celery, cucumbers and so on. Don't stop there, however.

Try different vegetables and greens along with your go-to selections. Just as with steamed veggies, mix and match accordingly. Don't be afraid to experiment. Remember that you don't need every vegetable in every salad. It's a lot of work to purchase and prepare the perfect salad every time. Keep it simple if you like and throw a few healthy veggies together. Your next salad can be an entirely different set of vegetables.

In the long run your body is receiving a wide range of nutrients. By keeping it simple you're more likely to continue your salad habit. Don't complicate it by trying to be a nutritional rocket scientist. It's *doing* that's important here, not impressing others with your knowledge. This is your personal battle and you're out to succeed.

Salads are good for lunch, dinner and snacks. The only thing allowed in your salad, other than vegetables, should be a *lean* meat, an egg, or possibly something that adds a little crunch to the texture. Try to keep the veggies the primary attraction in your salads. That way, if you overeat, you're still in control. You're okay, because it's all good, low-calorie stuff. Fill up on it and enjoy.

Salad dressings are the main weapon that will be used against you by that ole broom-riding menace. That witch will contaminate at every opportunity. If it's creamy, fatty or oily, then it's likely to be used against you. Nothing can destroy a salad more so than a nasty dressing. There are too many healthy low-calorie choices to be messing around with those fat-bombs. Look at the labeling and analyze the fat content. Remember not to trust the corporate peddlers and their shiny promises. They don't give a hoot about you, just your money.

"Oh, I only had a salad for lunch," I used to hear an acquaintance say. The only problem was she absolutely destroyed it. Fatty meats, loads of cheese, buttery breadsticks and a bucket of creamy dressing just obliterated it. Any hope of retaining its low-calorie value was done in by that deceptive beauty-queen wannabe of a witch. Put that mirror-bursting personification of ugliness on the next broom out of town. Do this by resisting her high-calorie temptations.

There are literally hundreds of options available as salad dressings. The majority of the commercial choices simply won't pass the test. Sure, they taste great, but that's the problem. They're composed primarily of fat or sugar or both.

The food manufacturers are very knowledgeable of human behavior. Appeal to the taste buds and the battle is won. That's their time-tested mentality and they're right. The average human relies on instant gratification and won't bother to read the content label. They'll rely on their satisfied palate for decision making without realizing it's going to pack the pounds on their ever-expanding waistline. Some simply don't care and others are operating on ignorance.

This logic applies to nearly every processed food item, but for now we're discussing salad dressings. A person may sample a particular dressing and say to themself, "Oh, that tastes great. I'll buy that." That's a big mistake. Further research is required.

Five seconds of analyzing the ingredients and the fat and sugar content will usually be enough. With practice you can master this skill. If you're serious about losing weight and getting fit you'd better read those labels. There's a lot of dirty laundry hidden away in that closet. Open it up and find it.

Don't limit yourself to the commercial choices. Some natural salad dressings include the trusty lemon and lime juices, red wine vinegar, picante sauce, hot pepper sauce and many others. To create something unique, take a half bottle of your favorite dressing and fill it to the top with red wine vinegar. Shake it up and you now have a one-of-a-kind dressing.

Regardless of the dressing you're using, try not to pour on huge amounts. Learn to appreciate the wonderful taste of healthy vegetables. They're a gift from nature. You may find you don't want anything diluting them, as they're great on their own. Whatever the case, treat those veggies with respect and don't ruin them with fatty additions. That's rule number one with salads.

Some people like a little crunch in their salads. It really adds to the mix and keeps boredom at bay. You never want to get so tired of an item that it's discarded forever. I've found that the shredded wheat cereal acts as a delightful crouton choice. Make sure you get the pure stuff and don't overdo it. The veggies are still the star of the dish. Keep them shining bright.

When ordering salads in restaurants you need to take special care. You're giving up a certain amount of control and you have to be on guard. Place your order deliberately and carefully. Order a light dressing and make sure it comes on the side. It wouldn't hurt to repeat the specifics of your order and make eye contact. That way he or she will remember it if a kitchen staffer messes up the order. Then you can send it back without any drama attached to it.

Those restaurant people love to drench everything with everything, so never risk the dressing directly on the salad. That piece of healthy spinach will be drowning at the bottom of the sea. Do it yourself and remain in control. You're on a mission and you're going to win. Others can't manipulate you into a corner where you can't back out. Never forget that you're in a war when you're in a restaurant. You're on their turf, their home court, their backyard. Play your best game and survive. Come out of it alive and well.

A healthy salad,
Calories low.
Keep it up,
Go, Go, Go!

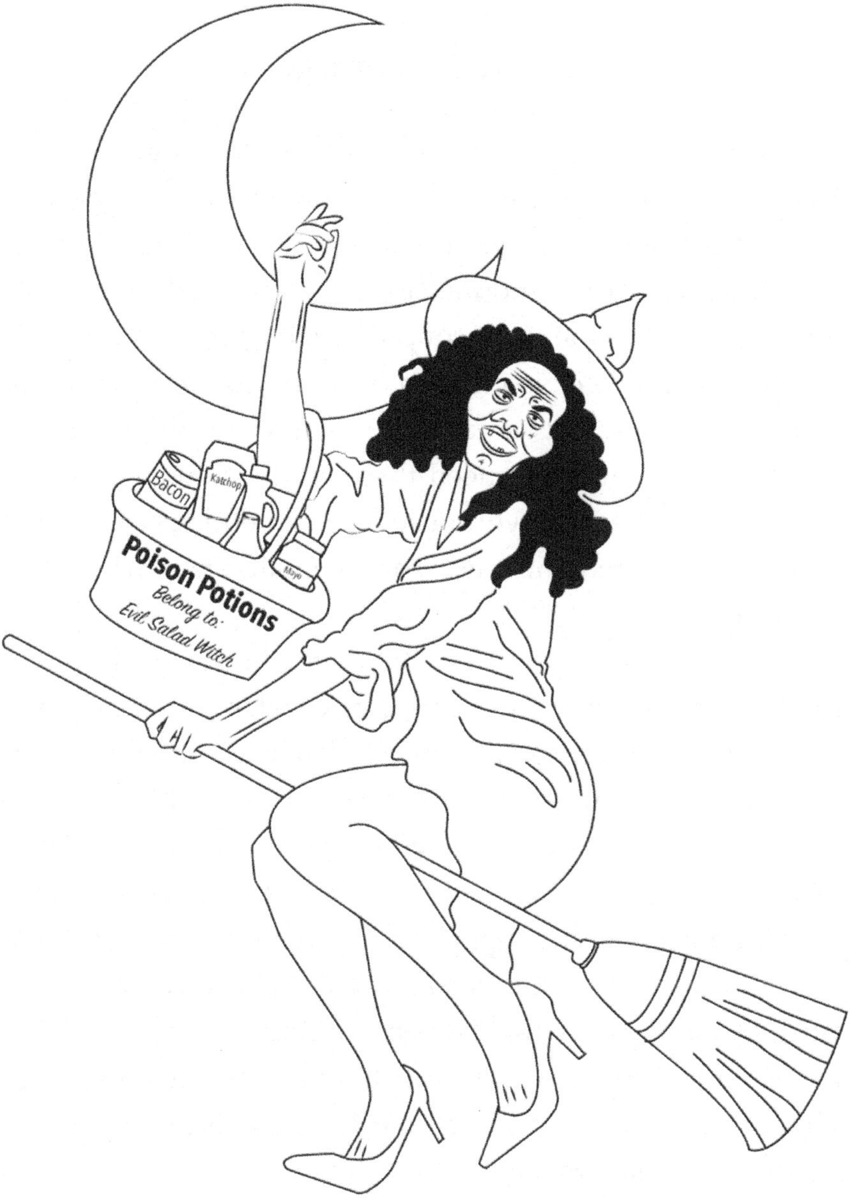
Bacon
Katchop
Mayo
Poison Potions
Belong to:
Evil Salad Witch

Prepared Vegetables IV

Let's move on to one of my all-time favorites, vegetable soup. As with all veggie concoctions, you can endlessly experiment with different vegetables and never tire of them. Vary the vegetables and the amounts of each one and it's possible you'll never have the same soup twice. It's infinite.

Chicken and beef stock are a common component of many soups and stews. If you can get past the conditioning factor you may find you don't need these at all. While they're tasty and relatively healthy, you need to be careful. Certain brands have added ingredients and many contain an overly amount of sodium.

There will be a recipe for this later in the book, but I'm going to sum up my favorite type of vegetable soup. It's based on a low-sodium vegetable juice. You may or may not add some water to dilute it for caloric sake. Add a variable, generous mix of veggies. If you like, throw in a little rice, lentils, or my favorite, quinoa. They add a boost of protein.

Experiment with peppers and spices for they add tons of flavor. Simmer it on low for an hour and you're done. Eat as much as you want of this fantastic, filling, low-calorie delight. You can't go wrong with this dish. I've found that even those hardcore meat-and-potato diehards seem to put up with it. That's somewhat amazing.

So, there we have it. Zarkoff Zucchini and his band of vegetable followers have paved the way for vegetable equality. Hopefully the trend will continue and vegetables will command the respect they so rightfully deserve. Enjoy those veggies!

Easy to make,
Tastes good too.
Veggie soup,
Good for you!

Lean Protein

To be strong and lean you're going to need protein. If you're trying to lose weight, fruits and vegetables will be your mainline defense against hunger. You'll strategically consume them throughout your day, but you must ensure you're meeting your protein requirements.

It starts getting tricky once you stray away from the veggie proteins. Lentils, soy products, broccoli, brussels sprouts, and several others are good sources of protein. Like many others, I choose to supplement my veggies with a more concentrated form of protein.

The problem occurs when you choose a protein source that contains substantial amounts of fat. Fat is your enemy at this point. You're trying to lose weight or at least maintain your weight. You can't aid and abet the enemy. That's treason against your body.

Meats are the principal deceivers in the protein chase. They contain the prize we desire, but attached is the killer of your fitness dreams, the dreaded fatblob. It doesn't have to be that way. You can avoid fat and have your meat also. Once again, it's an amazing simplicity behind the decision-making process.

Here it is. If it looks fatty, it's fatty. Can it get any simpler than that? I guess if you're blind it might pose a problem, but even then, you can ask someone else if they see fat on a targeted piece of meat. Ask a one-year-old, for they've already attained the necessary intellectual capacity for this incredibly easy observation. "Ooo, ooo, ga, ga, I see fat," they may reply.

Or they may coo back with a developmental milestone like, "The edible flesh of this particular domesticated, hollow-horned ruminant has been analyzed and I've cognitively arrived at an exemplary conclusion. This Bovidae mammal exhibits minimal esters of fatty acids and therefore is a superb choice for a low-fat, high protein consumption application. Now please give me back my pacifier."

You now see just how simple it is to analyze meat. If you see fat, it's fatty. If you don't see fat, it's not fatty. Don't fall into the trap of certain meats being grouped as fatty or lean. You have to look at those groupings in a very general way. Yes, chicken and turkey are overall leaner than pork or beef. They are usually wonderful choices in your lean protein dilemma.

However, there are many instances where it doesn't ring true. It depends on several factors, primarily what particular cut of meat it is. I've seen pieces of chicken that contain much more fat than a competing portion of pork or beef. Go with the leanest choice for whatever situation you're in at the time. Survival in your fitness war should be your only concern.

When it comes to meat, I do head for the poultry and fish first. Their leanest selections generally outdo the others by a long shot. I have seen some lean pork chops and sirloins and occasionally will change it up with those. Just do the right thing. Ask the nearest one-year-old if you need help. They'll know what to look for.

Eat those veggies,
Eat those beans.
When it comes to meat,
Keep it LEAN!

Lean Protein II

Family-and-friend barbeques can be a dangerous situation. And I'm not talking about that nasty relative that's always there spouting off political statements based in ignorance after a couple of glasses of wine. You know, he or she is the one always giving advice on morality and ethics, plus they're nutritional experts even though they can barely fit through the doorway.

The biggest threat at these barbeques is the guy with the white apron wrapped around his usually large body. Beware of the grill man, for he is in a power position, and he enjoys food. He can doctor up your otherwise healthy protein with some fatty substance that you don't want. You do not want to be on his bad side.

Befriend him as he rotates those sizzling chunks of meat. Bribe him with his favorite alcoholic beverage. Go retrieve one for him if you have to. Tell him your pretty friend thinks he's handsome. Compliment him on his grilling skills. Tell white lies and build upon this relationship.

Don't let this friendship backfire though. He'll try to reward you with his favorite meat-chunk. That would be the fattiest piece lying on the grill. "Oh, fat adds flavor to the meat," these guys like to pronounce. Well, he may be right, but fat also adds fat to your belly. Make a polite stand and opt for the leanest choice available.

The battle continues at the dinner table. Along with that mayonnaise-laden potato salad is another array of meats, some better than others. You have to stay the course as this war is forever. Fatblob ribs and other enemies are waiting to jump on your plate.

They're ready to slide down your esophagus and enter their version of the Holy Land. They so desire to transform themselves spiritually and permeate the heavenly confines of your intestines. Angelic beings will then guide them to your waist and buttocks areas, rewarding them with eternity in your heavenly abode. You'll pay the price by getting fat, but at least that rib is enjoying a holier state of existence.

That would be a wonderful gesture on your part to consume these highly-religious pieces of meat, but don't do it. Be a sinner and refuse to send them to their glorious destiny. Perhaps Aunt Sally or Uncle Rufus will take mercy on their souls. Fear not because you can bet someone will gobble them down. Animal fat is a hot commodity.

When it comes to lean meat, don't forget other options. Sushi is a favorite for many on the adventurous side. Wild game is another fantastic choice. It's not filled with those nasty growth substances the tricksters use to fatten up their animals. Do you really think that stuff could in any way be good for us? Of course not.

Now we've had our meat lesson. We know what types of meat to look for when we're making our choice. Don't get cocky at this point and blow everything by cooking your meat the wrong way. Stay away from the frying and preparing your meat in butter or oil.

Grilling, baking, steaming, broiling, and poaching are acceptable methods by which to cook them. And you know which toppings to avoid. They're usually greasy and slimy. Go find that one-year-old if you're having difficulty deciding.

Canned meats are a secret weapon when it comes to protein on the road. Take them along with a can opener and a fork and you're a survivor. Just open them up and eat right out of the can if necessary. A little healthy topping can add taste and eliminate some of the dryness.

You may ask why it is somewhat dry. That's because you made a wise choice when you purchased it. It was packed in water and was low in sodium. You also picked the leanest choices available. You skipped over those fatblob sausages and such. Your tuna, chicken or turkey was thoroughly analyzed by a team of one-year-olds and they determined it was suitable for you.

The next form of lean protein is one I highly recommend. Egg whites are one of the most pure and natural sources of protein that exist. They're low in calories and really pack an efficient punch in the protein arena. Although the yolks are packed with nutrition, they also contain most of the calories.

Lean and mean is the name of the game when it comes to egg whites. Body builders have been known to consume them by the dozen. Too much of anything is not good, but I think most people could benefit from a few egg whites daily. Mix in some high protein veggies and you'll feel energized all day long.

As always, beware of any destructive cooking methods. Don't ruin this low-calorie prince of a food with butter or such. A little healthy oil is okay if you're scrambling or lightly frying, but be careful. There's nothing tastier than a veggie omelet made with egg whites. Now that's a morning meal that will carry you through a long day. Don't ruin it by overdoing any cheese addition.

Hard-boiled eggs are a great way to sustain yourself calorically. Shell them, take out the yolk and feed the local birdlife. Birds love dining on this delicacy. Admittingly, there's not a lot of taste in egg whites alone, but you can add a dash of pepper or another healthy topping.

Try to develop a mentality of body maintenance, as if your body is a machine. Mindlessly make boiled egg whites a habit and you'll be glad you did. Consume them at intervals throughout the day. They're a clean fuel that keeps a geezer running smoothly and efficiently. Egg whites keep you well-tuned and sexy. Be that lean and mean senior machine. Strut your stuff.

Protein supplements are popular with many people. I'm sure they have their place, but I've placed them down at the bottom of my personal preferences. Although I'll occasionally snack on a protein bar, that's as far as I'll go. Protein powders and such aren't my thing. I'll leave that for the young dudes.

I prefer my fuel as natural as possible. It's all that hidden stuff that scares me. They've been known to contain sweeteners, toxins or contaminates. I like total control when it comes to what goes into my body. Those unknowns can strike you down later in life. Stay strong for the long run.

The bottom line is to keep your protein true and pure. Nuts and seeds, tofu and soy products, oats, cottage cheese, some of the other cheeses, milk, broccoli, quinoa, lentils, shrimp, brussels sprouts, they alone can take care of your needs. Make the right decisions. Be strong and healthy.

Roosters crow,
Cows go MOO.
Keep them lean,
It's good for you!

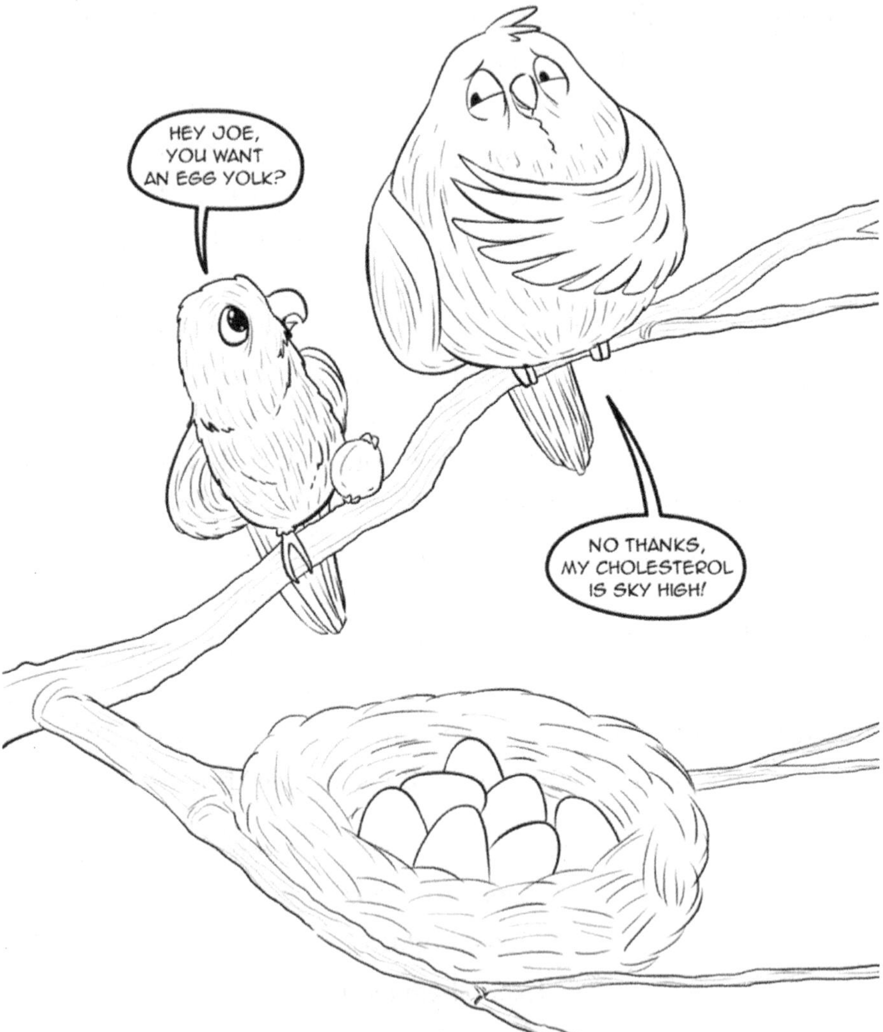
HEY JOE, YOU WANT AN EGG YOLK?
NO THANKS, MY CHOLESTEROL IS SKY HIGH!

Odds & Ends

Every day is an adventure whether you're trying to become fit or simply maintain a certain fitness level. New challenges arise on an hourly basis as you proceed through the treacherous waters of daily existence. Proper planning, knowing and understanding your enemies, keeping your nutritional weapons close by, and a warrior mentality are all necessary for survival.

There will be days when you'll feel overwhelmed. It will seem everything wants to drag you down. You're running against the wind and swimming upstream in an upside-down world. All you want to do is fall back into your comfort zone of your past unhealthy ways.

This is when your secret weapons come in handy. Step back, take a deep breath and relax. Just remember that you can get through it. Tomorrow will be a new day, a better day. Break out a secret weapon. And just what are these secret weapons? We'll get to that in a roundabout way after a moment honoring the great Zucchini.

Legendary Zarkoff Zucchini once stated, "A great man makes a great stand." Really? I personally don't think "A great man makes a great stand," is a grand example of oratory skill. It seems to me anyone can come up with that. Break out the one-year-olds and you'll find better quotations.

But what do I know? I haven't attained a God-like status like the Great One. I haven't become a historical figure in the world of vegetable rights. I am not the deeply adored and respected icon that was Zarkoff Zucchini.

His massive legion of followers, those who worship the very soil that begat his squashy butt, beg to differ with my lowly views. "A great man makes a great stand," therefore is now chanted at Zarkoff Zucchini memory-rallies worldwide. Banners abound flying his profound statement.

The point here is to not get caught up in petty quotation analyzation, but simply to take the great Zarkoff's advice. He may have been a womanizer, he may have been a hard-core drinker, he may or may not have secretly worn women's underclothing, he may have fathered fruits and vegetables across the land, but none of that should matter in the least. His flaws only made him who he was, an imperfect vegetable with a heart of gold.

No vegetable is perfect and the Great One was no different. Zarkoff Zucchini made his mark upon the planet and we should apply the principles of vegetable equality to our own hopes and dreams. I, for one, will worship the great Zarkoff forever, as there will never be a bigger name in the history of vegetable emancipation. He liberated vegetables worldwide and brought vegetable rights to the forefront of global awareness.

For that we owe Zarkoff Zucchini a plateful of gratitude and we should promise to never cover any vegetable with butter or greasy substances ever again. Zarkoff, you were so tormented. It's such a shame that you lost your life. Womanizing really cost you. Perhaps some therapy could have helped, or maybe another stint in alcohol rehab, but it's too late now.

I thank you, Zarkoff Zucchini, for if you were alive today, if you were to grace us with your presence for a brief moment, I would bow and show my genuine appreciation for all you have accomplished in the name of equality. Just stay away from my pretty little niece and don't touch the female tomatoes in my garden.

Booze and women,
Was the life he led.
Poor ole Zarkoff,
Now he's dead.

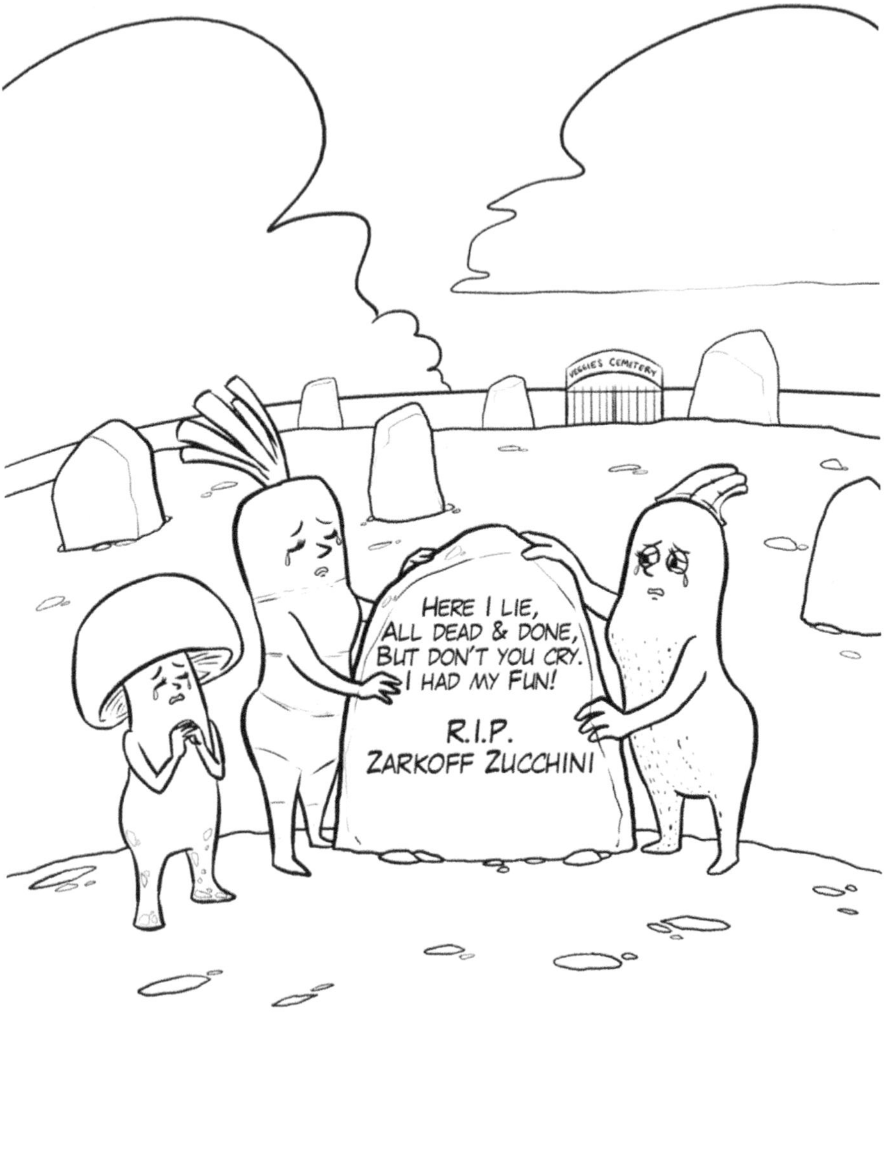
VEGGIES CEMETERY
HERE I LIE,
ALL DEAD & DONE,
BUT DON'T YOU CRY.
I HAD MY FUN!
R.I.P.
ZARKOFF ZUCCHINI

Odds & Ends II

Let's go back to the subject of secret weaponry in your quest to become fit. We were discussing that issue of great importance before Zarkoff's image-rehabilitation agency so rudely interrupted us. Your secret weapon is really yourself. Let me explain.

You woke this morning and you had a basic idea of your schedule. You planned accordingly and took three minutes to gather your emergency tools. These tools include a large bottle of water, not one of those showoff sipper-bottles the actresses tote around at the Oscar ceremonies. Really? There's not enough liquid in there to make an amoeba pee. No, your water bottle is a real water bottle. You'll drink from it all day long.

The next item you threw into your emergency kit was an apple, a couple of bananas and a little bag of any fresh veggies that's convenient to grab. Anything raw and fresh will do. There's no need to call cousin Bernie who is a physician and ask him which veggie possesses which nutrients. They're all healthy, so grab and go and don't be an over-analyzer. Over-analyzers are always running behind because they're late to the program.

This fruit and veggie mix is your first-line defense system to defeat hunger. During the day you may start to crave calories and your scheduled meal is an hour away. No problem, reach into your trusty veggie/fruit container dedicated to Zarkoff Zucchini and take a few generous bites. Wash it down with a gulp of water and you're good to go.

Maybe those little healthy treats didn't quite do the trick. Perhaps you're still hungry. That's where the next secret weapon comes into play. It's what I call a carbohydrate mix. There are countless healthy items that can go into this little container. I'll name a few including my favorites.

You're trying to lose weight or maintain your current weight so this decision is important. What we're looking for here are efficient low-fat energizers. You lose weight by eating, not starving. Fill your body with the good stuff and you won't be craving the bad stuff. Fatblobs are right around the corner awaiting an opportunity to jump into your abdomen and start blob-families. Before long they'll have a community center built within you and off to college their little blobbies will go. At that point you're doomed.

My favorite is so because it's quick and easy and I'm a touch lazy, or at least economically efficient in the energy department. It's a little container that contains a mix of spoon-size shredded wheat, maybe a few *unsalted raw or roasted* nuts, and a handful of raisins or another dried fruit. Go easy on the nuts in this mix even though they're a superfood in my opinion. What you're trying to get with the nuts is a touch of healthy fat to trick your body into satisfaction. You're trying to survive the day.

As always, go with your own style when you create your carbohydrate mix. Just keep it lean and mean. Those nuts can't be processed in oil or covered in salt. It's the same mindset with the raisins or fruit. If they're sweetened in *any* way, you're defeating the whole purpose. This precious container is meant to keep you alive and stave off those pesky fatblobs.

Fatblobs are especially prevalent in the workplace. Remember this, your friendly coworker who keeps offering fatty foods to you is not sincere. She's secretly hoping you'll fail, so you'll remain as fat as her. Refuse her offer to take you out to Big Butt's Diner for lunch.

Don't be afraid to be an individual, to be yourself. You make your own rules as this world will eat you alive if you don't. Politely say no to her offer of a crème cake snack. Win and do something extraordinary. It matters not that you're doing it via an unconventional method. We'll see who's laughing when you're strutting around showing off your new lean body, in a classy way of course.

One important rule with this is to eat very slowly and *wait* for a few minutes before grabbing something else to eat. Five minutes is usually enough for the body to receive signals that nutrition has arrived. Then the occupied-by-good-things flag is raised relaying the message to all fatblobs that they're not welcome. They can go invade someone else's innards and start major cities. You're not for sale to these sneaky opportunists.

Learn to use your weaponry and you'll be successful. Head off hunger at the pass. Timing is the key, so never allow yourself to *really* get hungry. You're walking a fine line between cutting calories and staying healthy. Go with your instincts and learn your one-of-a-kind body. You rule the body, it doesn't rule you.

Lean protein is an important weapon in your daily battle. The nuts can provide a substantial amount, but you may desire to add an egg or egg white, or possibly a can of tuna. You can take a bite right out of the can periodically throughout the day. This shouldn't bother you to do this in the presence of others because your new goal is to become as weird as me. I shouldn't have to remind you that the tuna is packed in water and low in sodium.

GEEZER ALERT!

Hold Those Eyes Open, You Tired Ole Geezer! It's Not Yet Nappie Time!

If you keep water, a few fresh fruits or veggies, your carb-mix container and a lean protein source handy at all times, you'll win. Now let's move on to some beverage weapons. They give your mind something to think about besides that bad stuff that lurks around every corner.

Coffee and tea can be a great help when you're trying to lose weight. They're super-low in calories while giving you something to consume besides food. They also take a considerable amount of time to drink, time that you're not concentrating on temptations.

Here's the problem associated with these great dietary weapons. Many of you want to contaminate your coffee or tea with sweeteners and heavy creamers. Don't do it. The only things that should be allowed should be a little low-fat milk, a bit of honey, or maybe a liberal pouring of lemon juice in your tea. Break those old sweetener and creamer habits and go basic with your coffee and tea. Grandma did it, mom did it, and that's the real reason you're doing it. Be strong and resist and start a new trend.

Sip your coffee or tea *slowly*. Remember these are psychological weapons more so than physical ones. They're time-stalling devices that allow you to concentrate on sipping instead of gorging on those pastries in the break room. You're trying to trick your mind and buy some time until that next healthy meal that's planned.

Don't overdo these as it's very easy to do so. Several cups of coffee or tea daily can be a lifesaver when it comes to food resistance, but don't let the coffee and tea consume you. If you catch yourself drinking more than three or four cups a day, try to rein yourself back in.

Remember that unlimited coffee and tea are temporary luxuries. They're crutches that get you through a crisis, allowing you to survive another minute, another hour, another day in this war upon temptation. Try your best not to abuse either one. A decaffeinated selection may be an option.

A quick note on sweeteners before we move on. Honey is natural and has been known to provide health benefits. It's an ancient remedy that's documented as far back as history takes us. Religious texts emphasize its sacred value. I intuitively feel there's something really special about it in ways that we're not aware. I think one day science will discover this. For now, use it in your tea or coffee and anything else that you may want sweetened. It's *absolutely* better than that big pile of processed sugar that sits in front of you.

Fruit juice is another possible healthy beverage, but a piece of fruit should always be number one. If you decide to go the juice route, make it a small glass. Use it as a pick-me-up to provide a healthy shot of quick energy. Be careful as juices do contain calories. You may want to dilute the juice with a sizable amount of water. I've been doing that for years. You're filled up and you still get that energy boost that you're craving. That's what these beverages are designed for, deceiving the body into satisfaction mode. Low-calorie verses high-calorie, that's the name of this game.

One last secret weapon in the daily struggle is about as simple as it gets. Do you feel yourself falling under the spell of ole Blubber Devil who floats around offices and workplaces worldwide? Nasty thoughts of fatty foods begin to flood your brain as he does his dirty deeds.

Fight him off by rising from your desk and going outside for a moment. You'd be surprised what a brief splattering of fresh air and solitude can do for your attitude. Any resistance from the boss should be met with a resounding, "Fitness and health are important to me, so please leave me alone for a moment." Show him who's the real boss. If he still resists, tell him you're exposing his affair with the secretary to his wife unless he shuts up and behaves.

There you have it. There are countless methods by which to win this war. Be creative. Put yourself into winner mode. Be somebody. Be you.

It's a battle,
It's a war.
You will win,
That's for sure!

CHAPTER 4

Bad Ways

"Winners change. Losers make excuses and talk like victims."
Trey Moffitt

Mean Ole Stuff

We're all flawed to a certain extent. Even heroes like Zarkoff Zucchini have a closet packed full of skeletons, and possibly some women's undergarments. There is a little-known book that's been making the rounds lately that depicts our iconic legend in a bad light. It's an unauthorized biography written by his longtime mistress, Cindy Celery. I, for one, am very disturbed at the revelations alleged in this hit piece of sensationalism. It reeks of greed, disloyalty and defamation of character.

I'm well aware that Zarkoff Zucchini was a flawed individual. From his constant womanizing to boozing it up, the vegetable had a zesty lust for life that was unrestrained. It's just that, in my opinion, Cindy Celery carried this way too far. Her book, *Zarkoff Zucchini, A Dirty Hero,* is a total disgrace as far as I'm concerned.

Ms. Celery is nothing more than a headline attention grabber. To suggest that Zucchini had an extramarital affair with a sausage biscuit is ridiculous. As is the outrageous claim that he was intimate with a bologna sandwich and fathered a hybrid processed meat. Fatty processed meats never turned Zucchini on, for he was a vegetable lover through and through.

Sure, Zarkoff loved the ladies that so beautified the produce sections of every city he visited. But to think he would stoop so low as to seduce a sausage biscuit is ridiculous. Although rumors abound of little meaty Zarkoffs, there is no way that he would ever propagate outside of his vegetable category, except for a pretty fruit here and there. This is purely an attempt by Ms. Celery to scandalize and capitalize.

My point here is that Zucchini, as flawed as he was with certain weaknesses, held true to his innate foundation of vegetable equality. And even if he did have affairs with female fatty meats, shouldn't it be the Great One himself to announce it. Zarkoff Zucchini, being a righteous, forthright individual would have been the first to claim, endorse, and love his preservative-laden, meaty child had it actually happened. His followers would have embraced their hero regardless. Anyone can make a mistake.

Let's not disrespect a hero who can't defend himself against this little vegetable strumpet so-called author. Long live the untarnished memory of Zarkoff Zucchini!

> *The rumors fly,*
> *Yes, they do.*
> *But Zarkoff says,*
> *They ain't true!*

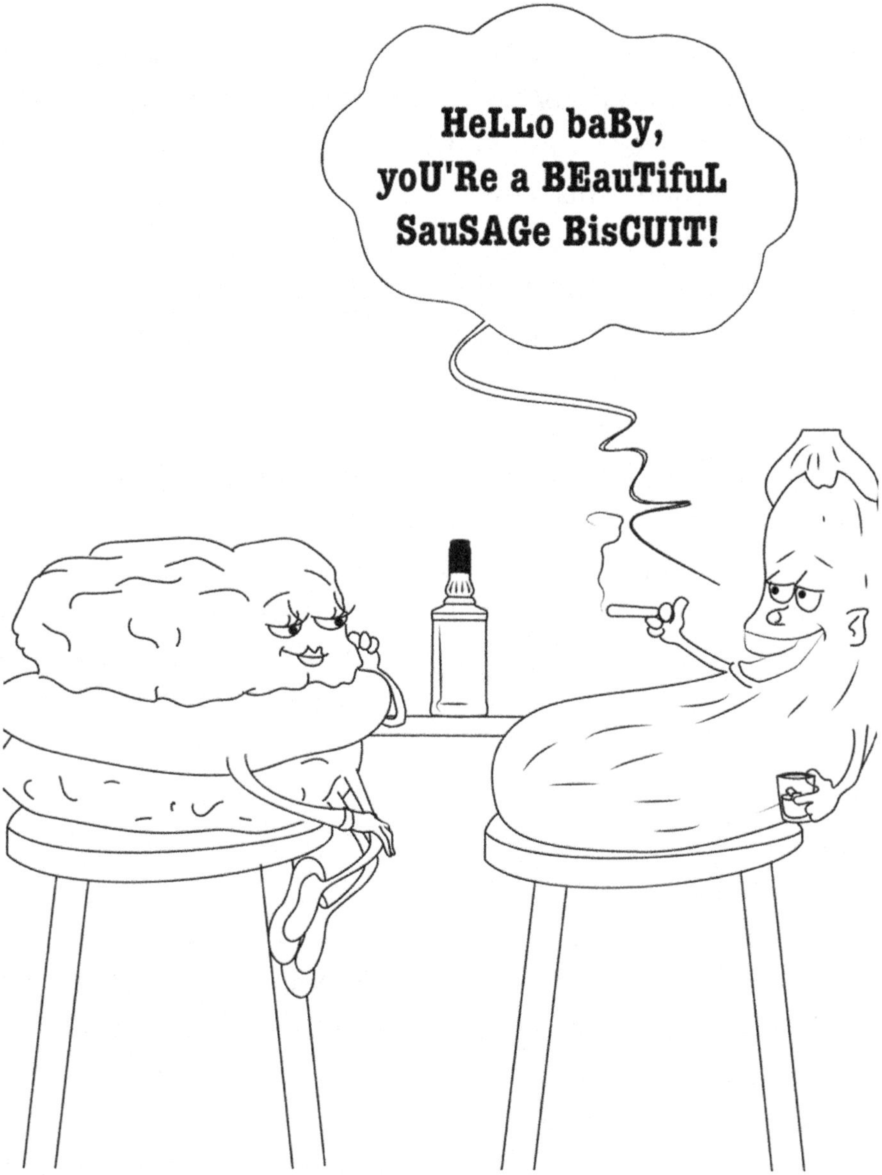
HeLLo baBy,
yoU'Re a BEauTifuL
SauSAGe BisCUIT!

Stress & Your Personal Life

Our return to sanity will begin with a discussion about a major root cause of obesity and illness. Stress is an assassin that kills and gets away scot-free as a framed patsy takes the fall. Rarely does this covert hitman who operates in the shadows ever get caught. We really need to pay more attention to stress and the incredible damage it causes.

Stress is an invisible killer that rarely gets the blame it deserves. That's because it's an underlying cause of so many issues. "Oh, he died of a heart attack," they may say. Stress could have been the real culprit in this case. There are countless ways the body reacts negatively to stress.

High blood pressure, heart disease, obesity, diabetes, and headaches are just some of the consequences of this covert killer. Stress symptoms may be affecting your health and you may not even realize it. Maybe you're blaming something else for the recurring headaches, frequent insomnia or your sudden lack of work productivity, when the actual cause is stress.

Stress doesn't just affect you physically, as it attacks you in a psychological manner also. You can experience sadness and depression, social withdrawal, irritability and drug and alcohol misuse. These are just a few outlets for stress to escape and rip you apart.

So, what's the answer? We're old and have been around the block, so we know stress-causing events will never stop. Experience has told us life never stops throwing punches at us. We wake up every morning to another day filled with challenges, some larger than others. It's not the daily obstacles that are the real enemy, it's our method of handling these crises.

It's all about attitude and proper mindset. Know those punches are going to be coming at you hard and fast. Be like a young Muhammad Ali and laugh at them as they graze your face. Tell those pesky attempts to knock you down that you're a pretty boy or girl and you refuse to lie down and give up. Beat them today and beat them tomorrow, and yes, they'll absolutely come gunning for you again tomorrow.

We know stress hits us from every angle. Many of us suffer financial stress. Not knowing how we're going to meet our monthly bills is always a major concern. Kids and grandkids seem to always be pushing our stress buttons. That will surely never change. Signing in to procreation of the species brings heartache along with all the joy. If your kids and grandkids turned out perfect, then watch out because something's lurking in the shadows.

Divorce is a whopper of a stressful event. Anyone who's gone through it knows that. Death of a loved one is about as bad as it gets. Yes, there are some major blows that cut deep into our souls. Once again, it's how we deal with it. There is no choice but to carry on. Get back on your feet, force a smile, and get on with the program.

One day this thing we call life will come to an end and we'll go on to the next level. As for this present physical existence, we're pretty much stuck in it to ride it out. Relief will come soon enough in the form of physical death. I sure hope the next level is a little more peaceful than the current one.

I'm hoping for a sandy beach, temperature around 75 degrees, maybe a pretty girl delivering me a cool craft beer upon my request, and we might as well throw in a nice cigar while we're at it. That's the dream, but for now it's all avoiding punches, dodging bullets, and struggling to make ends meet. Sooner or later, it will be our time to relax into eternity. Whatever your beliefs are, it's got to be an upgrade from our present situation.

While we're inhabiting this particular plane of existence, we're subject to the realm of the uncontrollable. No matter how rich and powerful an individual may be, there's no escaping this life unscathed. You know this as the tabloids scream it at you every day. Such and such a person lost control and feel off the deep end and their fame and fortune couldn't help them in the least.

There's a lesson in this for us all. It's no self-pity. Don't go around crying to others that you're a helpless victim and life dealt you a bad hand. All of us were dealt a bad hand, but just different cards. If there's reincarnation, maybe the cards will be different next time around, or maybe not. Who knows the answer, but the temporary fix is handling today's unique challenges. Get back on that horse and keep on trucking. Stress awaits and it's all about how we handle it.

Healthy ways to handle stress include reading, relaxing hobbies, listening to music, deep breathing, and spending quality time with family and friends. There are many others, just use some common sense and choose the right ones. Get the proper amount of sleep, don't use alcohol or drugs as a crutch, and above all, *eat right and exercise.*

One last note about coping with stress is to keep your sense of humor. This life wasn't designed to make sense, so throw a curveball back at it. Laugh as it swings and misses. Seriousness has its place, but sometimes it's your enemy.

For example, watch how you can disarm a potential conflict with a witty nonsensical comment. Leave yourself unassailable by muttering an outrageously stupid statement that is beyond deserving a reply. The response will be usually be a chuckle or a smile, and these are the antithesis of stress. So what if you're not solving the dilemma of who should be our designated leader. Hasn't that one been rehashed until it's charcoal anyway?

Some people thrive on arguing and this bit of defense can send them on the way to their next victim. Send stress packing right behind them. Make up your own silly Zarkoff Zucchini world and let it fly. Maybe it's not your cup of tea, but zaniness works for me. It's at least a better outlet than letting stress boil over and consume you. Regardless of how you channel it, use your own individual sense of humor. It's a great weapon against stress.

Life's gone mad, It's a mess. You be tough, Beat that stress!

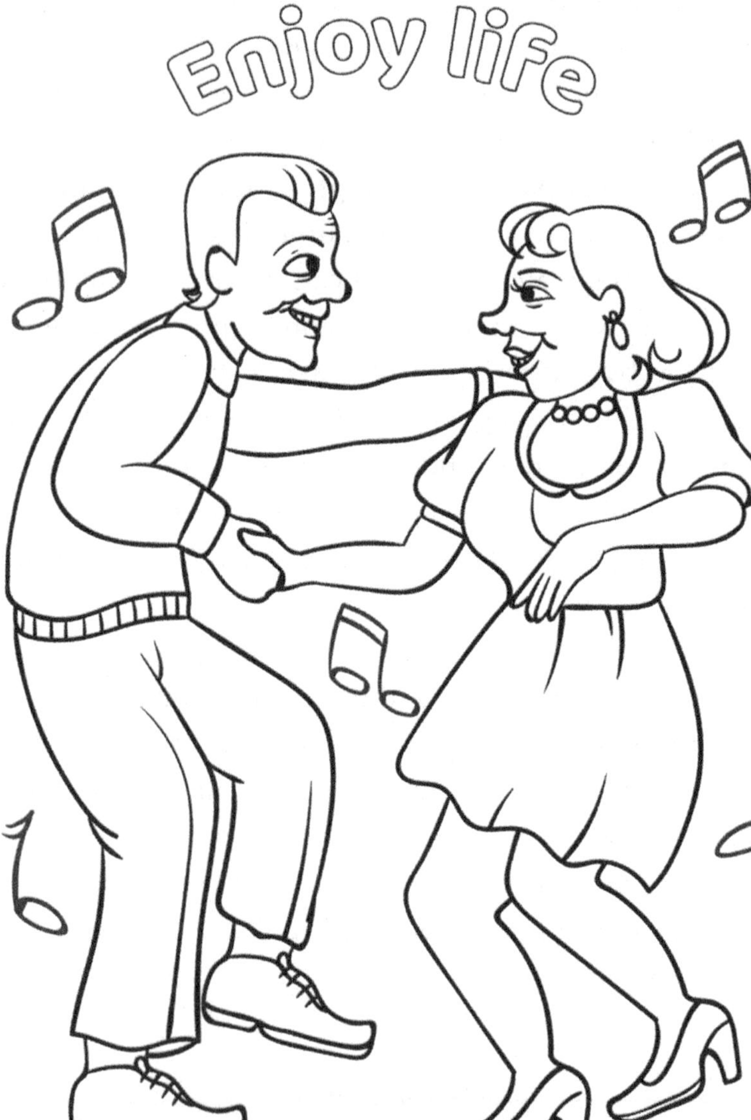
Enjoy life
Never too old to dance

Alcohol, Drugs & Cigarettes

We as humans love the easy way out. Often the easiest way out is no more than an escape. We block out our harsh reality by any means available. We numb ourselves so that the tough world doesn't seem so tough. We medicate ourselves with pills hoping that our inner pain will disappear along with the physical. We avoid the root issue and treat the symptom instead.

Escapism is a natural human trait. We escape through work, entertainment, television, video games and so many other ways. If we couldn't occasionally pull away from reality to unwind, we would explode. It might be an emotional explosion, but that can be as bad as a literal one.

Everyone needs a Disney sort of shelter every now and then. The problem occurs when the shelter becomes a permanent one. Hiding underneath a protective layer of fantasy doesn't protect you in the least. It's a deceptive mirage. A false sense of security is worse than no security at all.

Sometimes we sneak away from our healthy escapism and other outlets seduce us. Alcohol and drugs are the primary enticements that we grab onto for security. These substances are just fine when used correctly and in moderation. The problem is they can quickly become an easy fix to a much deeper underlying problem. Covering a hole in your floor doesn't fix the hole. You've actually double-downed on the problem. Now you may forget that a hole exists and you can step into it and break your ankle. Covering up problems isn't a long-term solution.

It's so tempting to enter that hazy world and never leave. It entices you and wags its little finger signaling you to come inside. You take a peek and it's so dreamy and cozy, so you step in for just a taste. It sure feels good. You like it and you return the next day for just one more look. Everything's bright and cheery and it's oh such a sunny day. You really like it.

You return each day until you decide to stay in your world on a permanent basis. Life on the outside doesn't seem quite so good anymore. This is so much better. Why bother with all those problems that lie just on the other side of the door? It's cold and mean out there and nobody seems to care. In this world I can be free. I can be me.

That's how easily it can happen. We can escape our pain as the problems pile up outside the door. When you finally open up the door to see if the world is still real, the problems come flooding in and they're bigger than ever. That hazy dreamland is shattered by reality and now you're more confused than ever.

Alcohol and drugs can sneak up on you and slowly take you away. Most people can handle them and keep them at bay in their proper place. However, there are many who fall deep into the abyss of true dependency. The drink or drug becomes more important than life itself. They've slipped into the chasm between reality and the dreamy escape upon which they've grown dependent.

At this point you're swimming in an ocean of fantasy. Reality is just a mirror that stares back and leads you nowhere. You've put yourself into an illusionary world that's no more a world than my fictional Zarkoff. Needless to say, it's time to seek help in a big way.

Cigarettes are a completely different type of enticement, but just as dangerous. Try to kick the habit before it kicks you. It will be a difficult task, but many have done it and so can you. I don't have to tell you what it does to your lungs and body. You've been around a long time and seen and heard it all. We've seen firsthand what it has done to others. Some of them may even be friends or family.

Today it seems to be prescription pills that cause many problems. Doctors recommend them and the cycle begins. I wish doctors would stop and think before they get out their little pad and start punching in a pill that needs a pill that needs a pill. I think all of them wish the best for us and truly want to help us. They're wonderful human beings. I just think common sense has been erased in many cases and mistakes occur. Treating the cause and not the symptom seems the best option.

I don't know the answer to kicking drugs, alcohol or cigarettes. Doctors and rehabilitation centers worldwide have struggled with this. The success rate isn't so high. The only thing I do know is *you have to want it*. You stand absolutely no chance at all of success if you don't truly desire it. Even then it's a tough road, but with determination and discipline you can do it. Good luck.

I wish I could,
Fly far away.
Gotta stay tough,
Deal with the day.

Sugar, Salt & Processed Foods

Profits drive the machine that is the food pipeline. They operate on consumerism and they learned a long time ago that sugar and salt sell. Somewhere back in industrial history a bright entrepreneur realized he sold more of a particular food item if it was sweet or salty. From that point onward our choices became limited. It's our own fault, as we could have resisted those first sweet and salty items.

The large food conglomerates react to our buying decisions as much as they are proactive. It really is an emotionless machine that can't be blamed. They're simply reacting to our consumer habits more so than any conspiratorial attempt to fatten us up with their tainted treats.

We're to blame by choosing these items. We pluck these blood pressure risers and diabetes inducers from the shelves and throw them into our carts with no thought at all. It's often the pretty face adorning the package that makes the sale. Don't be brainwashed. Sodas aren't necessary to sustain life contrary to popular belief.

The human body needs a certain amount of sodium as it plays a role in nerve and muscle function and regulation of body fluids. Many of us in the western world consume *much* more sodium than we need. This is where the problem arises. Too much sodium can cause hypertension that can lead to heart disease, kidney disease or strokes. How much fun is that?

All that processed sugar that we eat by the truckload is even worse. Our bodies can perform just fine without a grain of refined sugar. We get all the sugar we need from our natural foods. Sugar is a simple carbohydrate that converts into glucose and provides energy for us to watch television. Those reality shows can really tax our energy reserves.

The bottom line is our bodies do need sugars, but not the refined version that is added into virtually every processed food item. If people realized just how much sugar they consumed in a year they would faint in disbelief. That big white pile would make Scarface the coke dealer jump for joy. I hesitate to label processed sugar as poisonous, but I'm pretty close to doing so. In large quantities it's almost a match with cocaine. I'd stock neither one of them in the health food section.

Natural sugars found in natural foods are all we need to propel our bodies through an average day. Fruits, vegetables, dairy, and grains have provided mankind with energy for millennia. There was once a wise, great vegetable that very publicly pronounced, "Consume me and my mates and thou shall be pure."

Of course, it was the Great One, the iconic legend, the eloquent orator, Zarkoff Zucchini. He made that historic statement immediately upon winning his Supreme Court case. What a vegetable he was!

Start looking at the food product labels and you'll see what Zarkoff was talking about. Nearly every item has added refined sugar. Some of them have ridiculous amounts that border on insanity. There are many sodas that top 40 grams in one serving. Several have close to 50 grams packed into that harmless looking cutie of a can.

Why don't you do this? Run to your kitchen and pull out a bag of sugar. Measure out 50 grams and take a look at it. It will be a big pile of white powder, I promise you. Tony Montana would be proud. Now grab a spoon and start eating away at this delicious dish. After you sicken yourself and complete your task at hand, grab a soda can and compare the gram content to the grams that now float inside your intestines. Now what Zarkoff preaches about starts to make some sense.

Some people act as if sodas are a basic requirement of life itself. They start and end their day with cans of the stuff. Those sugary beverages are not necessary to sustain life. Caveman certainly didn't need them and neither do you.

Do you know someone who is obviously very unhealthy, maybe obese and sickly? They could even be your friend or family member. It's saddening to see them carry on with their habits despite knowing better. They're doing nothing more than dying a slow agonizing death. Take some time and quietly analyze their habits. Leave the preaching to Zarkoff because it doesn't work coming from us humans.

Odds are probable that person consumes a disproportionate amount of salt, sugar, and processed foods. They may start their day with a soda, continue on with fatty meats, sugary and salty treats, and so forth. Maybe they even drown themselves in alcohol washed away in a cloud of cigarette smoke. It's truly sad to witness someone you care about slowly commit suicide. Many have just given up.

Don't be one of these people. If you're bordering on this type of behavior, it's not too late. Learn as much as you can about nutrition and general health-awareness. The education part of this is easy. Then go cold turkey and turn your life around. The force lies within. You can do it, for there's a wealth of determination and discipline that's waiting patiently, lying dormant inside you. It's chomping at the bit to escape and show the world who you are and what you can accomplish.

Cut out or drastically reduce your consumption of salt, sugar and processed foods. You'll have reduced food cravings, improved memory, a healthier heart, prettier skin, weight loss, better moods, better sleep, less chance of diabetes, more energy, and maybe even a little Zarkoff libido boost. The benefits go on and on. Do it for you. Do it for those who love you. Do it for Zarkoff Zucchini. Just do it.

Love your sugar,
Love your salt.
All that stuff,
You must halt!

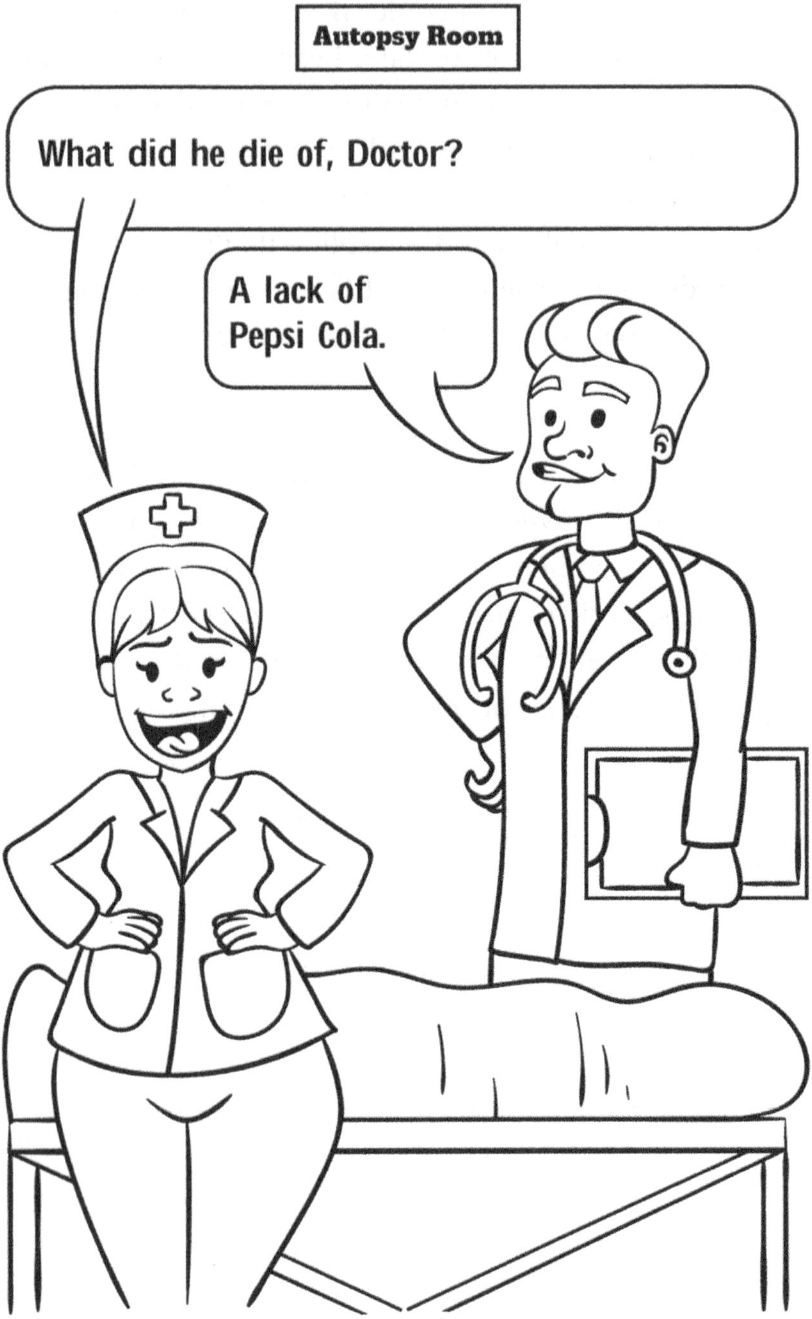
Autopsy Room
What did he die of, Doctor?
A lack of Pepsi Cola.

Fatty Stuff

Yes, the body needs a certain amount of fat. It was designed to burn it off on a daily basis, not collect it and carry it around like a ball and chain. Your daily intake of fat should be burned like a fireplace log, and fade out of sight like smoke from a chimney. An efficient body leaves no trace of yesterday's overindulgences. All those yesterdays can add up, and decades of them can leave you in an obese state.

Burn that fire log on a daily basis and send that fat out the chimney and into the wind. Disperse it into the sky instead of your hips and waist. Kiss that fat goodbye and welcome the next day's ration, for it will receive the same treatment. Fat in and fat out, that's the way we look at it. You ain't running no fat flophouse inside your body, as this southerner describes it.

It's all about being lean and strong. It's all about being fit and healthy and feeling that energy and confidence that radiate from within. The key behind being lean and strong is to choose the right foods and burn them away in an efficient manner. Be a machine and don't be a slug. Get it going and keep it going. I know you can do it.

Zarkoff Zucchini once made a statement that somewhat relates to our current discussion. He was addressing an audience at the annual Okra Appreciation Conference, where of course, he was the celebrity speaker. He was way down south, in the heart of Mississippi. Zarkoff always had a love for the southern states. As you may guess, it was more about the pretty southern belles than anything else.

"Greatness is great and that is good," were the magical words that flowed from Zarkoff as he took his place at the podium. The packed arena erupted in applause. Zarkoff must have possessed incredible charm, because most of us wouldn't achieve any acclaim whatsoever from such a nonsensical statement. But coming from the lips of the charismatic Zarkoff, "Greatness is great and that is good," brought down the house.

As he waited for the applause to die down, Zarkoff surveyed the audience. Oh, my, there were some pretty okra out there. These southern gals sure knew how to take care of themselves. They bundled up all that beauty and delivered it with a sexy southern smile. Mississippi was Zarkoff's kind of place.

Zarkoff launched into his speech, praising all vegetables, and okra in particular. He mentioned the Great Okra Massacre of 1884, where an entire field of okra was wiped out and replaced by a tobacco crop. He mentioned the Okra Advancement Act, a bill that had benefited so many okra, which he single-handedly pushed through Congress. He mentioned the overall progress that had been made in okra recognition, and how okra prejudices were slowly being eroded.

Zarkoff eloquently finished up his speech with a touching tribute to all native Mississippian okra. They had done so much and worked so hard to get where they were. Zarkoff told them there was much more that needed to be done, but there was no doubt they would accomplish their goals. He praised the Mississippians for their outstanding accomplishments and reminded them of their proud heritage.

There wasn't a dry eye in the house as Zarkoff ended his speech. He had touched on so many emotional issues. He walked off the stage amidst a thundering applause. The energy was electric as the vegetable hero waved back at the crowd. Once again, Zarkoff had proven why he was such an iconic figure in the world of vegetable rights. He was the one and only Zarkoff Zucchini.

Zarkoff slipped behind the privacy of the curtain. The crowd was applauding and giving him a standing ovation. Zarkoff felt very proud of himself. He sat down on a sofa to relax for a moment. He needed some time to regroup.

Then it happened. Zarkoff felt someone reach around him from behind. What the heck was going on! A rag was placed over his face. In a matter of seconds Zarkoff passed out.

"The chemicals worked great," said Pooches Peach. "Come on girls, let's drag this no-good vermin out to the truck."

Pooches and her two peachy accomplices quickly dragged Zarkoff's limp body to their pickup truck. They heaved him into the back and sped away. Not a soul witnessed any of it.

Zarkoff awoke a few hours later. He was so groggy. What the heck had happened? Where was he? Zarkoff realized he couldn't move. He had been tied and bound. And what the heck were these things attached to his arms and legs? He didn't know what was going on, but one thing was for sure, he was in a tight spot.

Someone entered the room. "Well, hello, Zarko the cheater liar man," a female voice called out. "How did you like those chemicals in your face? Did you take you a little nappy nap?"

Zarkoff's heart skipped a beat. It was Pooches Peach! Oh, no! This was not good. This was trouble!

"I followed you here all the way from your last speech in Atlanta," Pooches calmly stated. "You didn't really think I'd let you get away with cheating on me, did you?"

Pooches strolled closer to Zarkoff. She placed her hand on what looked to be an enormous metal box of sorts. "Do you know what this is, Zarko the cheater man? This is an electricity conductor and it's connected to your body. It produces 100,000 volts pushed by 100,000 amps of killer electrical current."

Pooches chuckled before she spoke. Her wicked smile pierced the room. "Do you know what that's going to do to you? Well, let me read from the manual."

Pooches opened up the manual and began reading. "Use extreme caution when operating this wattage/amperage unit. Accidental shock will result in severe pain, respiratory arrest, seizures, nerve damage, and severe burns. The heart ceases pumping, cardiac arrest occurs, and death is certain. Always use extreme caution with this unit. Never use around water, as water conducts electricity."

"Ha, ha, ha," laughed Pooches. "Take a look at your feet, Zarko boy. You're covered in a foot of water. How do you think that's going to make you feel when I pull the switch on this baby? HA, HA, HA!" Pooches reached out and took hold of the lever. She pulled down on it.

"Ohhhhhhhhh!" cried Zarkoff, as the current raced through his body. Zarkoff immediately went into convulsions. His body shook like a rag doll in a tornado. His eyes spun around in circles. He stopped breathing. His skin began melting away on his arms and legs. His heart began pumping erratically as electricity took control of his body. Pooches pushed the lever and turned it off.

"Did that feel good, Zarko boy?" slurred Pooches. "I hope so, because here comes some more!" Once again, Pooches pulled down upon the lever.

"NOOO!" screamed Zarkoff, as the current once again ravaged his body. Pooches watched with a big grin as Zarkoff sizzled. Again he went into convulsions. He stopped breathing and his heart stopped beating. Pooches laughed hysterically as fire exited the top of Zarkoff's head. She flipped the lever back, turning it off.

Pooches pointed her finger and wiggled it in Zarkoff's face. "That'll teach you to cheat on me! How do you like fire shooting out the top of your head? Are you just a little warm, Zarko boy? Do you have a fever? It looks like you're going to need a few skin grafts. You look good in melted skin. Goodbye, cheater man!"

Pooches exited the room, never to be seen again. Zarkoff was discovered the next week by a cleaning crew. There were no signs of life. One worker remarked that rigor mortis had set in. This was definitely a dead zucchini. Then another worker noticed some movement of the eyelids. Could it be possible there was some life left in this scorched vegetable?

Medics were called and Zarkoff was airlifted to a burn center. His body was burned beyond recognition. His entire skull had to be replaced with a piece of steel. All of his skin had melted. His heart was damaged beyond repair. He received yet another heart transplant. Both lungs were completely burned up. They gave him a single lung from a donor. Eighteen months of skin grafts ensued.

Eventually Zarkoff started looking like the old Zarkoff. He even had some females noticing him again. It wasn't long before he was back doing what he did best, chasing girls. It would be less than a month before he would land in the hospital again. This time six jealous strippers had used him as a shooting range practice target. He was shot over 200 times.

The moral of this story as it relates to your fitness program is this. Avoid fatty foods just as Zarkoff should avoid relationship confrontations. Most of us can learn from horrible experiences, but unfortunately Zarkoff was eternally doomed for failure. Use Zarkoff as a model of what *not* to do. Don't give in to your demons.

> *Fire came out,*
> *Of Zarkoff's head.*
> *Everyone thought,*
> *He was dead.*

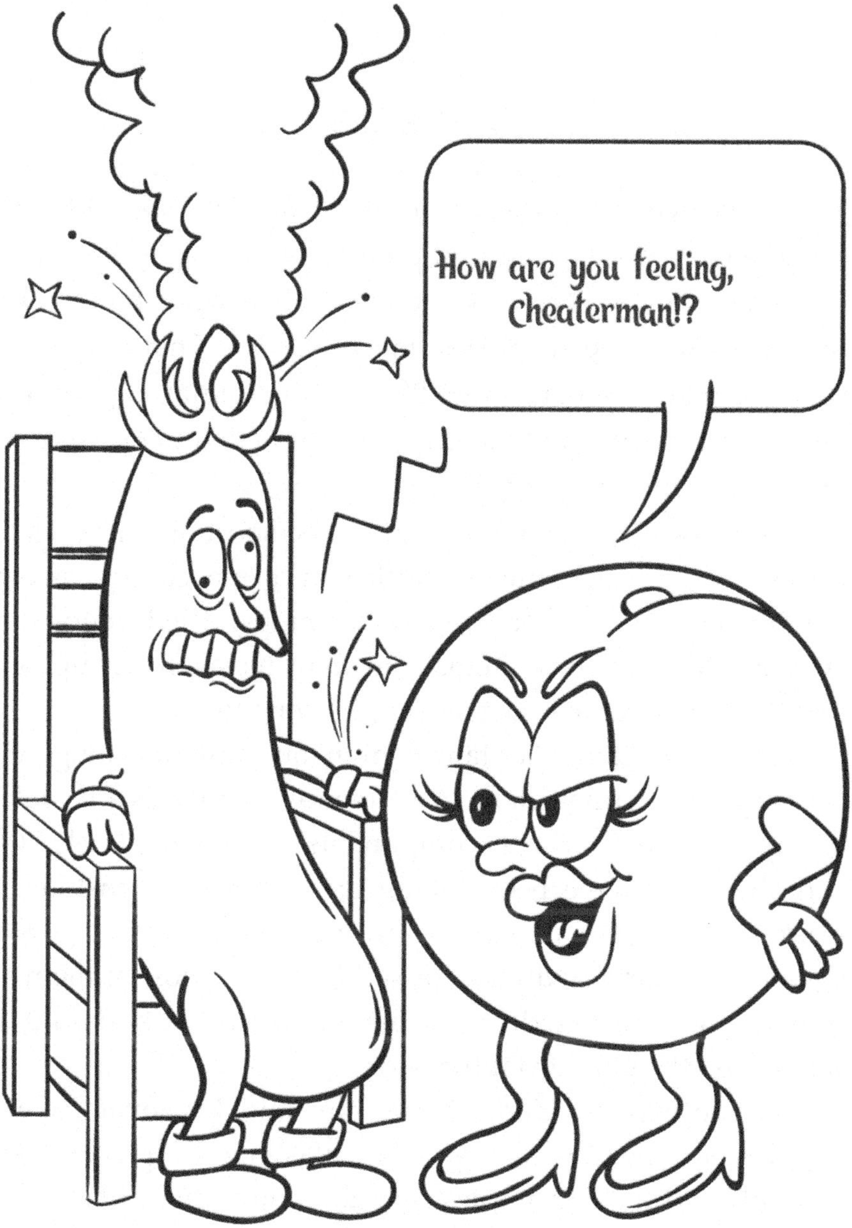
How are you feeling, Cheaterman!?

Fatty Stuff II

The body needs a certain amount of fat to sustain life. The body doesn't need a hundred pounds of excess fat. Worry not that one day you'll be in a situation where your body has to dip into a massive surplus of fat to survive. That situation is highly unlikely. What's more likely is that hundred pounds of blub will tax your body and organs and eventually land you in a state of major disarray.

What constitutes the fatty stuff? The short list includes the pre-discussed fatty meats, butter and margarine, sweets, mayonnaise and other creamy toppings, fried foods and cheese. Many of these items you may have grown up with and they've become a sort of comfort zone for you.

The above items contain a high fat content, along with carbohydrates and protein. We all know that foods are broken down into these three components. It seems lately that carbohydrates have been taking an undeserved bashing, at least in my opinion. I've heard people make the general statement, "Carbohydrates are bad for you." Most of them are lumping all carbohydrates together when they should be separating the good from the bad.

Let me explain. Zarkoff Zucchini and his loyal gang of veggies are nearly all carbs, a splashing of protein, and virtually no fat. Examples include zucchini, mushrooms, tomatoes, broccoli, cauliflower, cucumbers, celery, spinach, artichokes, and on and on. These are some of healthiest foods on the planet.

Yet I've witnessed dieters who refuse to eat these healthy items because they're mostly carbohydrates. What the heck! Really? As they're passing over these incredible weight-losing items, they're loading their plate with a Texas-sized chunk of fatty meat, spooning a swimming pool portion of butter on anything and everything, and eyeing that mayonnaise jar trying to figure out how to gobble it down in some manner.

It all defies common sense. They need to open their eyes and let a bit of reality seep in. In their delusional state they think that eating a diet of primarily fat will make them skinny. That makes about as much sense as drinking a gallon of liquor in an attempt to stop drinking, or moving to Manhattan to get away from people, or renting a permanent room in a brothel to stop sex-addiction. I apologize to Zarkoff for the last comment, as he struggled with this issue all of his life.

I know it's laughable, but it's real. Legions of people have drifted down this insane path to obesity. In a way, I blame a certain unnamed diet plan from years ago that swayed people away from healthy carbohydrates and into fat. A little protein was thrown in as a disguise for this masterful display of commercialism.

Give people what they crave and tell them it's healthy. Pull the wool over their eyes and sell them the Brooklyn Bridge or Eiffel Tower. What's next, a healthy dish of organic heroin, dotted with an aesthetic array of colorful barbiturates and tranquilizers, all glazed with a delightfully sweet cocaine paste. I honestly believe some people would fall for that one if they heard their beloved celebrity idol pronounce its beneficial attributes on TV.

Let's not stray too far from the issue of fat verses carbs and protein. You have three choices and three only. They are carbohydrates, fat and protein. The human body needs all three in different proportions. Nearly all the credible and ethical experts recommend around 20 to 30 percent of your dietary intake to be fat. Most of that should come from healthy veggie and nut sources. There are lots of options, just do a quick bit of research.

The problem is that people generally love the taste of fat, especially the bad stuff that I listed earlier. Many are brainwashed into thinking that carbs are the worst thing since Hitler. To lump carbs into a category with genocidal tyrants is incorrect. But in their confused state these people make decisions based on falsehoods of carb discrimination. It's no wonder veggies feel repressed and downtrodden.

People acquire a certain tunnel vision and they refuse to let go. These misguided unfortunates pass over the very healthy items they need to lose weight. They substitute with the worst choices possible and they think they're making the right choice. Then they're amazed that after all that dedication and discipline required to eat pure fat, they actually gained weight.

The bottom line with carbs is to acquire a brief education and then don't overanalyze it. Refined and processed carbohydrates are the enemies and the other ones are healthy unless you saturate them with grease and fat. Anytime humans take a natural item and start fooling with it, it's usually a recipe for disaster. Go natural. It's that simple.

Eat bad carbs,
You'll be sad.
Eat good carbs,
You'll be glad!

Fatty Stuff III

Onward with the fatty stuff and how to handle it. As I mentioned earlier, do your research and learn the good fats. That will take about five minutes of your time. Stay away from the fatty meats and the clumpy, creamy stuff. Yuck! Also included in this gangster family is butter and margarine, and the ever-present mayonnaise. Mustard is a wonderful option. If it's white and creamy, beware!

Butter is a tough one for a lot of you. The great Zucchini once remarked, "Butter me not, butter me no, butter's the enemy, butter's the foe." Even though this horribly misguided attempt at poetry has no literary merit in my humble opinion, Zarkoff made a precise and valid point.

Zarkoff was clearly aware of the detrimental effects upon his squashy vegetable matter. It is rumored he was buttered at an early age and never fully recovered emotionally. This could possibly explain some of his erratic behavior later in life. We should never judge any vegetables until we have walked in their shoes.

We should all heed advice and wisdom from the Great One. For many of you butter is simply a habit, no more, no less. You grew up slathering butter on your toast in the morning. It moistened your bread for you to gobble down as you trotted off to elementary school. As a youth you watched that cool clump of oily delight slowly melt away in your steaming baked potato. Oh, what wonderful butter memories.

Put a stop to buttery memories. This is especially true if your goal is to lose weight. The fact is that a small amount of butter may actually be beneficial to your health. The problem lies in the fact that it will make you fatter than those Sumo wrestlers if you keep buttering over a long period of time. Sumo wrestlers are known butter lovers. They're undoubtedly talented athletes, but you can obviously see the effects of butter on their physique.

So, there you have it. It's clear as can be. You have to give up butter, at least for now. After you've reached your weight goal, you can play around with it again. But even then, you'd better be extremely careful with this potent substance. It's basically pure fat, clings to your body, and bounces around when you dance. Those little fat rolls actually look kind of cute shaking around on a pretty woman, but most women prefer not to have them. This is according to a 2018 Dance Fat Roll survey where over 1200 women were interviewed.

Think of all the items that you may add butter to. Corn, vegetables, rice, and potatoes are just a few of these. Not only are you causing deep-rooted, long-term emotional stress to the vegetables, from which they will likely never recover, but you're also quickly moving forward to a career in Sumo wrestling. And we know that's not what you really want. Be a doctor or lawyer or maybe an aerospace technician instead.

There are many healthy and tasty alternatives to butter. Let's take a baked potato for example. Open it up and pour on some Worcestershire sauce, low-sodium soy sauce, picante sauce, or any number of hot sauces. Even some slightly sweet barbeque sauce will suffice. Anything beats a glob of pure fat.

You can also use the always dependable lemon or lime juice, mustard, black or red crushed pepper, horseradish or jalapeno peppers. The options are only as limited as your imagination. Don't be afraid to get your friends' attention. Being weird can be a lot of fun if you embrace it. And you know you're not really that strange, you're just determined to win at any cost. You'll get the last laugh as the pounds fall away while they continue their quest to become Sumo wrestlers.

When it comes to bread, people are programmed to think it has to be buttered. It does not. Toasted bread is so naturally tasty that it needs nothing added. A liberal pour of cinnamon does the trick if you desire a little added flair. As long as you don't go crazy with it, a touch of honey goes a long way in taste, especially matched with the cinnamon. Jams and jellies are packed with corn syrup and sugar, so avoid them at all cost. I don't have to tell you to stay away from the all-so-processed white bread, do I?

Butter is commonly used for dipping of various types of seafood. Sumo wrestlers enjoy their delicious Japanese seafood with a large communal buttering trough by their side. Approximately one gallon is allotted per wrestler per meal, according to *Sumo Weight-Gain Magazine*. This works for them, but your fitness goals differ from their objectives. As your dipping sauce you will use your creativity and innovate, maybe using the lemon and lime option or a seafood cocktail sauce. Go easy here because of the added sugar.

Cooking and grilling with butter are not good things. Pass on grandma's recipes and go your own way. All the aforementioned options apply here. Lemon, pepper, spices, healthy sauces, the field is wide open for experimentation. A healthy cooking oil *in moderation* beats butter any day. Open your mind to butter alternatives and give up the wresting career. Oh, and margarine is even worse, in case you weren't aware. Just say no to butter.

The next subject we'll address will be sweets. That one is quite the challenge for some of us. Those little tempting treats can be so addictive, sitting there adorned with a creamy crown and puffed up inside with some nectary, gooey delight. Sometimes it's even flowing out from the corners just begging you to take a bite.

The same problem arises with sweets as all the other iniquitous desirables. How do you like my new word *iniquitous*, impressive, huh? To save you the trouble it means not good for you. In other words, you'll get fat. The same strategy applies to sweets as it does to butter. For the time being, forget about those seductive temptations. You have to go cold turkey.

After you've attained your weight-objectives you may consume them cautiously, for they are tricky little connivers. These crafty rogues will seduce you back into fat-oblivion without your awareness of it. Seriously, sweets are dangerous terrain for a person trying to lose weight. Treat them as a formidable enemy. Don't give them a chance to wreck your well laid plans. It might require steely willpower, but you *must* avoid sweets to lose weight. Don't give them a chance to sneak back into your life.

Cheese is next on our hit list. That's another one that can be difficult to deal with simply because it's so damn good. Unlike butter and sweets, I suggest you keep it on your menu in *extreme moderation* while you chase your goals. It at least contains some protein and can really satisfy the cravings.

Never forget you're walking a tightrope here. Cheese is packed with calories and can really slow down your rate of weight loss. A bite here and there is about all you can consume. Don't worry, cheese will be back in your life after you reach your stated weight-goal and you've learned how to apply discipline to all these dangerous foods. Just like sweets, cheese can sneak in through the back door and lay waste to your dreams. Monitor your cheese intake very carefully.

Here's another trap to avoid for it can really pack on the pounds. It's fried foods. Stay away from an abundance of the fried stuff. That grease goes straight into those fat rolls that wobble and shake as you're doing the Watusi at your grandson's wedding reception. Shake it up, baby.

Frying is a painful experience for vegetables, so show some compassion here. A little-known fact regarding Zarkoff Zucchini's rich heritage pertains to his great-uncle. Tomas Pavel Zucchini, former czar of the Czech Vegetable Patch Republic, tragically lost his life in a frying accident at a Prague cookout. A statue stands in memoriam where he went up in smoke.

Just like cheese, a few bites of a fried substance will satisfy you. Just give yourself a few moments to absorb it before you go on a gobbling mission. Chill out and be cool. All that fried stuff isn't going anywhere. You're not going to starve in the land of plenty. As a matter of fact, let some other Watusi enthusiast consume it. You can sit back with a low-fat alternative and watch as the bouncing rolls provide entertainment.

So, there you have your fatty-stuff lesson. Go the healthy route and try to use healthy choices. Avoid the butt-shaker foods. Don't destroy the nutritious items in an attempt to make them taste better. Learn to appreciate their natural taste, or at least top them with a low-fat choice. Spices or a little heat work well. Cook them via the proper methods and above all, respect your foods. They're sacrificing a lot to provide nourishment for you.

I like butter,
I like being thin.
You can't have both,
If you wanna win!

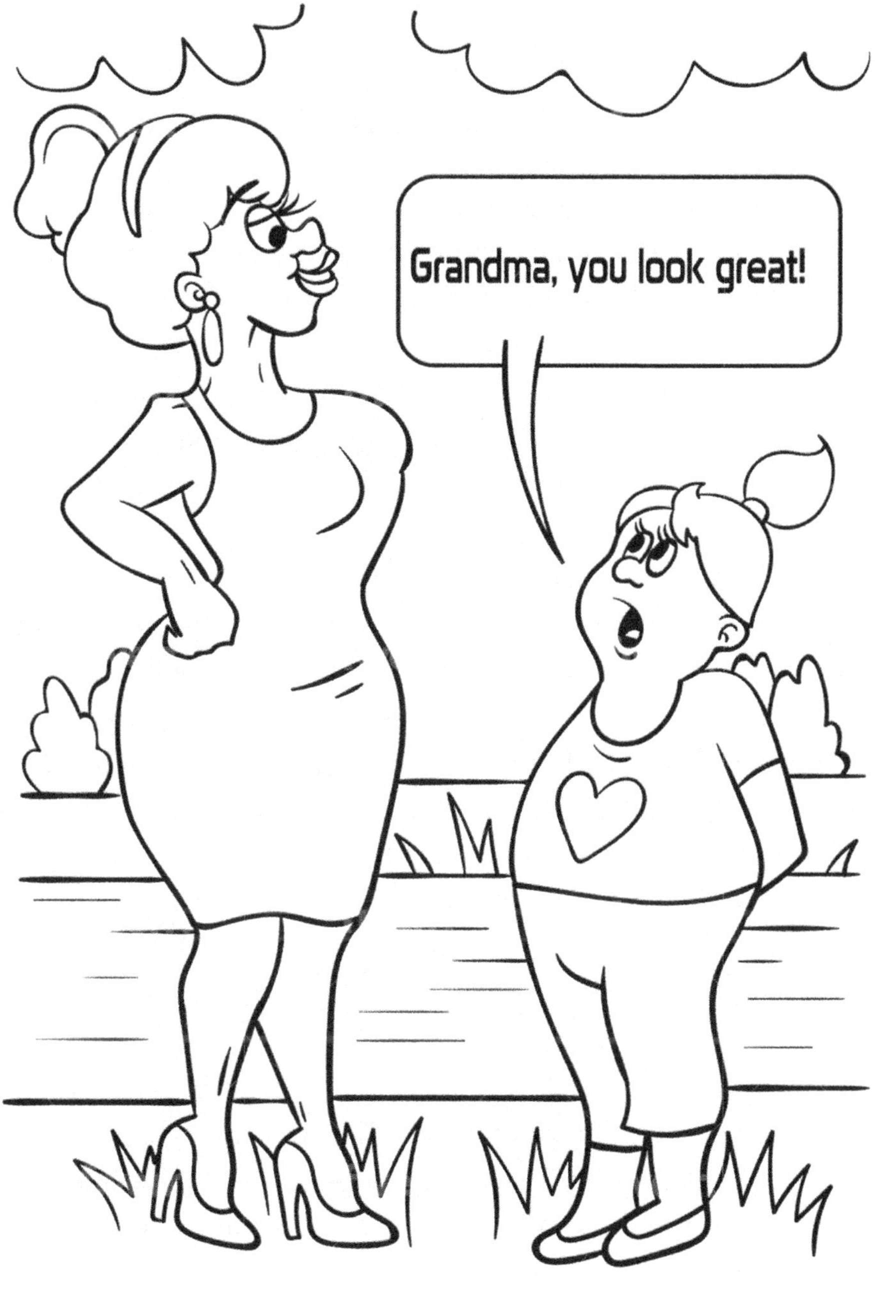
Grandma, you look great!

Distracting Stuff

Society is evolving more every day into one giant distraction. It's so easy to lose focus on what's real and what's not real, much less what's important and what's not important. We can't let this electronic haze of a culture take us over. Until they figure out a way to push a button to lose weight and get fit, you're stuck with the ancient technology that I'm promoting. Hard work, dedication, determination and discipline are what it takes.

But you know what? The wonderful thing about this, because it does require an expansive amount of work, energy and the ability to say no to certain temptations, is your competition falls by the wayside as the going gets tough.

Let them play with their high-tech gadgets and watch their super-sized, electronic marvel of a television. Let them turn off their lights by snapping their fingers or verbal orders. Let them save their precious calories because rising from the sofa requires too much effort. You just methodically grind out your daily routine on your way towards accomplishing something remarkable.

A day will come when it will become clear to others exactly what you're doing and why. That look in their eyes will give it away. They'll finally realize that you had a vision and you chased it with your heart and soul. Nothing can keep you from making your dream a reality.

The distractions that weaken your competition include television, computers and anything internet based. There are countless other ways to waste time. I'll try not to dwell on these as I've touched on them earlier. Just know they're a trap that's very difficult to escape once they've gotten a grip.

Television is the granddaddy of this abominable family. It is the founder and CEO of Atrocious Eating Habits Inc. Literally millions of pounds of annual blub can be directly attributed to eating while watching TV.

It's really quite humorous when you actually think about it. It's amazing that a group of humans can gang up and watch a little box for hours on end while mindlessly consuming a dizzying array of fatty foods. I personally think we're providing comical entertainment for aliens. It's mind control at its finest.

Set yourself some hardcore rules when it comes to television. You're not allowed to watch TV until your exercise is done for the day. Let it be some sort of reward if that's the mentality you need to succeed. Never consume anything but a low-calorie beverage while the television is on. You can devour a whole cow while watching television and never even realize it. That poor domesticated animal gave up its life and was never appreciated in the least. He or she deserves better.

Definitely avoid having the television on while your family is eating dinner. When you are watching the fat-box you are concentrating on the program instead of what you're plowing into your mouth. People unconsciously consume an unbelievable amount of food while their minds are off in that fantasyland. Try a little family conversation for a change. You might be amazed at what you can learn.

Bring back some of the simple pleasures that existed before the age of electronics. There are some very interesting people with some very interesting stories if you just take time to listen. Reality can be more entertaining than the fiction provided by the entertainment industry. It's healthy to talk and release the pressure valve of the daily grind. A blasting TV in the background is nothing but a psychological pacifier. Humans have an innate need to share their problems with others. Give them a chance to do so.

Never forget that television is nothing more than a habit. There are other options out there besides TV. Maybe you could enjoy some relaxing music with a glass of wine. Start a new hobby, write a book, give your mate some special attention so she doesn't run off with the pool guy, anything that gets you away from the seducement of television. Shut off that fat-box and enjoy some real life. Apply this to all the other electronic distractions as well.

I feel that a somewhat invisible distraction that people face is peer pressure. Humans have a basic desire to fit into their environment and be accepted. That probably helps to keep society running, but that same desire to be accepted can be detrimental to your fitness and nutrition program.

For example, suppose you're present at a social gathering with several of your peers. You've recently committed to losing some weight and becoming healthy. The host has prepared foods for everyone. Now let's suppose none of the options meet your new healthy requirements.

Everyone around you is indulging and raving about how delicious the food tastes. You may even be craving it on a primal scale. It's now critical decision time. Do you adhere to your new commitment or do you cave in and join the (probably overweight) crowd?

If you are naturally shy or an unassertive personality this can be an especially difficult decision. There are ways out of this dilemma. The choices include getting a small portion of the dish and pick at it until you can covertly throw it away. Another option is telling your host that you're simply not hungry at the moment. You could be completely honest and explain that you've recently committed to a low-fat diet.

Any of these solutions are better than giving up your nutrition plan, even if you're thinking it will be a one-time event. One time turns into two times, two times into three times, and soon you're back into your old habits. *Don't* let this happen.

You don't have to be a number in society. You don't have to be Ms. Fit-in-Perfectly and gobble down those fatty items just to make someone happy. You come first and never forget it. Figure it out, apply some social maneuvering, and cruise through this little mini-crisis. You'd better learn early because it's never going to end. You will constantly be challenged and you need to acquire the skills to handle these situations.

Social pressure from peers could possibly be your largest obstacle in the pursuit of fitness. Overcome that obstacle. Once you've asserted yourself in a couple of situations, it becomes much easier. Dare to be *yourself*. Get the job done.

If every day,
There's an excuse.
You won't win,
You will lose.

CHAPTER 5

Good Habits

"Excellence is not a singular act, but a habit. You are what you repeatedly do."
Aristotle

Habits Breed Success

Habit: a settled tendency or usual manner of behavior, an acquired mode of behavior that has become nearly completely involuntary.

As I write this sentence it's currently 4 a.m. That may seem an early hour to many of you, but to me it is my norm. They call that a habit. I rise early so that I can make time to write and exercise. I developed it several years ago and now it is nearly automatic.

At our age we're well aware of what we're doing wrong and doing right. It's not too late to make some changes and amaze someone. As a matter of fact, you'll make a much bigger impression at our advanced age than you would have earlier in life. It's not as hard as you think.

The key to all this is maintaining a proper mindset. Set a clear goal and go after it with every bit of energy and determination that you have. As you make the changes your body and mind will resist. Fight through those initial days and weeks and the body and mind eventually submit to the desire. Sheer desire prevails every time if it's the real thing. Once submission occurs a habit has been formed. Then it's all downhill from there.

Most of the habits described in this chapter are simple in nature. They're not difficult to understand. They're basically a simple "this or that" decision at a moment in time. One path leads to a lean and strong body. The other heads towards an overweight out-of-shape body. One of these simple decisions isn't going to result in a make-it-or-break-it critical result. It's a combination of many rights or wrongs that pave the way in either direction.

The main thing is becoming aware of that *exact* moment in time when a decision is in order. Allow your consciousness that's flooded with all that acquired wisdom to come into play. At that point it's nothing more than a split-second incredibly easy decision. The right way is obvious (sometimes painfully) and the wrong way is just as obvious.

Go the right way and you'll be so proud. You're on the way towards developing a good habit. Go the wrong way and you've just taken a tiny step backwards. That alone won't destroy you, but you've just accepted some failure. Many more consciously bad decisions and your brain will start slipping into loser mode. Catch those early bad decisions and don't let them lead you down the road to failure.

It's really that easy. Don't let that other book that you purchased with mine influence you the wrong way. You know which one it is because you can see it now. It's written by Mr. PhD and it's full of a whole bunch of highly technical terms and complicated programs. There's not a bit of humor in it and it's boring as heck. Just file it away in the bottom of your book cabinet and feel good about contributing to his Mercedes payment.

The point of this is something I keep bringing up. *Keep it simple.* Over-complicating matters does nothing but cloud the brain and induce a complete shutdown. Choosing between vanilla and chocolate ice cream is not a challenging intellectual process. You choose one and you're done. A hundred flavors in front of you is a completely different ballgame. The brain goes into chaos mode and panic ensues. You end up sampling eighteen of them and purchasing four.

Don't let the world decide for you. By this I mean block out all the distractions and focus on the task at hand. Never lose sight of your primary goal, your finish line. Take matters into your own hands and control your own destiny. Allowing a thousand little factors to influence you clouds the big picture. Always keep that image of a lean, strong and healthy you in your mind. This single-mindedness will pave the way towards success.

If I may, I would like to present an excellent example of how this works. It involves my personal hero and yours, the icon himself, Zarkoff Zucchini. There was a time, a few months before his tragic death, that the great Zarkoff was faced with a major dilemma.

His problem was an issue he had been struggling with his entire life, constant womanizing. His sex-addiction therapy had gone nowhere. Everything he tried resulted in dismal failure. Nothing seemed to work. Then he tried using minimalization and simplicity as a way to conquer this problem. He decided two was enough.

He got out a pen and a sheet of paper. He wrote down names of females with which he was currently having relations. He quickly had to add another piece of paper, then another. There was Lilly the hot red capsicum. There was sweet little Kaley Kale. There was innocent looking Becky Boysenberry who really wasn't so innocent.

Zarkoff's mind raced through them all. They were all special. Misty Mango was pure charm. Patty Passionfruit was a sensualist beyond description. Then there were the dancers working the fruit section. Zarkoff respected each and every one.

How did the great Zucchini handle this delicate decision of narrowing down his love list to just two? He blocked out all of the women in his life and let his subconscious decide for him. It was a quick and easy decision as he let his heart override his libido. There were two that stood out above the rest.

Candy Yam had been a longtime friend and lover ever since she arrived from North Carolina. She was sweet with a little touch of wickedness that excited him. She would make the cut. The other was Sherry Cherry with whom he had a wonderful relationship. She had a little California hippy-edge that drove him crazy.

That's how the great Zarkoff did it. That's how he simplified his love life and made progress with his sex-addiction issues. You can do it too. Simplify your life and don't let so many choices overwhelm you. Just make the right choice. It's so easy.

A word of warning here as I must be honest. I hope that you have more willpower than Zarkoff because he didn't adhere to his program for very long. Candy Yam caught him in a tray with Rhonda Radish two days after his sincere commitment. Only a hastily pulled-up plastic baggie separated the two. Zarkoff apologized, but all credibility was lost. He quickly drifted back into his lascivious lifestyle.

Let's move on to some good habits that you'll need to acquire in your journey towards a lean and strong body. We'll start with a common struggle for many people. We all need a certain amount of sleep.

> *Change your habit,*
> *Change your way.*
> *If you do,*
> *It will pay!*

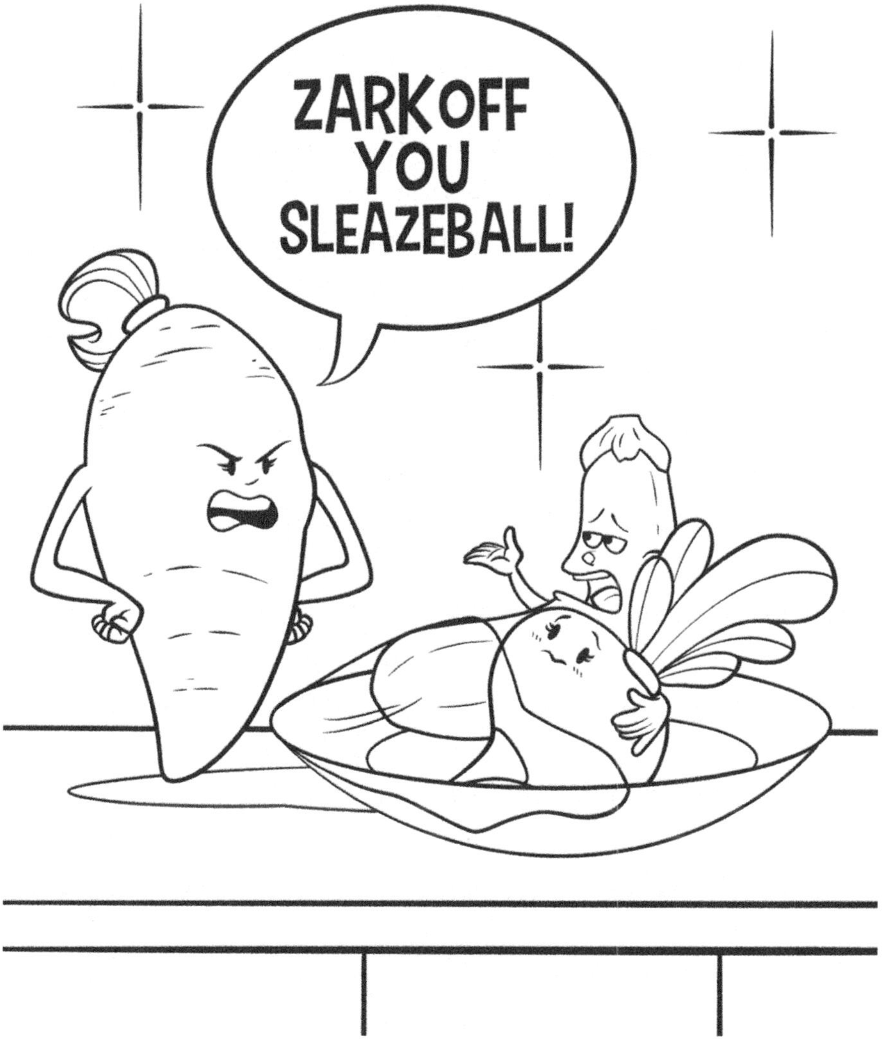
ZARKOFF YOU SLEAZEBALL!

Sleep

In the last section I mentioned that I'm an early riser. Many of you may operate on a different sleep schedule. It doesn't matter as long as you're getting enough rest. Go too long without proper sleep and you're going to pay for it.

At our age we're well aware of our personal sleep patterns. Most of us have somewhat of a routine that we're accustomed to. Now we have to budget time to allow for our exercise routine. An hour every day will have to be carved out and set aside for this. Occasionally you can cut it out of your sleep-time allotment, but you can't make a habit of it.

In Zarkoff's case, all he would do is eliminate a couple of sybaritic (go look that one up) beauties from his daily duties and exercise time would magically appear. For us it's not quite so easy. As always, television and electronic entertainment gadgetry should be the first sacrificial lamb that's tossed out to pasture. That usually frees up all the time you'll need.

Always be on alert during your first week or so of eliminating any type of electronic entertainment. The withdrawal symptoms can be devastating. Many people come down with severe cases of GWS immediately afterwards. Hopefully you won't be one of the unfortunates who perish, as some GWS patients die within hours after being diagnosed with this horrific affliction.

GarbageBrain Withdrawal Syndrome has been known to cripple a person's intellect beyond repair. The shock is just too much for these hapless souls. They are so addicted to their electronic devices that upon sudden deprivation their brains completely lock up. No longer can they sustain any form of normalcy.

Some cases are severe. All cerebral motor functions cease as they no longer know how to walk or talk. They can no longer feed themselves. Someone has to attend to their bodily waste needs. Breathing can become difficult and the heart slows to a crawl. Death is imminent unless the victim is treated with an enormous syringe filled with Facebook uselessness. This can temporarily stave off death, as the victim is getting the vital medication of uselessness that he or she so desperately craves.

GarbageBrain Withdrawal Syndrome is no laughing matter. If you feel early symptoms after eliminating a portion of your electronic entertainment, immediately turn on the television. Find the silliest, most ignorant show you can find and turn the volume as loud as it will go. Call 911 and start praying the medics can arrive in time to save you.

As you wait for help soak in as much of the TV show as possible and especially any annoying commercials that may appear. Hopefully this dose of utter crap will be enough to prevent immediate shock. Be aware that you will probably die, but no one will care because you've been a financial burden to them your entire electronic-addicted life.

Now let's get back to the program at hand. You need a certain amount of sleep and you need your additional time for exercise. It varies on an individual basis. Most of you know how many hours you need nightly to function properly. Slice out time wherever possible. Anything is better than simply sleeping less.

You will probably be going to bed earlier and rising earlier. It will take a while for your body to react to this change. It's okay to sacrifice a little sleep in the beginning. The worst thing you can do at this crucial time is skip your exercise. You're trying to develop a habit and it takes determination to succeed. Skip it once and you're heading down the wrong trail. Be serious about this.

Waking up well-rested is one of the greatest feelings. A geezed body needs that added focus. You can attack your day and be sharp and aware. Your exercise workout will be more focused and intense. You're less likely to stray away from your diet plan. Everything about your life will run much smoother than if you were creeping around rundown and exhausted.

Intentionally wear yourself out during the course of the day and you'll fall into that comfy bed at night and sleep like a baby. The next day you'll do it all over again. Get into this sleep and exercise pattern, eat right along the way, and before long you've got that lean, strong body that you crave. Sweet dreams.

Get your sleep,
Get your rest.
All day long,
Be your best!

Wake Up Hungry

Wake up hungry? By that I mean that you didn't gorge on late-night snacks so much that you're still full the next morning. It seems such an easy concept, but as many of you know, it's not always easy. Those cravings can really get to you at night, especially while you're engaging with our arch rival. That would be ole pesky television.

I fought the theory of late-night eating for years. I simply didn't believe it. I had read in several different articles that it's not good to eat before going to bed. My logic was, it is what it is, so it doesn't matter when you eat it. I was wrong. It *does* matter when you consume your food.

Studies have shown that eating during the daytime results in *less* blubber than consuming that same food before going beddy-bye. The body is a funny thing sometimes. It's programmed to efficiently process fuel when it's in action, rather than working overtime when it's supposed to be resting. I guess digestion runs on its own schedule.

The bottom line is to limit your snacking before you go to bed. If you must, hold it to something very light, maybe some fruit or another low-calorie item. Sometimes that doesn't get it done as far as the satisfaction scale goes. You're still looking for a little extra that keeps those pangs away.

One of my favorite weapons in this battle is hot-air popcorn. Alone it contains virtually no calories, yet can provide you with that feeling of satisfaction. I'm sure you know that buttering and salting it defeats the purpose. Don't do it.

Possibly experiment with some sort of spice if you absolutely need something.

The mentality you should have in this regard is that popcorn, or any other low-calorie snack, is a complete bonus. You have two options and two options only. One is to eat absolutely nothing after dinner. This is probably the best option. The other option is to be responsible and don't be stubborn with your old habits. So what if you've buttered your popcorn for sixty years. So what if your popcorn has always been of the salty variety. Come on, geezer!

Keep doing those things and you'll keep getting the same results. You know what those results are. That's why you're reading this book. You desire to have a lean, strong, healthy body. That's going to require some changes, otherwise you'll continue to add that five pounds every year. Year after year those pounds add up as I don't have to remind you.

Make those little changes, you wise geezer. Don't hold onto an old habit just because you feel it's the only way. It's not the only way. The world is full of many paths and this applies to your food habits as well. Be a maverick and break away from the traps that bind you. Let others swim in an ocean of butter and salt while you eat the same unbuttered, unsalted amount at a fraction of the calories. Your little tummy can rest overnight while they dream about monsters chasing them around.

Yes, some studies have shown eating just before bedtime can cause nightmares in certain individuals. What would you rather do? Would you rather sleep comfortably and wake up well rested the next morning? Or would you prefer bloodthirsty lizard-monsters chasing you down all night to devour you? That doesn't sound conducive to a good night's rest.

At times like these I always revert back to my personal hero. What would Zarkoff Zucchini do when facing late-night hunger pangs? He could order a pizza loaded with extra fatty meats and cheeses. He could opt for a large bowl of ice cream smothered with gooey chocolate sauce. Or he may decide on a bag of double-stuff cookies.

Zarkoff, with his infinite wisdom, unfaltering determination, and steel-willed discipline would always make the right choice. He and his girlfriend of that particular evening would analyze the situation. He would quickly realize that any food after dinner is a *bonus* and should be treated as so. The rule is to go light or not go at all.

There you have it. Zarkoff and his lovely babe would be munching away on unsalted, butter-less popcorn because he knows it's the right thing to do. He may not have always made the wisest choices when it came to his love life, but with food and nutrition he was always spot-on. What a guy, what a role model, what a legend. Long live the memory of Zarkoff Zucchini, activist, nutritionist, and sperm-donor extraordinaire.

Just a taste, ***Just a bite.*** ***No, no, no,*** ***Not at night!***

Eat Slowly

I'm sure you've read all about it. Every nutrition expert tells you to do it. Eat slowly and give your body time to react. There is a time delay between the act of eating and the satisfied feeling that comes afterward. Common sense tells us that if we eat slower, we allow time for our bodies to reach that feeling of fullness.

That means the feeling of satisfaction arrives before we cram down that last cheeseburger that's teasing us. The end result of this is a cheeseburger that won't convert into a fatblob somewhere on your body. No one wants a bunch of fatblobs, so slow it down. Send those Watusi butt-shakers down the road.

I've heard people say they don't have time to chew slowly and enjoy their food. They say they have to get back to work. Really? Is your job so important that you can't even take time to chew your food? Wow, you must be the most important person on the planet. I think it's more likely that you simply have a habit of eating too fast.

Try to change your style of eating if you're one of those people. Ease up and relax. Enjoy your meal. Your overworked digestive system will love you for chewing food before sending it down below. Thoroughly chewed food isn't so hard to break down. You're not one of those reptiles that swallows its prey whole. Give your stomach and intestines a break and let your teeth do the work instead. Be a smart geezer.

What's the answer to this problem? Maybe you should take a look at how much you're eating. Cut the portion in half, but take the same amount of time to eat it. If you're eating X amount of food in ten minutes, take the same ten minutes and eat only half the X. X's aren't that tasty anyway.

One simple idea is to adhere to an existing rule. This rule is called Empty-Mouth-First rule. It was originally proposed and brought before legislature by Zarkoff Zucchini several years ago. It was immediately voted into law on the merits of Zucchini's stellar reputation alone. When it comes to health and nutrition no one can top the great Zarkoff.

Zucchini's Empty-Mouth-First rule states, and I quote, "I will never put food in my mouth until all other food is swallowed." It makes total sense. Many people shove food into their mouths before they have swallowed the previous bite. Abiding by this simple rule will prevent this.

This alone slows down the process of eating. Make your dining experience a conscious event. It seems many people eat unconsciously, not realizing how much food they're piling into their mouths. Start respecting the food and savor every bite. Some animal or plant gave its life to sustain yours. You should at least honor it by not devouring it like a hungry lion. Treat food like the sensual gift it is, not like a chore that needs to be rushed through.

Do what you have to do to slow down your pace of consumption. Learn from the Europeans. They seem to eat their meals at a more leisurely pace than much of the world. They slowly progress through a meal rather than stuff it down in a heated rush.

Come up with your own ideas to slow yourself down. Place the fork down beside the plate as you chew. This keeps your deadly weapon at bay until that last bite has been swallowed. Maybe a liberal dose of a spicy sauce will slow you down. You can't take but so much of the hot stuff at one time.

Seriously, try to slow it down. No one is going to remove your food from your plate. It's not going anywhere. What's the rush? Show some class and have some etiquette. You never know who may be watching. You don't want to acquire a reputation as a slop gizzard.

Slop gizzards are about the most unsexy creatures imaginable. I once saw one in a Florida diner that disgusted me nearly to the point of purging my own food. I hope I never see another slop gizzard. This particular slop gizzard was female and even Zarkoff wouldn't consider intimate relations with her.

If you find yourself eating too fast, do something about it. Take time to enjoy your food. Food is one of life's greatest pleasures. Why turn it into a job? Relax, smile, and *slowly* enjoy your meal. Bon appétit!

Ate my lunch,
Way too quick.
Now I feel,
Like I'm sick.

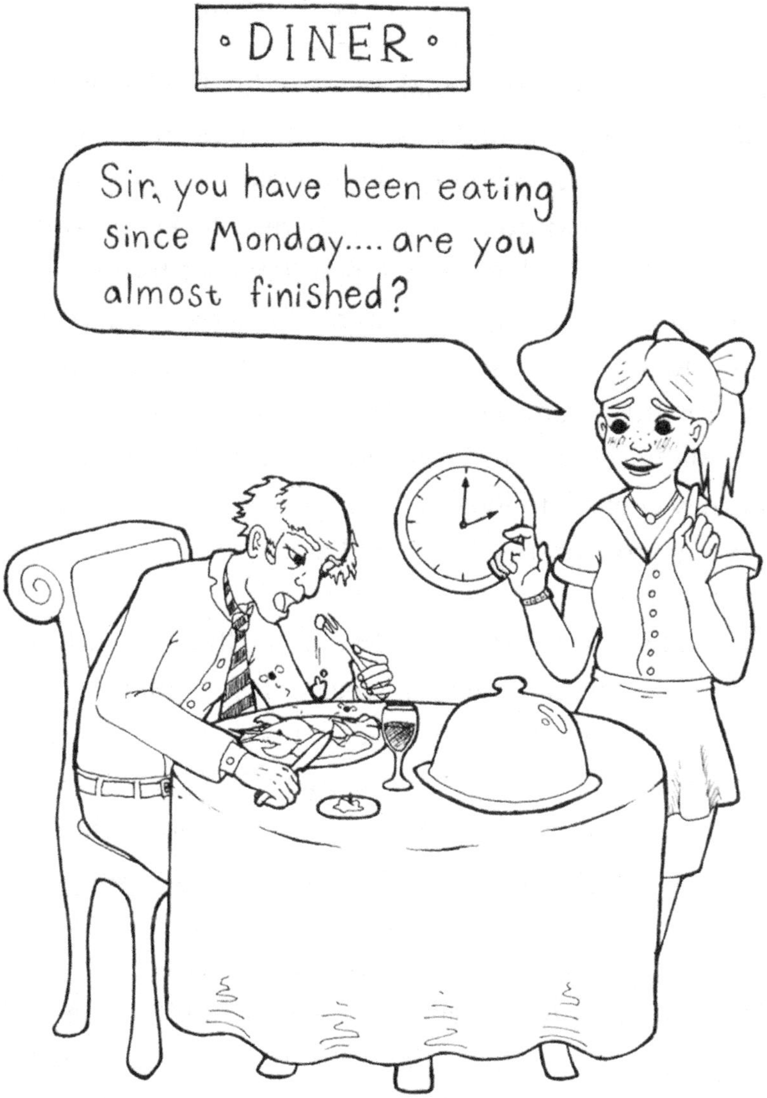

• DINER •
Sir, you have been eating since Monday.... are you almost finished?

Get Fresh & Read Labels

Be a freshness freak and make sure your food is in optimal condition. Look at your body as a machine that needs fuel. Make sure that fuel is top grade, not only as far as what you eat, but what condition it's in. Eat fresh to keep your body fresh. Geezed-up bodies need to be treated with respect.

Do you live near a grocery store? Most of us do, so there is no need to stock up on a ton of food every two weeks. The reason for this is simple. Fresher foods not only taste better, they actually retain more nutritional value. Not only that, but aren't they prettier to look at? Take a cue from ole Zarkoff and keep your food pretty. Just don't go getting aroused from a piece of lettuce as our hero might do.

Generally speaking, fresh food is healthier than food that has been around for days or weeks. Try to make a habit to shop often, every day if possible. Look at it this way, ten shopping-minutes a day is equivalent to seventy minutes a week. Wouldn't one big shopping expedition take seventy minutes? It's approximately the same amount of time. The big difference is your food is fresh all the time. You're maintaining peak freshness of your food on a daily basis.

Once you become accustomed to this, you'll never go back to buying fruits, vegetables, and meats in mass quantities. All they do is age and rot while they're stored in your refrigerator or cupboard. Pulling out and disposing of this nasty stuff is not my idea of fun.

This wouldn't please our late Zarkoff in the least. The spirit of the great vegetable rights activist has been rumored to come back and haunt vegetable abusers. He is said to hover over these abusers as they sleep and chant *boo* all night.

Sometimes an item is priced particularly well if you buy a larger quantity. If you go this route, remember this little freshness trick. Eat that item every day for a few days. It's okay to do this from a nutritional aspect as long as you change it up every few days. You'll still meet your nutritional needs. You're a wise ole geezer, so you'll make good decisions.

The body doesn't need every mineral and vitamin every day, just mix it up periodically and you'll be fine. When that particular item is depleted, move on to a different fruit, vegetable, meat, or whatever food group you're dealing with. If you're feeding two people, do you really need food for sixty people in your house? I think not, unless you regularly entertain the front line for the Pittsburgh Steelers.

When buying produce, don't be afraid to analyze the fruits and vegetables very closely. Choose the freshest looking ones. The same goes for milk, meat, eggs or any similar items. Look at the packages towards the back of the cooler. Sometimes they're as much as a week fresher than the more visible selections.

Check the freshness dates on the containers. Always pick the absolute freshest package available. Leave the older items for the shoppers who don't care. You know who they are. They're the ones rushing through the store so they can scurry back to their televisions. It would be sinful if they happened to miss a rerun of *The Beverly Hillbillies*. Granny might get angry and start chasing them around with a frying pan.

The same mentality applies to canned goods, cereals, bread, condiments, *everything*. Start making a habit to check and compare freshness dates. Your body will love you for it. Get fresh and stay fresh. Make Zarkoff Zucchini proud. You know he's fresh, just ask his girlfriends.

My food tastes fresh,
The way it should.
Yummy, yummy,
It's so good!

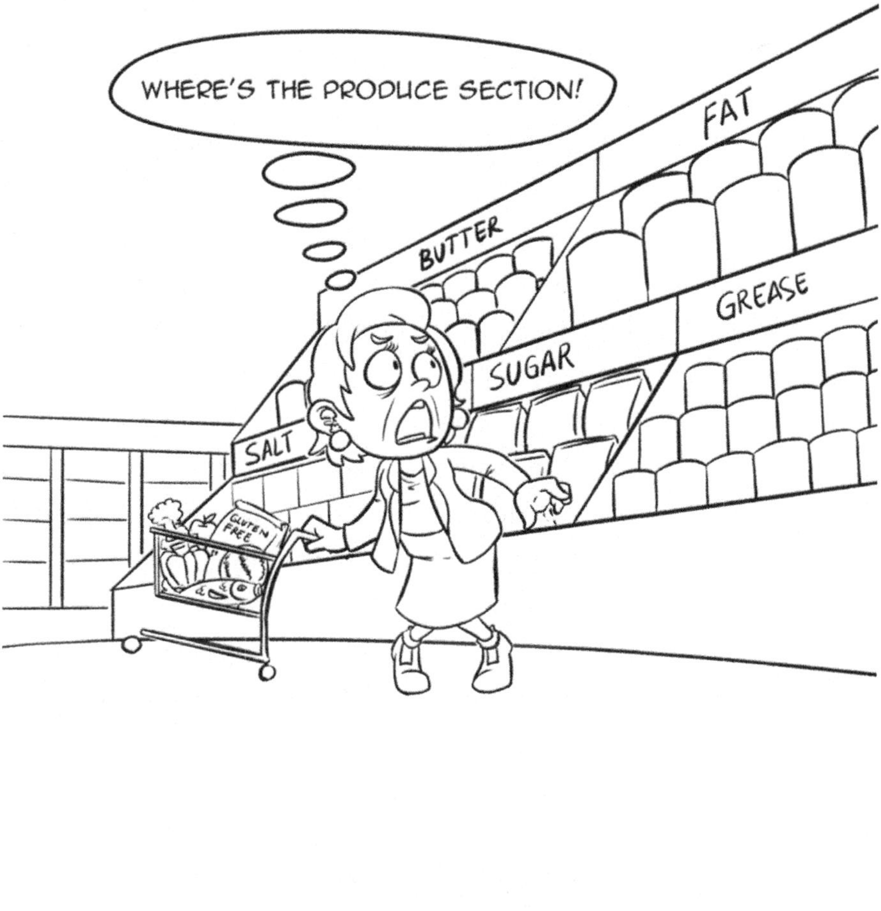
WHERE'S THE PRODUCE SECTION!
FAT
BUTTER
GREASE
SUGAR
SALT
GLUTEN FREE

Get Fresh & Read Labels II

The previous subject easily flows into the next one. Reading and understanding labels on food products is of prime importance. There is no set formula to understanding these labels, but by repetitively practicing this habit you'll quickly grasp it. The main thing you need to look for is any deceptive trickery that the big companies use to sell products.

Don't just go by the glitzy pronouncements shouting at you on the packaging. That's corporate manipulation at its finest. They're experts at staying within the law, yet totally deceiving you. Their team of marketers and attorneys are out to sell products any way they can legally do so.

Learn to delve into the fine print. That's the area where all the good stuff hides, the facts and figures that pertain to your health. It's all in the details. It can make the difference between being lean and strong or a wobbling fatty. Wouldn't you rather be lean and strong?

So, what do you look for? The first thing you need to do since you're an old geezer is go to the eye doctor. Buy some new glasses. You're going to need them because those nutritional labels are in nano-print and they're intended to be that way. Those guys don't want you straying off into that area. That's their worst nightmare.

They want you to read that big, black, bold print on the front of the package. You know what I'm talking about. It's screaming some silly slogan that's designed to make you pick up their product and place it in your cart. Then you move on down the line and repeat the process.

After Doc Eyeman has provided new eyewear for his geezed patient, you can begin studying your nutrition labels. What do you look for? Mainly we're looking for fat and sodium content. We're also looking for sugar, corn syrup or any sweeteners they may try to slip in there. The ingredients should be listed in percentage-of-product order. If the first or second item listed is bad, then beware of that particular product.

Most of us don't have time to run through all the minerals, vitamins, and such listed on these things. They're there to pollute the waters with distracting mumbo-jumbo anyway. They figure if they can hide their little ingredient secret inside a mountain of scientific jargon, you'll never see it. Just have a general awareness of vitamins and minerals and you're fine in that department.

Serving sizes muddy the waters even more. Learn to understand the labels on the foods you most commonly purchase. If a serving size is tiny, then the amount of the bad stuff doesn't seem so terrible when it's spelled out on the label. The problem here is you may eat twelve servings not knowing this critical information. Use some common sense and estimate what their declared serving is verses your wisdom-induced version. Sometimes I think they model their serving sizes in an unrealistic manner.

From now on, every time you're in a grocery store, take some time and study various nutritional labels. Pay special attention to the basic foods you'll be eating. These include canned tuna or chicken, canned beans, milk, rice, condiments, sauces, *anything* that has been processed and packaged.

Luckily, with most of our foods, we don't have to look at labels. When it comes to meat, we're mainly concerned with freshness dates, although you do need to watch for tricky sodium and sweetener additions. As far as fat content, remember the basic meat rule. If it looks like fat, it is fat. It's as simple as that.

Fresh fruits and vegetables are basically unprocessed, so don't be concerned about the fat content of these items. Just remember they're all full of various nutrients and the fat content is minimal. Rotate your selections and you'll get your balanced diet.

Go the organic route anytime you can, unless you love the taste of poison pesticides. Always assume *all* fruits and vegetables have an invisible layer of poison coating them. Wash off that toxic mess at the first opportunity.

Start becoming conscious of everything that goes into your mouth. Nutritional labels can educate you once you learn to interpret them. Keep processed foods to a minimum. You're not going to lose weight eating that crap. Research every label as if your life depends on it, because in a way it does. Pay special attention to "calories from fat" and keep it low. This is a very telling detail. If you let that one slip by, you'll risk becoming one of those wobbly gut-slingers that hobble around various retail outlets shopping for oversized clothing.

Stay fresh and read those labels. Monitor every bite that makes it to the fork and spoon. Always remember, honor, and salute Zarkoff Zucchini as you enjoy those fruits and vegetables. Any one of them could be an offspring from one of his numerus flings. They deserve respect for their royal heritage.

There's bad stuff,
In your food.
Read the label,
Make it good!

Dine Right

There is no doubting the refined, suave personality that was Zarkoff Zucchini. Such sophistication and culture placed him in some high-brow establishments. Hobnobbing with the elite of the vegetable and fruit establishment was his norm. The urbane, polished Zarkoff naturally excelled at the art of fine dining.

The following episode happened early after he became famous. At the time it was scandalous, but Zarkoff's future mishaps would progressively usurp the previous one. Zarkoff Zucchini had a knack for the spotlight, whether he wanted it or not.

Always sporting a beauty by his side, heads immediately turned when the Great One strolled into a room. On this particular summer evening Zarkoff was with his date. Candy Apple had just been pronounced Miss Fruit Universe. The two celebrities were the stars of the evening. Dining at trendy Le Vegetable Marlowe's, Zarkoff was eloquently placing a dash of caviar into his mouth when a disturbance occurred.

Two tables down were the French Ambassador of Agricultural Equality and his wife. Red Ruby was a stunningly beautiful, red tomato. She had just been proclaimed tomato of the year for her prodigious fund-raising talents linked to over a hundred charities.

Suddenly Red Ruby got up and walked over to Zarkoff's table. Without saying a word, she picked up his glass of Burgundy and proceeded to throw it in his face. The other patrons watched in shock as she took his plate of mussels and smashed it upon his head.

Red Ruby snatched a bowl of onion soup from a nearby table. She poured it down Candy Apple's dress. She gave the table a violent kick, sending a knife flying. It lodged in Zarkoff's throat. Out popped his Adam's apple. It rolled onto the floor.

At this point the establishment's owner raced over to subdue the distressed woman. She shouted obscenities at Zarkoff as she was being dragged away. Medical staff was called in to attend to Zarkoff. Red Ruby was truly a tomato gone mad.

Needless to say, it was quite the embarrassing scene for the elegant and refined Zucchini. The tabloids were immediately all over it. Some called it his worst moment ever. Little did they know this episode would be a mere footnote compared to future coma-inducing exploits.

Red Ruby had been a past girlfriend of Zarkoff's. They even had a brief encounter after she was married. She could never let him go as she was totally obsessed with him. Sighting him in the restaurant with another woman was the final straw. Zarkoff Zucchini was her man and no one else could take him. She went delusional and lost all control.

The point of this story is dining should be a quiet, pleasant experience. This is a prime example of how *not* to dine. Altercations in the middle of a meal are about as bad as it gets. Let Zarkoff's horrible moment be a lesson for us all. Let's learn from it. Don't run around with ambassadors' wives and always enjoy your meal in a quiet and relaxing manner.

> *Don't dine wrong,*
> *It's not right.*
> *Don't you stress,*
> *Don't you fight!*

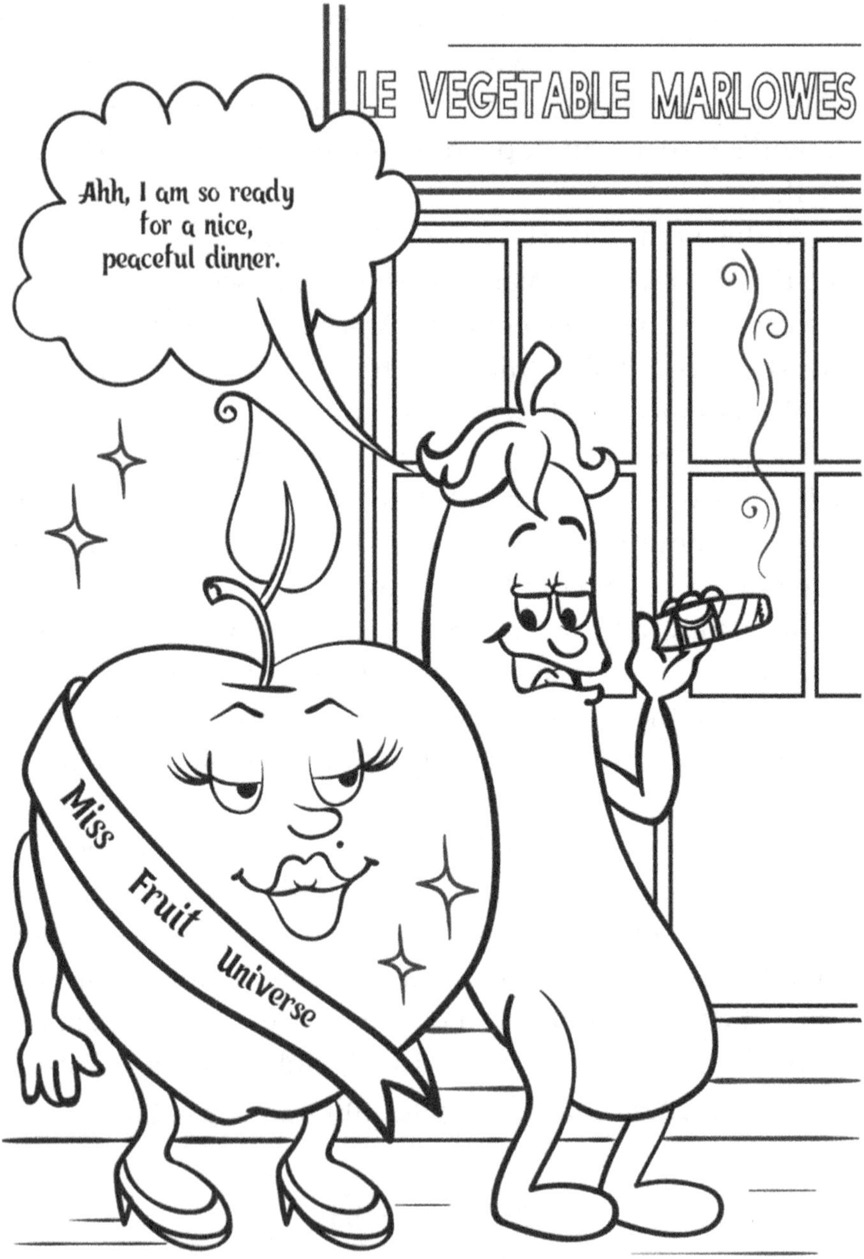
LE VEGETABLE MARLOWES
Ahh, I am so ready for a nice, peaceful dinner.
Miss Fruit Universe

Dine Right II

Zarkoff's misadventures never cease. Thankfully, our dining challenges aren't so dramatic. Day-to-day obstacles include phone calls, roaring TV's, annoying music, crying babies, and such as that. These can be troubling though, especially if they're ongoing in nature. Interruptions during meals cause you to lose focus, allowing bad habits to creep in. Set yourself up for success through preparation and adhering to a few simple rules.

Here's an example. Let's say you've arrived home after a pleasant day. You've been eating healthy snacks and small light meals throughout the day. You've accomplished your exercise routine and you're feeling very good about yourself. Now you're finally settling in for a well-deserved healthy dinner.

Your phone rings as you place that first tasty bite into your mouth. It's cousin Natasha calling from Colorado. She *always* has a good story to share and is a delightful conversationalist. You reach to accept the call and quickly realize something. That first bite of food disappeared down your throat and you never even realized it. You certainly didn't take time to enjoy it. It was just calories unconsciously slipping into your body.

Now it's decision time. Accept the call or don't accept it are your two choices. If you don't accept it, you run the risk of not reaching her later. Cousin Natasha is a wild child always in search of her next adventure. That's what makes her stories so delightful and entertaining.

However, if you take the call and listen to her, all that food is going to disappear within you. You'll have consumed it without enjoying it and possibly barely chewing it. You may even reach over for some additional snacks before it's over. Natasha has been known to share some rather expansive stories. It's not conducive to your new health and fitness program and you're certainly not going to lose weight that way.

What do you do? The answer is an easy one for a wise geezer. You decline the call and mute the phone. You tell yourself from now on the phone will be muted every time you eat anything. You will become stubborn as a mule and never break this ironclad rule.

Of course, there are emergency situations that arise in life and there are exceptions to everything, but you're wise enough to not turn everything into an emergency. Years of living have taught you that. Nothing will disturb your well-deserved dinner.

That's the warrior mentality you need when you sit down for a meal. *Nothing will interfere.* Nothing will get in the way of your quiet, peaceful, healthy meal. Let everyone know your new rules and how serious you are. Many of you have your meals at certain designated times. Your friends and family will be made aware that these are not good times to try to reach you.

Meals were meant to be relaxing, a time of pure enjoyment. Polite conversation is a nice accompaniment to a healthy meal. Some light music in the background is okay if that's what you like. Learn to love the quiet as you dine. Pure silence is bliss as you concentrate on your delicious food.

Television is out of the question, even a muted one. All those subliminal flashing advertisements can get into your head and you won't even know it. Let nothing lead you astray from your stated goal of becoming lean, strong, and healthy.

Eat slowly and think positive thoughts. Don't let the worries of the day seep in as you eat. This is your time. After you finish you can carry on battling the world as we know it. As we've discussed earlier, problems will never cease. Give them their due, but don't let them cross into your territory.

Mealtime is your time and you're going to defend it at any cost. The war will be an ongoing one and you're going to win. If some weird situation arises during mealtime, deal with it in a calm manner and move on. Strong emotions are detrimental to good digestion.

This leads us into a different type of dining situation. Eating in restaurants always poses dilemmas. It's usually one right after another. You really have to be tough to survive this gauntlet of attacks. It becomes much easier once you've gained experience.

As you ease into your fitness and weight loss program you should really avoid most restaurants. There's nothing to gain and a lot to lose. Losing weight means taking control of the situation. You can't hand that control to the burger-man behind the counter. You're the boss, not that well-intentioned fryer back there clogging everyone's arteries.

You can frequent all the restaurants you desire after you reach your goals and learn how to maintain. If you're serious about losing weight, try to stay out of them for now. However, there will be times when they pop into your life. Here's where some little tricks will apply.

Let's pretend you're a month into your fitness program. A social situation arises where your presence is absolutely required at a dining affair. You can't let this derail you and slide off the tracks. If at all possible, sneak in a healthy meal *before* arriving at the location. Yes, eat a whole meal before dinner.

When you're full of your good stuff, all that fatty bad stuff won't seem so appealing. Then you can simply order a beverage or possibly a small salad. Remember that the primary goal of restaurant salad-makers is to drench healthy vegetables in a mountainous volume of creamy, fatty dressing that could fill the Grand Canyon.

They are trained at chef school to maim as many people as possible by fattening them up to the point of death. The best chefs can kill upwards of a thousand people per year, more so if they get their own TV program. To all you chefs out there, and especially my chef friend, please realize I actually love you. I sometimes get carried away in the silly fiction department.

If you have a favorite restaurant that serves some healthy dishes, enjoy them. Just be beware of attacks that will keep coming. When you are dining out, always remember you're in enemy territory. You're behind the front lines and they're gunning for you. You're on the hitlist, so don't get caught up in the crossfire.

You have to take charge of every detail, otherwise that chef and his loyal underlings will slice you to pieces. Some waitstaff will look at you as the lowest form of life on the planet. You will be total, absolute scum in their eyes. You're asking them for a low-calorie dressing on the side, grilled fish with no heavy oils, brown rice instead of white. You're returning the bread because it's buttered, doing the same with a potato due to a fatty substance that saturates it, and so on. The list is limitless.

You are a living nightmare in the eyes of your waiter or waitress, not to mention the professional killers behind the scenes preparing the food. If I were you, because you have more money than I do, I would apply some good ole palm-greasing.

Upon arrival at the restaurant, walk around and disperse twenty-dollar bills to all the employees. The head chef gets a hundred. Slip the owner another hundred. Grease everyone's hand in sight. Bribery carries a lot of weight and can keep killers at bay.

Inform them that you have mental issues. You're on the verge of being committed to an institution and prone to violence. You are an out-of-control, unstable geezer, one who is very demanding about food. Show them a signed statement from your psychiatrist stating that you are full-fledged crazy and subject to breakdowns. Make it known that you're loose with your money, but extremely fragile emotionally and mentally.

At any moment you may fly off the handle and do things you'll regret. Let it be known there's more money for everyone if the meal goes according to your demands. There will be cash bonuses for all involved if you walk out of that place happy.

That should do the trick. It will be an expensive meal, but you'll have made it through the crisis. That is what you have to do when you go out to eat. It's not easy when someone else prepares the food. If you make them angry, well, I've heard some stories of what they can do to your food. They're not pretty by any means. Handle the situation. You have to win at any cost.

All around,
Things distract.
Eat in peace,
Be relaxed!

CAFE

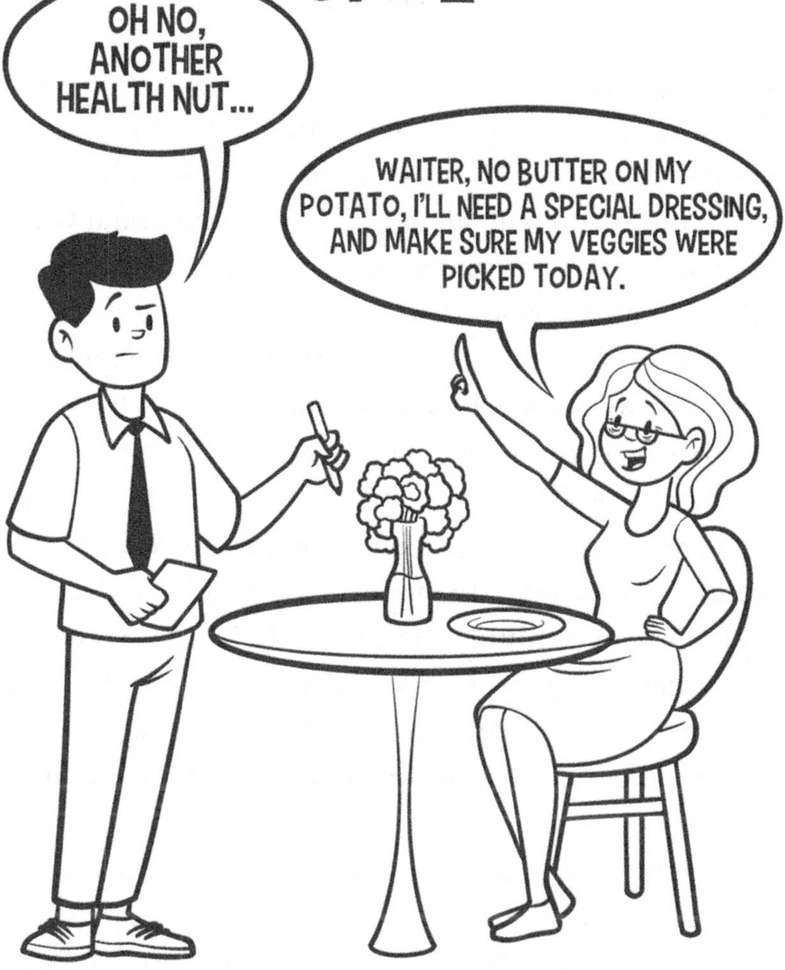
OH NO, ANOTHER HEALTH NUT...
WAITER, NO BUTTER ON MY POTATO, I'LL NEED A SPECIAL DRESSING, AND MAKE SURE MY VEGGIES WERE PICKED TODAY.

Attitude

It's you against the world, one lonely geezer swimming against the tide. As you progress through your fitness plan it will seem everything is an obstacle, intentionally placed in front of you so you will fail. It can overwhelm you if you let it. You can prevent this with the proper attitude and outlook.

It's all in how you approach this war. Getting physically fit is more of a mental affair than physical. Remember from earlier what we spoke about. The mind controls the body, the body doesn't control the mind. That brain of yours is the control center of it all.

The reason you have put on a few pounds is because your mind allowed the body to overeat. The mind decided to sit on the sofa instead of hitting the treadmill. Now you're going to use the mind to get back on track. Your body is pushing you to take the easy way out. It's trying to persuade you to lie back, put your feet up, and watch that handsome-hunk TV star fight bad guys.

The mind is the boss though, and the body will submit every time the mind issues a command. It's a combination of intellectual activity and pure willpower. Remember that quote from earlier on. It was from one of the greatest winners in sports history. "You can do anything you want to do if you want it bad enough," he simply states.

To accomplish something remarkable requires commitment. It's a vision from the mind, effort from the body, and most of all, an outpouring of heart and soul. It has to come from within. Gyms and fancy workout clothes aren't going to get the job done. *You* get the job done. Why go through life and just exist? It's never too late to make a change, a big change.

One day at a time, that's the only way to look at this fitness project. The need for immediate gratification is what stops most people. Many people put a month or so of dedication and discipline into diet and exercise, yet they see little visible results. They ask themselves, "What's the use in doing this? I'm not getting anywhere." Then they quit.

That's where the vision comes into play. When you see the big picture in the back of your mind, the little steps become easier to plow through. You grind through your exercise routine thinking only of today. "I have to get it done today," you say. "I'm not worried about tomorrow or next week or next month," you tell yourself. You focus on the task at hand.

The same goes for the daily struggle to eat right. Whether you're trying to lose ten pounds or a hundred pounds, the strategy is the same. You're accomplishing your goal through a series of small steps, not one giant leap. Every single day is a challenge. Every minute can bring an unexpected temptation that requires addressing.

Maybe you're at the end of your emotional rope one day. Everything seems to be going wrong. Then your neighbor knocks on the door bearing a box of steaming fresh doughnuts. You're at your weakest moment, but you say no and politely send them back with her. You truthfully tell her that you're going to get fit. You tell her you're not allowing yourself to consume sweets at this particular period of your life. You just made it through a critical moment. You're staying strong.

Expect the unexpected. What happened yesterday has nothing to do with today. You're proud of making it through yesterday, but that doesn't mean a thing today. Who knows what will happen tomorrow? You deal with the *now*.

After you've conquered enough *nows*, you'll have gradually trained yourself to fight the temptations of the wrong foods. You'll also learn to avoid the temptation to take a day off from your exercise routine. It's so easy to say, "not today," but don't do it. Get out there and get it done. You'll be so proud of yourself. Don't let those *nows* control you, you control them.

In the beginning you can't afford to look past today. When you wake up tomorrow, you'll be proud of what you accomplished, but another today is ready to attack. Get ready to deal with it. Time will pass. In one year the whole world will marvel at what you did.

Another important aspect of maintaining a proper attitude is the ability to innovate. When it comes to eating right and exercising, being open-minded is a huge asset. It allows you to be creative in order to accomplish your immediate task. Winners make it happen.

Your bottom line is to get the job done. Nobody's going to pat you on the back for getting it done. Nobody's going to console you if you don't get it done. It's all you and it has to come from within. If you're in this fitness program for daily cheers, you're doing it for the wrong reason. Pat yourself on the back and move on.

Be creative. That's what it takes to get it done sometimes. Try a new fruit or vegetable because it may become a favorite. Experiment with a new way of eating your foods, especially in particularly demanding situations.

Picture this situation. You're in a location and it's lunch time. For some reason you didn't prepare and there's nothing on hand to eat. There's a market close by along with a fast-food establishment. Instead of surrendering to the grease-pit option, you walk into the market. You pick out a couple of fresh veggies. Let's pretend one of them is a green pepper.

You take it to the restroom and wash it. Those deadly pesticide chemicals are worse than the embarrassment of being seen washing a vegetable in the restroom. It's all about pure confidence and an ironclad belief in yourself. You'll show those who may snicker at you. That's the type of tunnel-vision it takes to win. That's step one.

Now you pay and walk outside with your pepper. You began eating it as you would an apple. More looks and chuckles ensue as you are doing something out of the norm. You watch as meatball-shaped human beings exit the burger place across the street. A couple of them see you eating your pepper and they point and laugh. You simply smile and wave, and the meatballs roll back home to their televisions. That's step two. Congratulations, you're making progress in the weird department.

Before long you'll actually enjoy this twisted game of being different. I admit I'd rather fit in, if possible, but sometimes a little touch of madness is required to succeed. I've done it all because madness comes easy to me. Eating tuna directly out of a can is nothing new. I've used two twigs as chopsticks when there was no other option for spooning it out.

All this may seem odd and comical to the masses and I suppose it is. Really though, it's all about determination and the will to make it happen. If you want to be a meatball, that's fine and dandy. Go your own way and enjoy the rotund life. There's nothing wrong with that. It's just not for me. I'd rather walk than roll.

When it comes to exercise there's no limit to how weird you can be. You can really put on a display of comical entertainment in this field. It's much easier to maintain control of your weirdness in the eating department. All you have to do is prepare and possess some healthy snacks. With exercise it's not always so easy.

Temporary situations will arise that can prevent you from exercising. However, you can still make it work if you've got a touch of showman about you and can handle the unwanted attention. They'll laugh for sure, but they're usually meatballs anyway.

I was once traveling cross-country in an RV. I stopped at truck stops along the way for my showers. Before showering I would lay out my mat in the parking area and do my exercises. I'm sure I provided much entertainment and joy to my trucker audience. Who knows, maybe it even inspired one of them to start a fitness program.

I've also had a rainstorm halt my walk. I took shelter just outside a conference center. It was packed with construction industry people. They sure got a kick out of watching me doing jumping jacks in soaking wet clothes. There are many other examples of creative workouts that I won't bore you with.

Just remember that you *can* get it done. Lok at the world as one big gymnasium, a playground for exercise. Find a way and a place to walk, jog, run in place, swim, perform calisthenics, do push-ups and crunches, dance around and act the fool, *anything* to get that heart beating. Turn a rock into a dumbbell, a lake into a swimming pool, or a parking lot into a jogging track. Innovate to eat right and exercise. Just do it.

Gotta stay fit,
Every day.
You can do it,
Find a way!

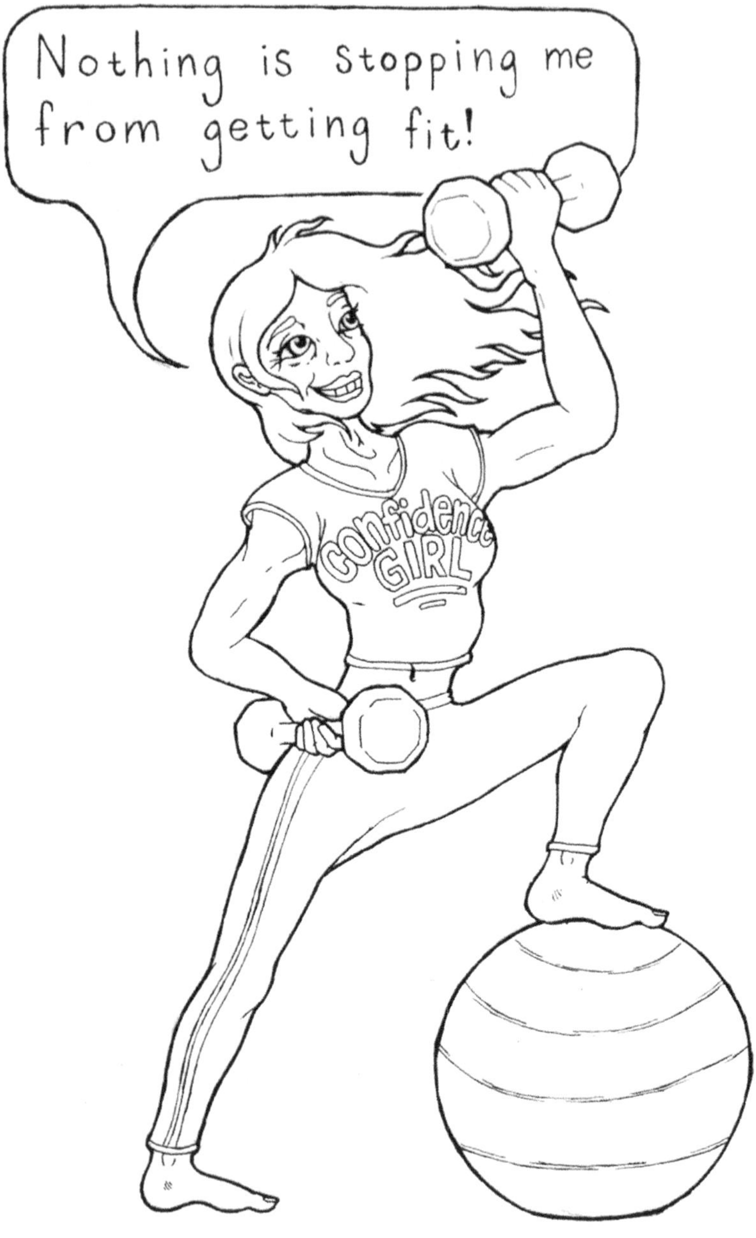
Nothing is stopping me from getting fit!
Confidence GIRL

Attitude II

Let's address another attitude adjustment. I call it macho-man syndrome as I'm speaking to the males here. I'll go out on a limb here and suggest this affliction is a direct result of societal conditioning. From birth we're programmed to think the perfect male specimen is a giant muscle-bound action TV hero. "Bigger is better," they're constantly shouting at us through all sorts of media.

Rippling muscles that literally burst out of shirts, bulging arms that are big as redwood trees, backs and necks that look like they're layered with steel pillars, this and more is what we're bombarded with every day. That's barely attainable by even the most fit young kid. Come on, don't be a delusional geezer.

My God, we're old as Methuselah, so how are we expected to carry on like this? I'd bet that ole biblical patriarch didn't lift a single barbell in his nearly thousand-year existence. He didn't need to bench press the equivalent weight of Cairo to prove himself to the world. He probably ate and exercised sensibly and let fate take care of the rest.

Here's the secret tip, guys. You don't have to be a massive, muscle-bound weight lifter to be in good physical shape. You know, the guys that we see on TV and magazines who are so pumped-up they don't even look human. If you don't believe me, go ask a random selection of females which body type they like on a man.

You'll find that very few actually prefer the oversized body-builder style. Most like a well-toned, muscular male who looks somewhat normal. Sigmund Freud would tell you that's all you need to know to be successful. Please the girls and it all falls into place as far as he's concerned. I'm in full agreement with this libido expert, as would the great philanderer Zarkoff Zucchini, if his presence still graced us.

Many guys are overly concerned about appearing super strong. Get over that bit of conditioning and stop worrying about it. A lean, strong aerobic machine is just as good. It's better in my opinion. Walking, running, biking, swimming, etc. are all excellent workouts. Combine one or more of these with a simple dumbbell routine and you'll have a complete body program.

There's no need to compare yourself with Hercules or the latest action-movie hero. Mister action-hero probably eats anabolic steroids by the boxful. That may work for him in the short run and make his muscles larger, but it's causing severe damage to his body. He'll pay the price in the longer term.

Not only that, but it's been rumored that these steroids cause tiny wees. Do you really think Zarkoff Zucchini would approve of such nonsensical behavior? What good is a massive body if wee shrinkage occurs? The payoff verses risk factor just doesn't add up. Zarkoff says no to miniature wees, as he's rumored to suffer from this affliction.

Many men jump on fancy weight machines and start blasting out heavy duty reps. They're filled with hope of instantly converting decades of fatblobs into muscle. Sorry, but it doesn't work like that. Years of cream puffs and cheap beer doesn't just fall off the body and reinvent itself as rock-hard chiseled muscle. Going slow is the only option at this point for two reasons.

Number one is *you are old*. You're a *geezer*. Do you really think your body is going to respond like a twenty-year-old? Do you really think those muscles that have lifted nothing more than a liter of beer over the last forty years will like being pushed around like that?

Of course they won't like it. They'll resist the only way they know how. They'll break, tear, or shut down completely. You'll pay for that big mistake. You'll be out of commission until they decide to heal, and that's no time soon. There's no doubt about it.

Reason number two for progressing slowly on the weight-lifting program is the fact that fatblobs should be the focus at this point. Even if you did gather some muscle on your body, it would be covered by fatblobs. It's best to concentrate more on steady aerobic exercise in the beginning. Every week add a tiny bit more to your strength program. Then it will all come together at the right time.

Your muscles will strengthen and fatblobs will shrink accordingly. Maybe at that point you can actually see some shaping taking place. Be cool, for it will happen. Don't blow it early in the game. Let those steroidal little wee-weeers enjoy their brief time in the limelight. You're in this to win in the long run.

Get away from other aspects of the macho man mentality also. It's okay to turn down an alcoholic drink. You're not proving how tough you are by downing a shot at 11 a.m. It's okay to pass on a fatty piece of meat. "Forget a salad, that's for women and wimpy men," you may say. Keep up that attitude and you'll see who has the winning edge. It won't be you.

Never would a macho-head think about *walking*. When it comes to walking off a couple of layers of fat, the macho mentality resists this at all costs. That's for girls and girly types. Never would a macho-head be caught in a brisk walk that's burning calories and using muscles in a sensible manner.

No, no, no, he would rather burst a disc in his lower back lifting the maximum weight on the weight machine. A few doctor visits later and a pain pill addiction away lurks total disaster. Walking would have been so much better, but at least he'll have the perfect excuse for not exercising. "I hurt myself lifting the maximum," he can brag. Well, that doesn't go very far in the fitness world.

A macho man looks at a pretty girl and tells his buddy how he could satisfy her deepest desires. Unfortunately, it's all a pipedream of sorts, a fantasy that will never happen. The truth is his stomach could literally crush her and he has the stamina of a sloth on barbiturates. Miss Pretty Girl doesn't want him. She wants that lean, strong, toned dude down the street who exercises in a sensible manner. He does pool work on the side.

All of us men have at least somewhat surrendered to the societal macho-man programming. We can't fall so deep inside that hole that we can't climb out. We have to realize that stuff is for the kiddies. Those young guys haven't acquired our wisdom, so they're really susceptible to the big-muscle trap. They have yet to learn that wee shrinkage is not a good thing. They have yet to learn that macho behavior isn't conducive to longevity.

Let's learn from the women. In a lot of ways, they apply more common sense than we do. Males don't need to go around proving themselves superior over other males by lifting more weight. Prove yourself superior by another method. Using the brain is a good start. Let's relax and accomplish our goal of becoming physically fit.

If some goon-head laughs and mutters an obscenity-laced comment towards you as you aerobically walk down the street, smile and wave to him. Goon-head doesn't have a clue, doesn't have a life, and the pool guy keeps his wife company while he's at work.

Goon-head would also laugh at your lunch selection and the low-calorie salad dressing you order on the side. He thinks you're a big wussy as he wolfs down his deep-fried animal smothered in a rich animal-fat gravy. Don't waste any brain cells on Goon-Head. His job is to appear macho and die several years before the average woman dies.

That's right, it's a documented fact that women outlive men. There's a reason for that and the reason is stubborn male ignorance. We're so stuck on pretending that we can't see who we really are. Let go of that machismo and wise up. You'll be healthier and you'll start seeing less of that pool guy hanging around.

I'm a macho man,
Oh, so strong.
I broke my back,
What went wrong?

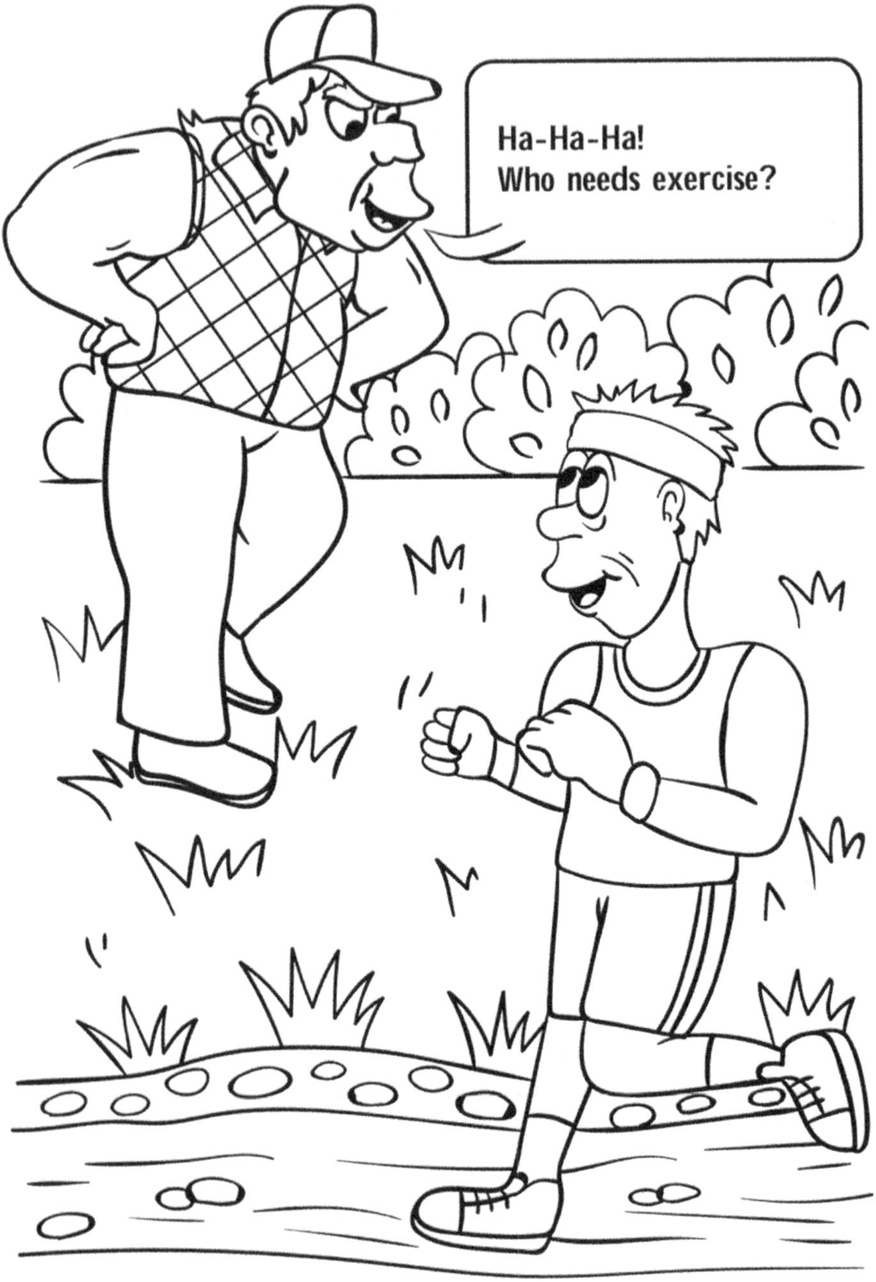
Ha-Ha-Ha!
Who needs exercise?

Attitude III

Many people think that eating healthy requires a lot of special attention and effort. They feel that because it's healthy it's not a natural part of life. That's how far we've fallen in our perception of nutrition. It's a myth that eating right takes more time than eating the bad stuff.

It's actually the other way around. You need not use convenience as an excuse to eat junk. Remember the scenario earlier, the one where fast food was compared to reaching into a small container and grabbing a healthy snack. That's exactly what applies to this subject.

Let's say you're going on a day-outing and you're figuring out your meal plan. You can take five minutes in the morning to pack your fresh fruit and vegetable mix, protein source, and a container of a simple carbohydrate mix. Your protein could consist of canned tuna or meat, or maybe a boiled egg or two. You could use some leftover lean meat from your previous meal if you have some.

Your so-called carbohydrate mix could contain shredded wheat, nuts, raisins or another unsweetened dried fruit, and possibly some high-quality crackers. Watch the fat and sodium content on the crackers. It's really an easy and quick preparation to throw this together.

This little bit of effort should take five minutes at the very most. Three minutes would be a more accurate estimate. Now let's compare three minutes to our other option, visiting a fast-food establishment that in actuality isn't so fast.

First of all, you have to drive to the restaurant. This could be one minute or thirty minutes. Then you're either waiting in line to order or waiting in the drive-through lane. There's more waiting as the babies cry in the background and the knucklehead behind you spouts his political views in between uncovered sneezes. And don't forget the wannabe rap star beside you that's blasting his eardrums out on the latest musical device. You can hear every vulgar lyric as blood pours from his ears.

You finally get your food. The order is messed up and you don't get exactly what you want, but you take it anyway. You wolf it down because it's the law. Section 236, Article 21, of the Fast-Food Regulatory Commission manual states that all fast food must be consumed within ten seconds. Otherwise, you have committed an act of felonious consumption which is punishable by death.

You can choose your own method of death upon conviction. You can select being drowned in an oversized soft drink or being thrown into a vat of hot frying oil. Most slow eaters choose the oil option, as it is quicker and less painful. They say only the first few seconds hurt.

If you're a fast eater and survive the always present Eat-Fast enforcement officers who work undercover pretending to be vagrants, then you've just saved some time. Now you burp a few times and head back to the car. You drive back to your destination and settle back into whatever you were doing.

Now you see how fast food isn't always so fast. When you arrive back at your destination, you see Johnny taking a nap. He was the smart one who brought his own little collection of healthy items. He ate them at a leisurely pace and still had time for a siesta. Whose meal was the most convenient? Who had the most relaxing meal? Whose arteries still flow without burger blockage?

That's just one example of the fast-food myth. The real key to this is that little bit of preparation before you leave home. You can take these simple creations virtually anywhere. They're lifesavers when your body needs fuel. They're great for the workplace. Snacking on them periodically during the morning can actually free up your lunch break for something else.

That leads into a creative possibility. You've just discovered extra time for whatever activity you may choose. Are you struggling with finding time for exercise? This could be the solution.

Lunch breaks provide an excellent opportunity for a brisk walk around the parking lot. Don't let any shyness or timidness stop you. Embrace it and be a trailblazing role model for others. You may be surprised how others react in a positive manner. They might even join you. You could be the spark they need to start their own exercise program.

I once knew a fellow who worked near an upscale apartment complex. He would slip into their pool on his lunch break and swim for forty minutes. His co-workers thought him to be a bit strange, but he didn't care. He later found employment as a pool guy working for their wives, always scheduling appointments when the husbands were coincidently away.

At your home it's even easier to apply the healthy-is-convenient method of eating. Many foods are ready to eat instantly or in a matter of minutes. If you notice, many fancy recipes are doing nothing but taking a naturally delicious, healthy item and converting it into a fat-bomb. Why not just save all that time that's spent destroying good food and eat it the way it was meant to be eaten? You can then use that extra free time to clean your own pool.

The fact derived from this is eating healthy can be extremely convenient. All you have to do is keep the good stuff around. Keep the processing to a minimum, as less-is-more applies to so many foods. It can still be very tasty. Above all, don't go around telling people that you eat junk food because it's more convenient. That's simply not true.

A major part of becoming fit is your general attitude and making it a priority. We touched on this earlier. So often financial concerns outweigh fitness and health objectives. But should they really? Re-prioritize yourself and shed those keeping-up-with-the-Jones' money pits. Simplify and concentrate on a healthy body instead.

Long gone are our yuppie dummy days when we competed strictly in the financial arena. We now realize being healthy and feeling good are what it's all about. Days filled with doctor visits, surgeries, chemo-therapy, dialysis, and all that dreaded stuff are horrible.

Much of it can be avoided, or at least delayed, by practicing and abiding by the simple concept of eating right and exercising. The sooner you start the process, the less likely the days are consumed by all that medical crap that we abhor. Play golf instead of sitting in that dreary doctor's office. Enjoy a nice lunch instead of getting blood work every other day. Swim in your always-professionally-maintained pool instead of hanging around the cardiology wing of the hospital.

Let's get back to those important food decisions, especially the spontaneous ones. One little mental trick that seems to work is the substitution rule. You're reaching for a snack because it's a life-long habit. Maybe it's not such a healthy snack. Take a moment and think. Is there anything similar I can eat that's considered healthier? There usually is an item that can replace it and taste just as good or even better. With repetition you can easily make this a habit.

Use that geezed-up brain. An example of this substitution mentality could be that bowl of ice cream that you eat every day. Make the switch to a low-fat, low-in-sweetener yogurt or maybe some other creative option. Do you pile the butter or sour cream on your baked potato? Consider salsa or a lighter less-fatty option. A little sweetness is probably better than the pure fatty stuff if you're trying to lose weight.

Every time you consider a certain food, ask yourself if you have a healthier option. Be conscious and aware of what you're eating. Educate yourself on all of your food choices. There are unlimited healthy and nutritious items out there to choose from. Surely you can find a few that you enjoy. Substitute good for bad.

Here are a few of the hundreds of potential substitutions. Create your own.

THE USUAL & THE SUBSTITUTE

Whole milk – low-fat milk

Sweet, salty snack – hot-air popcorn

Ice cream – low-fat frozen yogurt

Two eggs – four egg whites

Cookies – cereal

Butter – salsa

Mayonnaise – mustard

Croutons – shredded wheat

Husband – pool guy

Make right choices, All day long. They add up, Don't be wrong!

CHAPTER 6

Get Yourself Ready

"Luck is when preparation meets opportunity."
Lucius Seneca

Prepare for Battle

War is hell, and that's exactly the way you need to look at your fitness program. If it were easy everyone would be lean, strong and healthy. A quick glance around tells you that's not the case, but that's exactly what's going to make you special. You're going to accomplish a remarkable feat. Then you're going to maintain it, because your foundation will be built on a solid support system, not some flimsy, gimmicky, quick weight-loss scam.

Prepare yourself mentally. This will be one of the biggest challenges of your life. Losing weight and getting in shape is not easy. You have to fight hard, as you will be attacked from all sides. Temptation will surround you, constantly nipping at your heels to submit. You'll have to rely on your iron will to succeed.

Your friends will resist due to jealousy. At times it will seem as though the whole world is against you. Fight it out, for you cannot cave in. You can't give up early in the game.

Make it the first month and things will start to become a little easier, but by no means easy. You have to keep struggling and learn from any mistakes you make.

Be as stubborn as you can and stick to your plan, for the plan works if you work. Make any necessary sacrifices to make this a success. If you do this, you'll win this war, but always remember one thing. This war is never over. It's an ongoing war where you'll constantly have to be on guard. The enemy can slip behind you at any time and ambush you. If you master the basic principles, you'll survive. As long as you don't get cocky, over-confident, or lazy, you'll persevere.

You need to plan this as seriously as Zarkoff Zucchini plans his monthly carousing schedule. Going into battle without a well-laid plan is asking for defeat. A loose plan with holes is a ship sinking in the ocean. Have definite concrete rules and abide by them.

One slip is okay, but you had better punish yourself emotionally and make sure it doesn't happen again. Failure in the fitness game can be a gradual process. Allow mistakes to continue and one day you'll wake up and find you've reverted back to your old ways. That's not going to happen. Set your mind to it right now.

This is your personal battle. You don't have to announce it to the world. You're doing this for you, not for recognition. Don't worry, you'll be recognized and you won't have to say a word. Your lean body will speak for itself. You may choose to make those closest to you aware, or you may decide to tell no one of your fitness plan.

You may not realize it at the moment, but this will become an inner awakening, born of desire and confidence. You will take back control of your body from the theoretical demons that have hijacked it. It's your body, not theirs. This will be physical, emotional, and intellectual in nature, touching your very soul. It's not going too far to label it a spiritual experience.

If it were easy, then we would all be walking around fit as a fiddle. What fun would that be? You're not in this to become another number. You're out to become someone special. Appreciate the fact that this is a difficult task, because that's what will separate you from the flock. Follow your vision. Let the sheep be led as you plow ahead with determination and discipline on your path to success. Visualize the finish line and let nothing stand in the way.

You're ready to take this on. That's the biggest step of all. If you've read this far, you're already a success. You know what's required of you and you're ready to step into the front lines and do battle. The nuts and bolts of the program are simply something that you'll plug into. You'll ride the program into success. The key to everything is what's lying in your heart. You are the key that unlocks the gate.

The next chapter will lay out the actual food plan and the timing behind every bite. You'll have to use a bit of creativity to personalize it to your schedule. Everyone's situation is different. Maybe you're retired or you may work, possibly even two jobs. It matters not because you're going to make this happen regardless of the circumstances. The tough always find a way.

You'll make your particular situation work out. There are no excuses. If you want it bad enough, you'll make it happen. It's a personal challenge to yourself. It's something you have to prove to *you*. You were given one body and whatever shape it's in is your reality at the moment. Your schedule is what it is and you can fine tune it to be successful. Be positive and make the change to your body. It starts and ends in the mind. Excuses are for losers and you're no loser. You're a winner.

For simplicity this eating and exercise plan is based on a 9 to 5 work schedule. Other commitments may interfere with this. Don't panic, simply make adjustments to fit it into your schedule. If your 9 a.m. is in reality 2 p.m., then adjust accordingly. Rearrange the food consumption times to fit your needs.

Be realistic and allow time for what you're doing. Be serious as you lay out your plan. *Write it down*. This is a very important step. You want something to look at to guide you. That little piece of paper will become your boss for an indefinite time period. Spice it up with some happy faces or little thin stick figures. They might give you that extra push of inspiration or motivation you may need one day.

Without the proper plan, you set yourself up for problems. Even with complex schedules you will manage to do it. You just have to be creative. If you constantly travel, it can become very tricky. You didn't live this long by being a dummy, so you'll figure out a way. Determination is the answer.

Are there any items that will be particularly difficult to give up as you proceed with this program? If so, choose *one* and allow it in extreme moderation. Yes, *one* item only. Maybe it's a sweet of sorts or maybe it's a craft beer at the end of your day. Abuse this privilege and the penalty will be total avoidance. You'll be sent to vegetable and fruit prison for being a naughty little lad or lass. All the vegetable inmates will belittle you. The fruits will abuse you. You were a bad carbohydrate.

If you feel you can't manage a taste of your treat without going overboard, then don't even attempt it. You'll have to go cold turkey as you're doing with everything else. All your goodies will have to be shelved until you're deemed responsible enough to touch them. The fitness gods will let you know when that happens. Until then kiss them goodbye.

> *There's no limit,*
> *To what you can do.*
> *Nothing can stop,*
> *You from being YOU!*

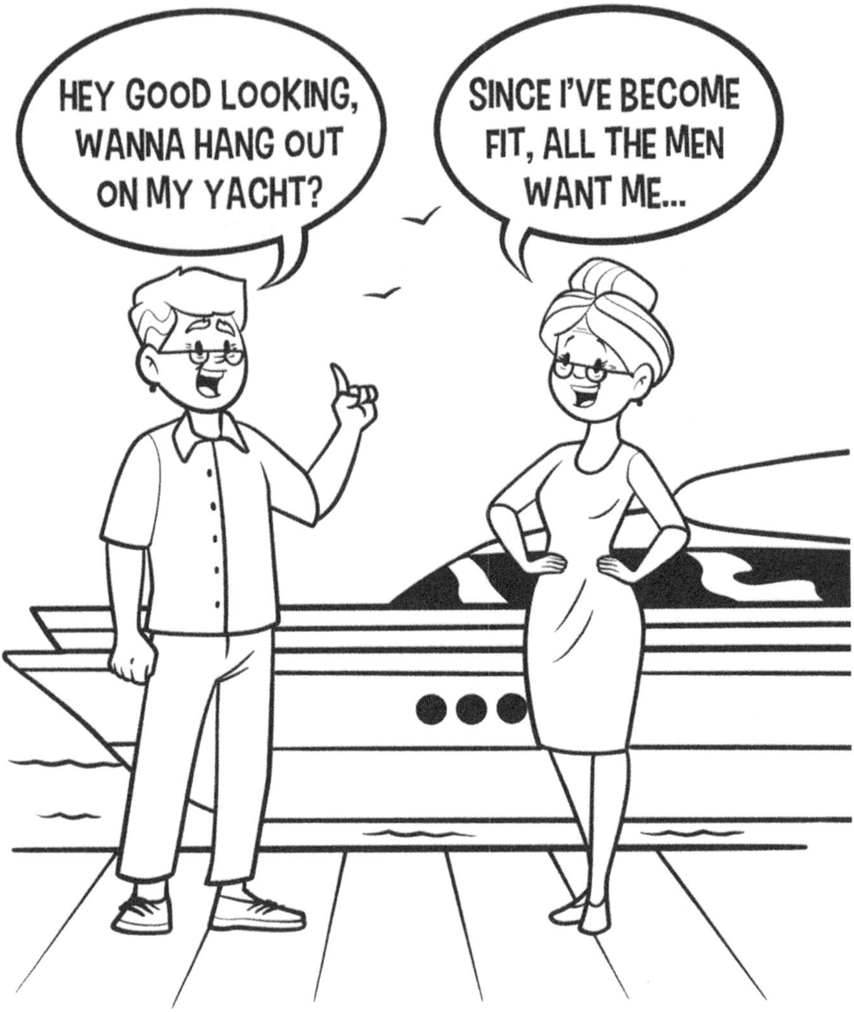
HEY GOOD LOOKING, WANNA HANG OUT ON MY YACHT?
SINCE I'VE BECOME FIT, ALL THE MEN WANT ME...

Prep It

This is it. There's no turning back. You've decided that you're going to get fit and you have a plan. You don't just jump into it without having all your weapons in front of you. Go ahead and gorge on all the fatty crap you desire for they'll be gone indefinitely. A couple of days of this is okay, just don't go Porky Pig crazy. You're transforming yourself on your start date.

Set your start date and get on with the program. Make sure you have no major commitments on that day. You don't want distractions of any kind. Don't be changing your starting date. You can't get into those wishy-washy habits before you start this intense project. You'll certainly be doomed with an attitude like that. Don't even think about celebrating with alcohol the night before the big day. Exercising with a hangover is no fun.

A couple of days before you begin battle you should stock up on your weapons. Unless you think you can get by without it, you'll need a container of some sort to carry your fruits, vegetables and such. I suppose a thermos jug may work. A tiny cooler with those re-freezable packs works well. Always remember to place your ice packs back into the freezer on a daily basis.

Don't take this buying decision lightly. Your cooler will be your best friend. I'm sure your friends will joke about you and your best buddy, the cooler. Go with the flow and beat them by persevering with a slow and steady commitment to your fitness goal. One day you may see them toting around a similar cooler because they want to accomplish what you've accomplished.

If you walk out of the house for thirty minutes, take it with you. Thirty minutes can turn into four hours. You know that as your ancient wisdom reminds you. *Do not* get caught without your healthy snacks. This is surely inviting disaster. You may get away with it the first few times you try it, but like anything else of a nefarious nature, you'll get caught at some point. Believe me, I know.

When it happens once, you're on a wayward fork in the road. Like everything else, once becomes twice, and you're heading in the wrong direction. You shouldn't leave the house without your cooler any more than a soldier would go to battle without a weapon.

Get caught in enemy territory without a defense and you're at their mercy. You'll be gunned down and stomped on by greasy, fatty, caloric entities that thrive on your demise. They want you to die a slow, torturous, obese death. They're heartless creatures that feed on the weak. Be strong. Don't let them have their way with you.

Your body needs fuel and without a supply of goodies it will seek out anything that is filling. Immediately make a habit of carrying your cooler everywhere. Maybe place a large handwritten reminder note above the exit in your home. That should do the trick. It will give your guests something else to laugh about when they visit, but you'll show them. One year from now they won't be laughing.

Always carry a water bottle. This is incredibly important. The body needs water and it can't come in the form of soft drinks or other unhealthy beverages. The only possible added ingredient would be a touch of pure, unsweetened fruit juice. If you haven't the skills to consume pure water, then learn now. Slam it down like those ole cowboys do their whiskey when they hit the saloon after a long month on the dusty plains.

Whatever it takes, you'd better acquire a taste for pure water. If you can't, tell your best friend to chain you up in a basement without food and water. Tell him to turn the heat up to a hundred degrees and leave you. Within two days I'll guarantee you'll be begging for water. Friends don't let friends drink sodas. Learn to carry your water bottle *every-where* you go.

A small can opener is another item you'll need. You may not like it, but sometimes you may be forced to consume canned meat. Tuna, chicken and turkey are great options here. Always choose the ones packed in water, no oil. Make sure you get the leanest of the lean by analyzing the labels. Your goal is to provide protein without excess fat. Becoming lean and strong is what you're looking for, right? Equate lean with lean meats, and strong with muscle. Lean unadulterated protein is the answer here.

Spend a little extra money and get a quality can opener. Your ancient fingers and hands aren't as nimble as they were in your youth. You don't want to become discouraged early on due to can opening issues. The good openers are smooth and easy. Don't let a cheap opener throw a kink in your fitness program. Okay, you tight-asses?

Another weapon you may choose for your dietary arsenal is a hot-air popcorn popper. This is a secret weapon in late-night advances from the enemy. A small bowl of this extremely low-calorie snack can keep those pesky cravings away. Always beware of Butterman though, for he loves to sneak by the bowl and contaminate everything with fatty butter. He knows when to strike and he knows a weaker human can't resist. Give Butterman a kick in the butt and send him on his way.

You may also want to purchase a vegetable-steamer insert. It's very simple and inexpensive. Steamed vegetables are a lifesaver option of preparing vegetables. Indulge in them at least once or twice a week. Butterman has been known to frequent areas where steamed vegetables are present, so keep a watchful eye out for him.

There will be other tools of the trade you'll buy along your journey to become fit. Experiment and see which ones you like. Never stray far from the basics, because the root of all this is simplicity. You're out to win this game. Make it work.

Now it's time to stock up on your primary food weapons. Get a little of everything, but not too much. Remember that freshness is what you're always striving for. You can overstock slightly on the non-perishable items. These include canned goods, dressings, sauces and such.

Do not overbuy on fruit, vegetables, milk, eggs, juice or any perishable items. Butterman's spouse, Rosey Rot, tends to hang around these items. She loves to make them wilt, mold, smell and generally contaminate your cupboard and refrigerator.

Butterman and Rosey Rot have a strong marriage and are very committed to obesity and putrid decay. They exchanged vows inside a fabulously decorated rotten watermelon. It was one of the most sought-after invitations in all of decomposed high-society, an affair to be remembered.

That should motivate you to stay fresh. Rotate your fruit and vegetable selections regularly. Take note of your weekly grocery bill. This healthy-eating lifestyle is actually considerably less expensive than the processed route. It's time to purchase some healthy foods. Always go with unsalted and unsweetened if you can. Stay organic if possible. Let's go.

Food Choices

All vegetables, all fruits, all lentils

Brown rice, quinoa, potatoes, corn, steel-cut oatmeal

Eggs, low-fat milk

Unsalted raw or dry roasted nuts

Lean meat

Canned tuna/chicken/turkey

Spoon size shredded wheat, raisins, hot-air popcorn

Low-fat, healthy sauces/toppings/dressings

I'm all ready,
Ready to go.
I'm so ready,
GO, GO, GO!

Mental Prep

Your body is now your temple. Nothing enters it without clearance and a background check. Most items in today's processed society won't make the cut. For many of you this will be a major change. We've all been bombarded by the salty, sweetened, greasy products that push their way into our lives.

This will be such an undertaking for you that you'll almost need divine guidance to get through it. I think a motivational quote from the Great One is in order here. Zarkoff Zucchini was no stranger to adversity and challenges. Those moments were when he rose to his greatest heights. Zucchini seemed to thrive on extreme adversity. It brought out the heroic qualities within him that us lesser beings can only dream of. What courage the little green vegetable possessed.

"We do what we do because we do what we do," stated the Great One on that eventful January morning. Once again, I see no great literary relevance in that particular quote. Any of us could come up with that in our sleep. However, because it passed through the lips of legendary Zarkoff Zucchini, that simple declaration became a piece of history.

It is now the most famous statement ever attributed to the iconic vegetable. It is written above the entrance to the Vegetable Hall of Fame located somewhere deep in a beet field in Ukraine. The story behind "We do what we do because we do what we do," is one of tremendous courage and exemplary heroism.

It all started on a cold, snowy evening deep within the Himalayan mountains. On top of Mount Kangchenjunga were two stranded young cucumber lasses. They had somehow made it all the way to the top of the 28,000-foot-high peak. The pretty little cucumbers were now facing extreme weather and blizzard conditions.

Temperatures were expected to dip below -40 degrees. The young girls stood no chance of survival. The locals at the bottom of the mountain had already written them off as deceased. There was nothing that could be done to save them.

As fate would have it, Zarkoff Zucchini just happened to be in town. He was scheduled to give a speech at the base camp of Sikkim to a group of orphaned radishes. Early in his display of eloquence he was interrupted and informed of the tragedy unfolding high above him. Without hesitation Zarkoff rose to the occasion. He apologized for canceling his speech and quickly donned his arctic attire.

"I'm going to rescue the girls," Zucchini calmly pronounced as he strolled out of the room.

"Don't go, you'll die!" pleaded the crowd that had gathered for his speech.

"I must go," Zarkoff replied. "Pretty girls must be saved."

Zarkoff began making his way up the mountain. It was cold and dark and Zarkoff disappeared into the night. The townspeople began weeping as they watched their hero walk off to a certain death. They immediately began planning a memorial for their beloved icon. He had certainly just entered his last courageous act of an illustrious life.

To everyone's surprise Zarkoff appeared the next morning with his two beauties in tow behind him. His story of courage and bravery astounded the townspeople. No one but Zucchini could have pulled off such a feat. His reputation reached stratospheric heights.

It had not been easy. Constructing a makeshift sled from some scrap metal, Zarkoff placed the distressed girls onto the device and proceeded to pull them to safety. He began the treacherous journey back down the mountain in total darkness. Zarkoff trudged through the night, not letting thirst or hunger interfere with his focus. Pretty girls had to be saved.

Finally, exhausted beyond description, Zarkoff arrived and immediately collapsed. A medical team quickly attended to him and the girls. Zarkoff waved to the cheering crowd as they carried him away. "We do what we do because we do what we do," he muttered just before he passed out.

His followers couldn't believe what had just happened. It was a feat no one thought could be done, not even by the great Zucchini. The fact remained that he *did* do it, and the girls were safe. His reputation for bravery and courage expanded throughout the vegetable community. The media worldwide quickly grabbed onto this heartwarming tale of heroism. The global vegetable community applauded Zarkoff Zucchini and his latest act of courageous selflessness.

Zarkoff decided to stay an extra month in the village. The owner of the local inn provided a suite for Zarkoff and his two new girlfriends. They were spotted around the local watering holes drinking nearly every night. It was all celebration and good times.

It all came to an ugly end when a conflict with Sikkim's mayor occurred. Zarkoff had one drink too many and made inappropriate advances toward the respected mayor's wife.

Both of his girlfriends, along with the mayor's wife, became incensed at his behavior. It was not a pretty sight.

One of the young cucumbers began beating Zarkoff with a mud brick that was lying nearby. The other smashed a dumpling bowl over his head. The enraged wife pushed Zarkoff to the floor and violently plunged a stick of Yak butter down his throat.

Local authorities were quickly called to the scene and Zarkoff was dragged away to safety. Arrangements were immediately made and he was hastily whisked away on a private plane out of the country. The nasty event tarnished Zarkoff Zucchini's reputation forever in the town that loved him so. "We do what we do because we do what we do," was the only public statement Zucchini would ever make on the embarrassing event.

That's how we have to look at our new challenge to become lean, strong and healthy. "We do what we do because we do what we do," should be your guiding statement from this moment on. Although it didn't end well, nothing can change the fact that Zarkoff accomplished what he set out to do. He rescued those young girls. That's the iron-willed mentality it will take for you to survive in the war to become fit.

You are you,
One of a kind.
You can do it,
It's all in the mind!

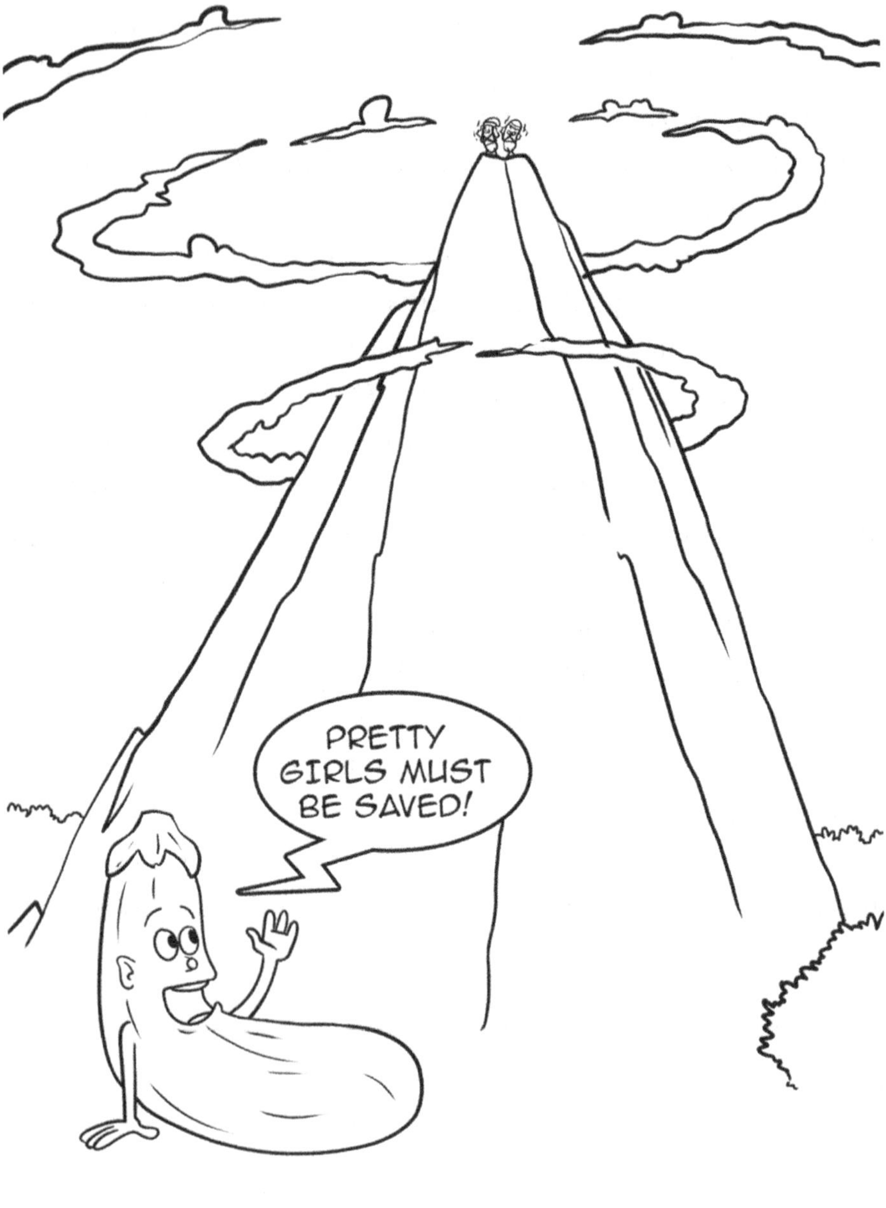
PRETTY GIRLS MUST BE SAVED!

Mental Prep II

Losing weight is likely a major goal for many of you. Believe it or not, the exercise plan will not be so difficult. Start small, add a little every day, and before long small becomes substantial. You'll do it so gradually you won't even notice it. Watching what you eat won't be as easy.

You will need extreme discipline to overpower those established habits that have been ingrained for decades. The first step is to determine what you will eat and how much of it you will eat. Then the difficult part begins, sticking with your program. Temptation will be around every corner and you should expect it. Declare war and defend your territory.

Your territory is your body. Everything that enters your body does so through the mouth, at least everything edible. This was mentioned earlier, but bears repeating. That little hole in your head called the mouth is the key to survival. Control that small piece of real estate and the game is over. You'll win. It's that simple.

Manage the mouth and the body has no choice but to lose weight. Simplify it down to a child's terms. Your mouth will always be near you, so you don't have to worry about it going away. It's small, so there's not a lot of area that needs protection. You and you alone feed it. No one else physically pushes items into it. Mental activity is required to place a fork into the mouth. Control that mental activity and monitor that fork.

An unhealthy item can make it to your lips, but unless it actually passes into your mouth, you're a winner. Imagine this. You have armed soldiers guarding this restricted area. *Nothing* passes without clearance. Automatic weapons and ten levels of security await anything that makes its way to your lips.

Only one item is allowed total clearance and that is water. Everything else is strip-searched and analyzed for contaminants. Fat, salt, sugar and all other bad-guy intruders will be handcuffed and whisked away to a maximum-security food prison. There they will receive an unfair trial, because you're the judge, and will be executed in a timely fashion. Some items won't even be granted a trial, for they will be shot on sight.

Fried foods, butter, mayonnaise, soft drinks and candy are just a few of the hundreds of items assassinated by your mercenary killers. Your kitchen floor will be littered with bodies. A more gruesome scene could not be imagined. Show no mercy to these evil-intentioned intruders. The enemy deserves no slap on the wrist. They need to die for their traitorous act of betrayal.

Slaughter them and make an example for all others who may even think of entering your mouth and sliding down your throat. Imagine what a Baby Ruth bar would think if he saw a Snickers lying dead on the floor. He would likely run back to a safe domain and forget all about trying to sneak into your mouth. He would head to the closest television and select someone else. Those unconscious viewers make for easier prey.

Other items are thoroughly searched and questioned before being granted access to your innards. Vegetables, fruits and lean protein can enter if they are of legal size and are not contaminated by butter, sugar or salt. Any contamination means instant death and they are shot immediately, twice just to make sure. Make sure you leave one severely wounded, wailing and shrieking in pain. This will serve as a warning of undoubtable suffering to any bad guys awaiting on the outskirts.

Yes, it will be a bloody scene around your mouth. Death and destruction will reign, but that's the way it has to be. Inside your stomach, however, it will be a peaceful, relaxing, enjoyable scene of tranquility. Fruits, vegetables, and other healthy foods will be mingling and socializing and having a great time. All's cool without all the riffraff, rabble and other social undesirables hanging around.

Without grease, fat, butter, and sugar crashing the party, everyone's happy. Thank God for those armed guards providing security and keeping criminals at bay. Life's a blast inside the safe zone that is your belly. As long as that mouth is guarded freedom and justice will prevail.

There will be liberty and good times for all healthy foods. There will be a quick and decisive death to anyone who thinks they can ruin the fun with fatty contaminants. Attempt to penetrate the border and you'll end up like those unfortunates littering the kitchen floor. Death to all perpetrators is the clear message here. Don't let the bad guys inside. *Guard that mouth.*

Now let's move on. As you know this fitness program is a one-year minimum startup. Don't even think of speeding up your expectations. Just grind it out and let the dedication and discipline take care of the rest. Since losing weight will likely be your goal, it will be very tempting to jump on the scales every five minutes to see if you've made any progress.

This is a very bad idea. At the early phase of your program your body is in shock. The scale is your worst enemy at this point because it plays head games with you. After you attain your desired weight, the scale becomes a dear friend. Let me explain.

Many expect immediate gratification, especially after truly committing to eating right and exercising. Here's a scenario. You start your program and for three days you do everything perfectly. You're feeling really good about yourself. However, three days of doing all the right things might not be rewarded by a number on the scale. It's highly possible you may not lose any weight at all. It's even possible you can *gain* weight.

That's because there can be a sort of delayed reaction between what you do to your body and how it reacts to this action. Put yourself in your geezed body's position. After decades of having junk food plowed into it, it became accustomed to the abuse. Three days of healthy eating is not going to instantly convert you into Thin Lizzy.

Your body is dazed and in shock. It is so confused that it could take weeks to adjust. After years of candy bars, it has no idea what a carrot is. It is so accustomed to fried foods that it's stunned by the sudden change to grilling and steaming. "Water instead of soft drinks! What are you doing to me?" it may scream.

Here's the big issue with all this. Suppose you eat healthy and begin a nice exercise routine. For a month you apply yourself and you're proud as a peacock. Jumping on the scales, you can't wait to see how much weight you've lost. You watch in horror as the number appears.

"One pound!" you shout. "All that work and discipline and I lost only one pound. To hell with this torture, I'm going back to my old habits." This is a very common occurrence. You must exhibit patience and look at the scale as an enemy at this point. Wait until someone *genuinely* tells you they think you've lost weight. Then step on the scale. It may take a matter of months, but this ensures that you won't become disillusioned and totally abandon the program, kissing all your hopes and dreams goodbye.

Your body needs an adjustment period. Remember that it put up with all the abuse you gave it. Now it's your time to suffer. Don't risk getting discouraged by stepping on the scale too soon. Eventually you *will* start losing weight. When that happens, your metabolism will speed up and the pounds will steadily fall away.

You have to view the big picture here. Let the other weaklings give up and latch onto another pipe-dream, gimmicky, weight-loss scheme that will surely disappoint. You're going to continue with a common sense, long-term program that will have permanent results.

Everyone will lose weight at different rates. Simply change your eating habits, start an exercise program, and don't worry about your weight. After a comment or two about your noticeable weight loss, then it's safe to get on the scale. Now you are truly on your way to becoming Thin Lizzy.

Now you have confidence. As you continue to work hard towards getting to your desired weight, step on the scale once a week. The scale has transformed into a good friend. It is now an indicator of your dedication and discipline. It is now a confidence-builder and will encourage you to become even more determined to accomplish your goal.

Finally, you have reached your goal. Your weight is exactly where you want it. Through this long, tough battle you have gotten in touch with your body. You know what it needs and when it needs it. Don't let it slip away. The battle is a continuous one.

At this point use the scale every day if you like. A pound or so difference isn't going to mean anything, but you want to catch any major weight gain and head it off at the pass. Fight back and revert back to your prime methods of losing weight to get yourself back on track. The scales don't lie. They're like a true friend who tells you the nasty truth even though it might hurt. Get thin and stay thin by turning the scale into an ally, not an enemy.

It takes time,
To lose weight.
If you're patient,
You'll look great!

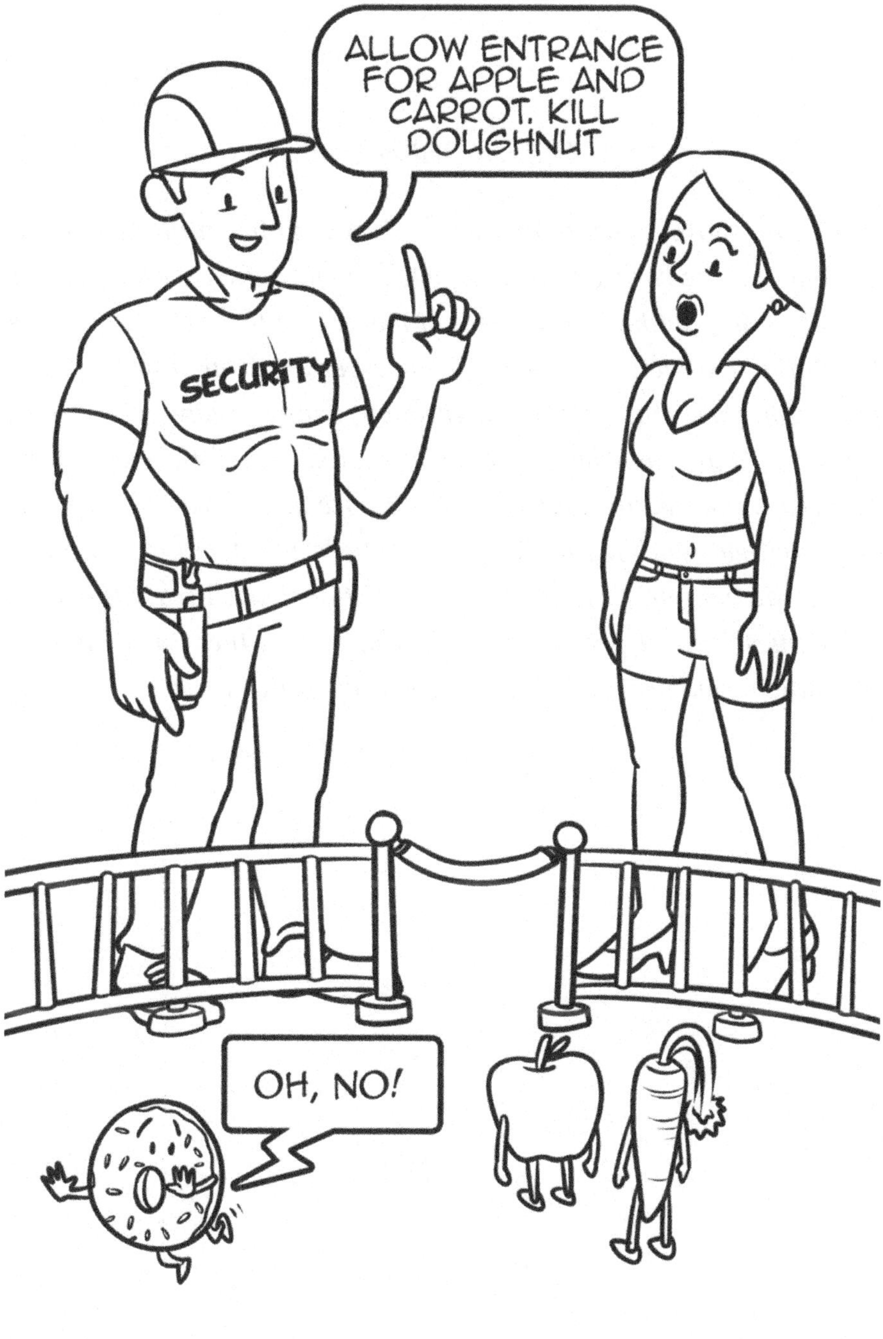
ALLOW ENTRANCE FOR APPLE AND CARROT. KILL DOUGHNUT
SECURITY
OH, NO!

Hidden Dedication

There are countless books that are dedicated to the author's mother. It's really quite boring to be completely honest. That's why this one is hidden deep within the recesses of mounds of text. My mother has faithfully stood with me through some very difficult times, all my fault. She has stuck with me through trying emotional periods, bailed me out financially due to my fiscal stupidity, and totally believed in me every single day. Never once did she lose faith in me. And she had good reason to do so, believe me. I put her through some arduous times. Her love is unconditional and I truly think she is the most special person in the world. I am a lucky soul. Phyllis Dixon Johnson is an Angel. This book is dedicated to her.

Mental Prep III

We also touched on the next point earlier, but I would like to expand on it. Eat before hunger, that's so important. You have to get mentally prepped for this and not allow cravings to rule. A bite of something good can stave off twenty bites of something bad. It's sort of a cat and mouse game with your body and your mind.

It's really an acquired skill, but you can learn it quickly if you get to know your body. Through trial and error, you will eventually learn when to eat a healthy snack to prevent overwhelming hunger. You will also learn what type of snack to eat and when to eat it.

The right mix of fruits and vegetables, protein, and complex carbohydrates will work, especially if you time them correctly. For maximum weight loss, fruits and vegetables should be your main weapons. You'll still need a certain amount of protein and complex carbohydrates.

If at all possible, learn to like egg whites. The calories-verses-pure protein ratio is as good as it gets. Your goal with all protein is to get it into your body as lean as you can. So much protein is wrapped with layers of fat. It's sort of an unwelcome package deal. It doesn't have to be this way. Egg whites are the great escape in this department. Earlier in the book we discussed them, but here are a few more important details. This is vital stuff.

At strategic times during the day, you can quickly consume an egg white. I realize that a boiled egg white is about as tasteless an item as can be imagined. However, you have to look at the finish line and what you're going to accomplish. You're not into this to enjoy the tastiest, most flavorful food. That's not your goal. Your mission is to *do what it takes* to lose weight, become lean and strong, and show yourself and others that you are a remarkable human being.

Here's what you may have to do. Mindlessly eat that little egg white and forget how tasteless it is. Throw some pepper on it or spice it up with something if you like. Look at it as medication that will transform your body into what you envision at the finish line.

In reality, you're being punished for all those high-calorie, high-fat goodies you've enjoyed in the past. You were bad and naughty and now you have to confess your sins and repent. Every time you take a bite of something relatively tasteless, think back to your wild, reckless days of irresponsible actions. Rely on those memories and realize you've had your fun. Now it's time to get serious and take care of business. Gobble down that egg white and don't complain.

Methodically eat these little lifesavers at strategic times during the day and you'll provide your body with its daily requirements. Four of them will result in very few calories in relation to the protein your body receives. They're muscle builders and toners. All the serious body builders know this.

A few egg whites, a few handfuls of a carbohydrate mix, a small ration of unsalted, dry-roasted or raw nuts, and heavier consumption of fruits and vegetables should be enough to snack your way through the day. Mix each category throughout the day. Try to always start your snacking with a few bites of your fruit and veggie mix, then proceed to your protein, and lastly the complex carb mix. Those first few bites of fruits or veggies can go a long way toward satisfying that craving before it gets a grip.

It's really an art, managing the little mind game that's being played out between your cravings and your doses of healthy snacks. It actually can become fun once you're into it. Fine tune your consumption to fit with your particular body. Never let yourself feel too weak, but also never allow yourself to attain that completely full sensation.

Ride that fine line between lean nutrition and caloric overload. Above all, avoid gluttony. Those days are long gone. A *new you* is on the horizon. You're going to soar so high you can see the future. You'll ride high on confidence and that fantastic feeling of accomplishment.

Your goal with this is to give your body what it *needs*, not what it *wants*. Once you determine where that line is drawn, you can reach optimum efficiency in weight loss, yet retain your strength. Negotiate a truce with your body. Both entities really want the same thing, a lean, healthy machine that looks good, feels good and runs like it is brand new. Strive for that and get as close to that dream as possible.

This will not be easy, but good things never come easily. You know because you're as old as the hills. Use that been-around-the-block wisdom and apply it to your own body. Learn it, master it, and keep that body right on the edge. Be that mother bird feeding her hungry chick.

That chick is always crying for more and more, but wise ole mom gives it just what it needs. Fat, slow birds don't survive long in the wild animal world. They're the first prey to be gobbled down by the predators. Lean, mean and healthy are the keys to surviving our ruthless human jungle also. The sooner you learn to beat hunger *before* it reaches you, the easier it becomes. Rule your jungle.

I'm fat and slow,
And I'm oversize.
But I'll be fit,
Cause I'm wise!

CHAPTER 7

The Food Plan

"Overcome obstacles and criticisms with supreme confidence."
William Rago

Let's Do It!

A great vegetable once stated, "Greatness is always great." As you know, words as those could only have come from the mouth of Zarkoff Zucchini. Only he could say something so simple and meaningless and get away with it. "Greatness is always great," is just a plain dumb statement, but that doesn't stop Zarkoff followers worldwide from spouting it at every opportunity.

Annual Zarkoff rallies always start with a traditional chanting of "Greatness is always great." This is supposed to create an inspirational environment in which the rally will thrive. I personally think it's kind of silly, but once again, who am I to judge?

I'm no Zarkoff Zucchini. I'll never be remembered for eternity. I'll never go down in history as an iconic hero who literally saved the whole vegetable race. I'll never go down as the vegetable who conquered over a hundred STDs and eventually became immune to antibiotics.

"Greatness is always great," will be our guiding source of inspiration for this important chapter. We'll be discussing the actual nuts and bolts of the food plan. Hopefully your mindset is that of success through hard work, dedication, and discipline. That's how you'll attain your goals.

If you begin to falter and doubt yourself, revert back to one of the dumbest statements ever and try to take it seriously. "Greatness is always great," should motivate and inspire. Use this to provide a much-needed boost during any troubling times ahead. If that doesn't work, then just mark Zarkoff off as a sex-crazed, overrated veggie celebrity who somehow managed a following. Then follow your own guidelines and inspirational motivations and get it done.

Okay, here we go. Seriously, if you're not mentally prepared, back off and don't start yet. The mental aspect of this cannot be underestimated. A quick, unprepared entry into this means an early exit. Then you're back to where you were and it will have been nothing more than another failed attempt at becoming fit.

Then you'll lump me with all those gimmicky fitness promoters that I so despise. Please don't do that. Apply yourself and make it work. Start this program with the right state of mind. Make sure you're looking into the future with no expectations of becoming fit overnight. It never works like that no matter how those glitzy ads present it.

Those smooth-talking showboats may get wealthy overnight, but you'll be left behind in worse shape than ever. Back off now if you're not ready. Go back, get your head together, and then go for it. That's how to make it in this brutal endeavor. It's an undertaking of enormous commitment, so don't dive into shallow water and break your neck.

If you're ready, then let's progress onward with the food plan. You'll start your war. It may be the biggest battle of your life. You may feel like a drug addict kicking your addiction. The first weeks, even months, may feel like absolute torture. You'll get through it though.

Finally, you will reach your desired weight. You will add certain food items back into your life, appreciating them more than ever. You will *not* fall to pieces at this point. You will let the scale be your friend. If you find yourself weighing three pounds more than you like, you'll report back to the torture chamber for a few days. You will lose weight quickly.

After this happens a couple of times, you'll begin to instinctively know your body. Be careful not to lose *more* weight than you desire. Eventually you will stabilize your weight and maintain it at your desired level. This will keep those torture chamber visits brief. You *will* stay in control.

This is *not* a diet. From this point on, if anyone asks, you are *not* on a diet. A diet is temporary and this is permanent. Sure, this is highly restricted in the beginning, but it's only the first step towards complete control of your body.

Step by step, you'll slowly change your eating habits. You will likely start out sacrificing most of what you eat now. By the time you've reached your desired weight, you will have learned to appreciate healthy foods. Then you should eat many of the items that you have given up, but in moderation.

You'll be amazed at what happens next. You will find yourself eating the healthy stuff even though you have a choice. French fries, pizza, cheese, sweets, mayonnaise, etc., will be back in your life. The difference will be they won't *control* your life. You will control them. You are changing your eating habits for life. *You are not on a diet.* Are you ready? Let's go.

A change for life,
Starting now.
I'm gonna do it,
Cause I know how!

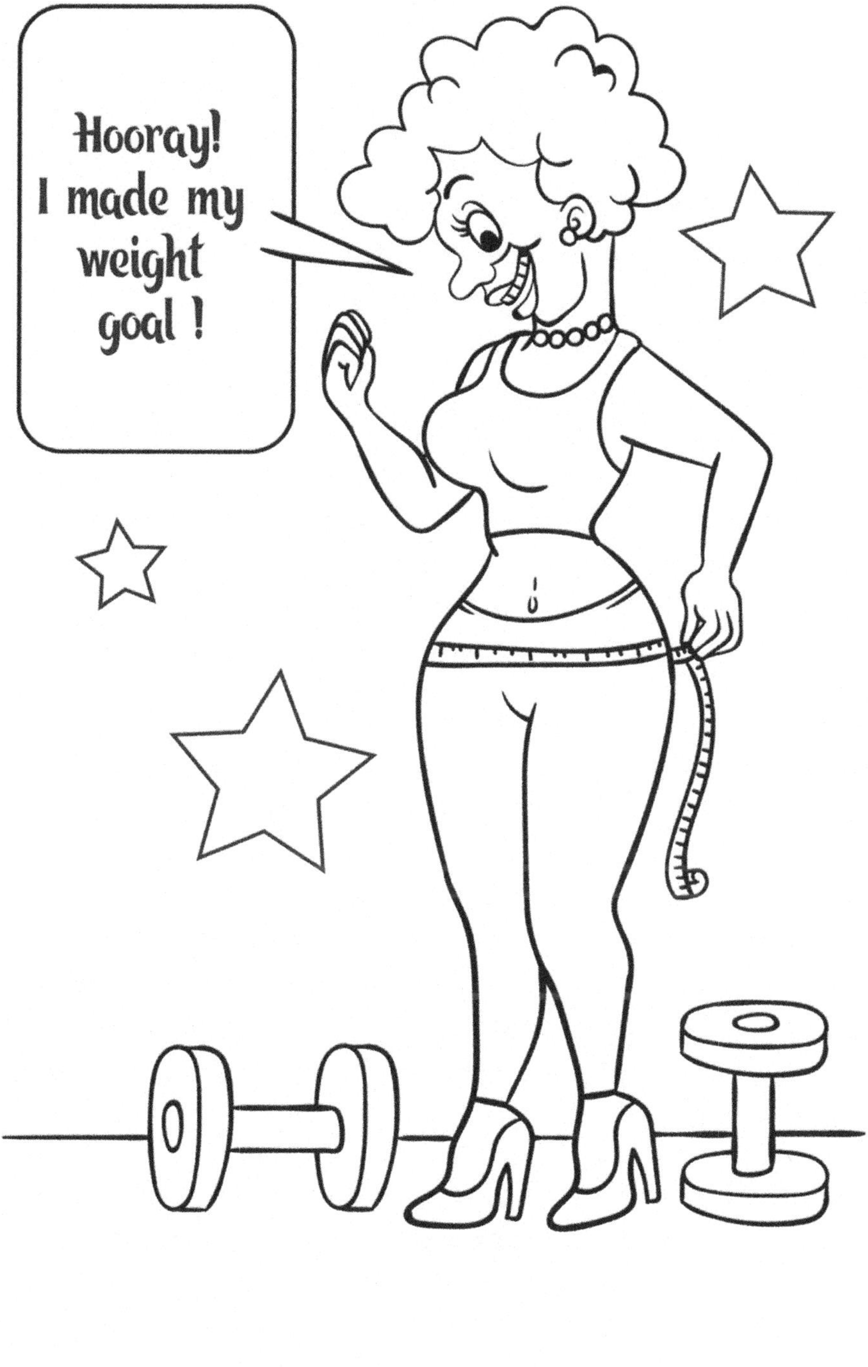
Hooray!
I made my
weight
goal !

Let's Do It!

The following plan will work. It has been tested and it's safe and healthy. You'll receive adequate nutrition as long as you don't skip any of the steps. Fight through it and you'll come out the other side a winner.

This is war. Are you ready for battle? It's time to forget the gimmicky diets because they simply don't work in the long run. You know because you've experienced it. To lose weight you have to cut back on calories. It's that simple.

This will hurt, but this will work. So here it is. Read very carefully and pay attention to the important notes. If you stumble, put it behind you and continue to move forward. Don't worry, Zarkoff's spirit will be guiding you in times of weakness.

NOTE: Don't skip any part of this plan. All of it is necessary. Your body needs protein and carbohydrates.

NOTE: A word about measurements here. Measure your food amounts only once or twice, then estimate it. A *little* more or a *little* less will not be a problem. Don't cheat intentionally as you'll only be cheating yourself. From a psychological point, measuring your food is not good. You will feel trapped. Don't measure your food.

NOTE: Mix and match your protein sources if you like. Compare your primary protein sources and calculate accordingly. Two cooked egg whites contain approximately the same protein as one third of a small can of tuna, around 9 grams, give or take a couple of grams. You'll need to do a little math if you're using other lean meats. A little more or a little less isn't important as long as you keep those protein calorie counts low. Choose lean.

NOTE: This is a *very* tricky one! For simplicity, this is basically a 9 to 5 based model. No time is provided for other commitments or obligations. *Personalize it to fit your own hours.* Rearrange it to make it work. *This is important!* Get your personal schedule right *before* starting. For all of you, you *will* make time for exercise. See the exercise plan chapter.

NOTE: Make sure your last meal of the day isn't too heavy. Rearrange the prescribed dinner into lunch if possible (switch number 10 with any earlier number.) You'll have to rearrange the other timed snacks to be proportionate and accommodate for this. The only reason I have dinner listed as the heavier meal is client feedback. The latter part of the day is the only time to prepare a meal for many of them. As you know, I'm always trying to be practical and realistic. I don't want you to get frustrated and consider total abandonment. Regardless, it's *always* better to ease into the night with a belly that's not stuffed. Go to bed slightly hungry.

NOTE: *Nothing* else goes into your mouth. Armed guards are stationed at your mouth.

Gonna eat right,
That's what you'll do.
Eating right,
Is Good for YOU!

The Plan

1: Rise from bed at 7 a.m. (we're using this time for simplicity purposes, so adjust this to fit your schedule.) Drink at least 4 ounces of water immediately. Have a large cup of coffee or tea if you like. Add nothing more than 2 to 3 ounces of low-fat milk. Absolutely don't add any sweeteners or artificial creamers. A small amount of honey would be the only exception here. Boil one or more eggs for later or plan another protein source.

2: 7:15 a.m. – Eat all the fresh, unsweetened fruit you want, just act in a sane manner here. Mix and match often. Veggies will work here also. Eat very slowly. Exercise now?

3: 9 a.m. – Drink at least 4 ounces of water. Eat a boiled egg white or an equivalent protein source. Exercise now?

4: 10 a.m. – Drink at least 4 ounces of water. Eat a boiled egg white or an equivalent protein source. Exercise now?

5: 11 a.m. – Eat a quarter cup of oatmeal or unsweetened shredded wheat. Steel-cut oats are the least processed. Add a couple of ounces of low-fat milk to your shredded wheat if you like. Add a few raisins or another unsweetened fruit to your oats or cereal if you like. A touch of honey is fine. Exercise now?

6: 12 p.m. – Drink at least 4 ounces of water. Eat a boiled egg white or an equivalent protein source. Exercise now?

7: 1 p.m. – Snack on all the raw fruit and vegetables you want and a handful of your carbohydrate mix. This mix consists of shredded wheat and/or healthy crackers, dried or fresh fruit, a small amount of raw or dry roasted nuts, unsalted and unsweetened of course. Exercise now?

8: 3 p.m. – Drink at least 4 ounces of water. Eat a boiled egg white or an equivalent protein source. Exercise now?

9: 5 p.m. – Snack on all the raw fruit and vegetables you want and a handful of your carbohydrate mix. Have beer, wine, or a cocktail if you like. Cocktails can't contain sugars or creamy substances. Exercise now? If not, it's getting late!

10: 6-8 p.m. – Eat one of the meals provided in the recipe chapter OR snack on your all-you-can-eat fruit and vegetables and a handful of your carbohydrate mix. Remember this is your last meal of the day, so *keep it light*. Did you get that? *Keep it light!* Feel free to improvise and create your own meal, but if you stray from the basics, you're looking for trouble. *Eat very slowly.* By now you know what's allowed and what's not. Cheat and you're only hurting yourself. Drink only water with your meal.

11: Nighttime – If you absolutely need a snack, it must be raw fruit or vegetables or possibly a small amount of hot-air popcorn. No salt, oil, butter or additives are allowed on the popcorn.

12: Forego that last reality show and go to sleep. Get at least seven hours. You've got another grueling day tomorrow. You are in the process of laying down the foundation for the future. You will *absolutely* get tired of this schedule every day. You will curse me and hate me for steering you into this program. You will even consider ditching my program and exchanging it for the latest con-man special. You'll quickly come back to your senses and realize I'm right. You will stay on track no matter how rough the waters get. You'll learn to like natural foods. You will like me in the end. Congratulations on surviving another day.

All day long,
Into the night.
All I do,
Is eat right!

Maintaining

You did it! You've struggled and fought and you reached your desired weight. Go enjoy a simple celebration evening because you deserve it, but don't think for a second that your work is over. This is a critical time and you have to realize it. This is what separates the gimmicky programs from the ones that actually work.

All the hard work, dedication and discipline has taught you something about yourself. You're beaming with confidence so much that you glow when you walk into a room. Others can see a brilliance about you that wasn't there before. You're the star of the show and you like it. You're not about to let it all slip away.

This reminds me of another famous Zarkoff Zucchini quote. You know, those generic nothing-of-any-substance statements that flow from the mouth of our loose-lipped hero. Yes, those childish little mutterings that are looked upon as great philosophical declarations by his loyal following.

"A vegetable is a vegetable forever," was what the audience heard on that humid evening in south Florida. Zarkoff Zucchini was in the midst of delivering an eloquent speech at a Donators for Disabled Datils event. The arena was packed, a large number of them being the fiery datil peppers, a vegetable with a reputation for its unrestrained emotional character.

The captivated audience was completely under his spell when he uttered these now famous words. The crowd erupted in applause the moment the last syllable passed through Zarkoff's lips. A standing ovation spontaneously occurred which lasted over twenty minutes.

It soon escalated as emotions took hold. A crowd-control security team had to be called in to manage the overwhelmed assemblage of Zarkoff fanatics. Datils were especially affected. Several of them, racked-with-emotion and weeping uncontrollably, had to be carried away on stretchers. Two of them were so shaken by Zarkoff's heartfelt proclamation that they suffered coronaries and died on the spot. Local Miami officials were so concerned that they brought in the entire police force and the city's mental health officials.

At one point they were worried there would be a mass suicide. This was after one crazed-with-emotion datil stood on a chair and began chanting "Return as Zarkoff! Return as Zarkoff!" He thought that if everyone died on that particular evening, they would all be reborn as the great Zucchini.

The disturbed datil was well on his way towards convincing the crowd when a trained team of mental-health advisors arrived on the scene. Several from the crowd had already woven makeshift ropes from their ties and were getting ready to hang themselves. They were transported to the asylum.

"A vegetable is a vegetable forever," had so stirred emotions that it was impossible to quell the crowd. It finally took Zarkoff himself to bring order to the building. He pleaded with them to remain calm. Most of them reluctantly settled down.

A small group of Zarkoff fanatics remained, having lost total control. They were arrested after they tried to blow up the building. They were trying to build a better datil society by sacrificing the audience to be reborn as baby Zarkoffs. They were stopped just as the bomb was about to explode.

What can we learn from this? Let's take this statement, "A vegetable is a vegetable forever," and let it guide us in maintaining a successful nutrition program. It's probably not going to help us in the least, but why not? Pretend you're a vegetable and that you will forever be a vegetable and use that mentality to maintain success. Let's give the great, charismatic Zarkoff Zucchini some well-deserved credit and recognition. If nothing else, he's the quintessential issuer of meaningless statements that are perceived to be meaningful.

We'll simply use the Great One's sheer magnetism and presence for inspiration. You're shining bright and riding high after winning the battle to attain your desired weight. Everyone openly or secretly is amazed at your accomplishment. You should be really proud of yourself.

> *You did it,*
> *You lost weight.*
> *Lose to win,*
> *That's your fate!*

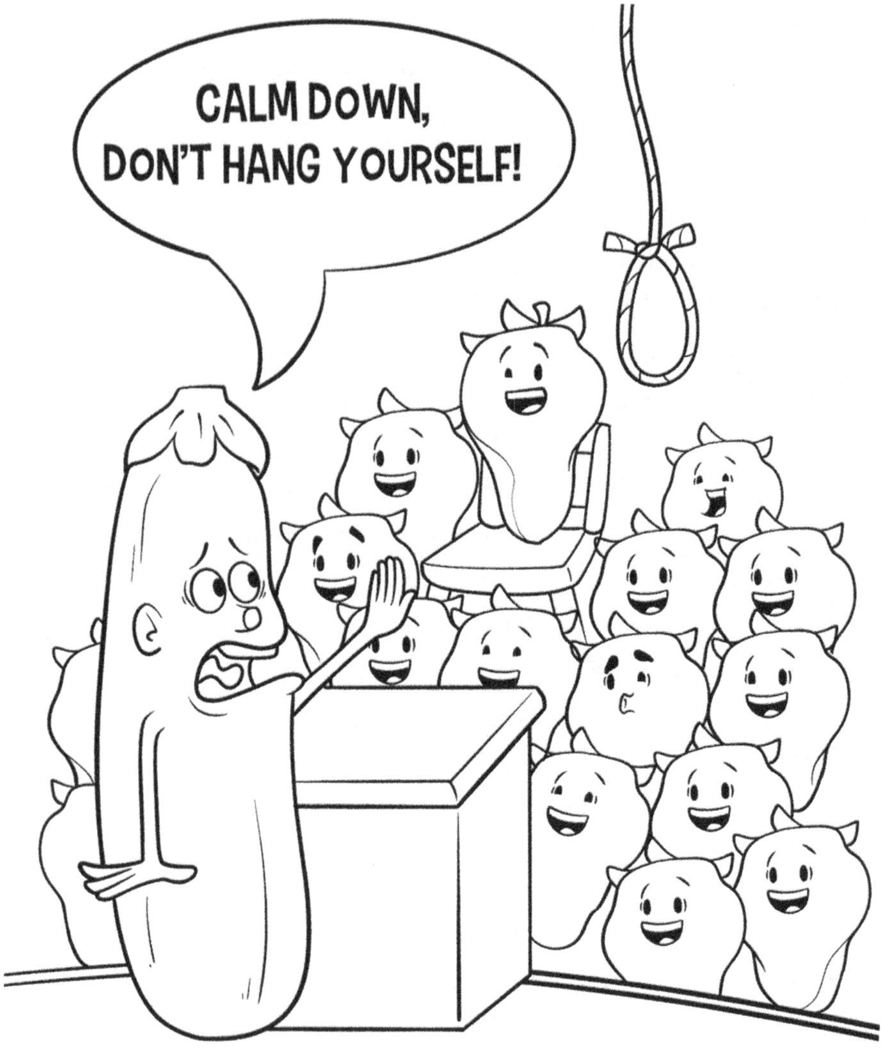
CALM DOWN,
DON'T HANG YOURSELF!

Maintaining II

As you well know, because you've probably been through it, maintaining success is crucial. Remember when you started and looked at this as a one-year-minimum project to become fit? That's the same long-term mentality needed to maintain.

Fast forward to another year into the future. Do this as you stand before a mirror and look at yourself. The mirror reflects your success. Next year you'll look even better because you'll continuously become more toned.

Close your eyes and let the image settle within. Envision yourself as being one year older and better than ever. Ingrain it into your mind and let it burn into your psyche. Soak the image into your soul and spirit. Make it such a permanent part of your being that it becomes impossible to dismantle. You *will* continue to be the amazing person that you are.

Be a role model for others and show them that it's an ongoing process. It's not a prove-yourself-and-move-on little piece of your ego. It's the *new* you and you intend to keep it that way. You like being on top for you've earned it.

You intuitively understand your body. You're in touch with its finer nuances at a cellular level. You know its needs and desires, when it's happy and unhappy, and how to coexist with it in harmony. It's all a bundle of electricity where every electron affects the whole.

You and your body are a team that is stuck with each other through the good and the bad. There is no other option. It's the nature of the physical and all its influences. It's a tangle of genetics, emotions and ambition. It's a lifetime of habits, some good and some not so good.

Everything is interwoven and you've mastered the assemblage of it all. You're the captain of a complex cast of characters that are the influences of your unique whole. Pure unadulterated desire placed you in the leadership role of your willing subjects. You've earned their respect and now these influences willingly submit to your desires.

The power of pure determination should never be underestimated. There is no limit to what can be accomplished when the mind wants it bad enough. You can take it as far as you want. Only a lack of imagination can hold you back. Unleash your dreams and set them free. Nourish them with raw desire and send them soaring to the heavens.

Apply these principles to your health and fitness goals and fly as high as you want to fly. Soar into the future and peek back into the present. Let the future guide the present towards the magnificent and remarkable. With this positive outlook you will never go back to your unfit ways.

You will never be fat again, never let emotions rule you, never have to deal with insecurities that destroy. You're a supremely confident individual who understands the concept of looking within for the power, energy and force to reckon with challenges and stated goals.

In this situation you'll use that knowledge and willpower to maintain your desired weight. You'll keep eating your basic foundation foods as you've grown to accept them and embrace them. You'll also moderately consume any other items that you loved from the past. The difference is you control them just as they used to control you.

In moderation you can enjoy meats, pizza, desserts or whatever it is you want back in your life. However, they won't wreak havoc like the old days. They'll behave because otherwise they're evicted forever from your life. Your mind is the issuer of all the rules, the dictator of what is allowed into your body.

You're going to maintain your weight. Always opt for the healthier items when you have a choice. Don't stray too far away from the nutritional foundational foods. Fruits, vegetables, oatmeal, low-fat milk, brown rice, uncontaminated potatoes, lean meats, and egg whites still constitute the mainstay of your diet. They are still the center of your life. You'll always prepare them in a healthy manner.

You'll constantly keep a close eye on your weight. The scale is now your best friend. When you see a slight weight gain, you'll go back to the basics. You're an old pro at reining it all back in. Never again will you gain more than three or four pounds. If that happens, you simply shift into raw determination mode and take it off.

Every time you do this you continue to build self-esteem and confidence. Finally, you'll get to the point where you just *know*. You'll intuitively do the right things for your body without even thinking about it. It will be completely automatic.

All of your friends now know you as a winner. Keep it that way. You've placed yourself high on a peak. You're a big success in the minds of your peers. You know what they say, the bigger and higher you are, the harder you fall. That term is absolutely applicable in this situation. It can be precarious if you allow it.

Don't even let the thought of failure enter your mind. You're well aware that this is a never-ending war, but the hard part is done. Eat right and exercise regularly and you'll stay on top. Congratulations and cheers!

Riding high,
Full of success.
Keep it up,
Be the best!

Maintaining Tips

This section will provide a few pointers on how to keep your dream alive and flourishing. Your core confidence will carry you through it, but you can never let your guard down. You've reached your desired weight goal and you've earned the right to *slowly* bring some of your favorite foods back into your life.

You have to treat this as if you're hiking across a frozen lake. The ice is very thin and apt to break at any moment. You're tiptoeing across the lake, praying that the ice holds up until you reach the other side. One little misstep and you're doomed, left to die in the freezing waters. That's exactly the way you need to look at the situation as you slowly bring your old foods back. Treat this lightly and you'll be just another statistic, another weak loser who lost weight and then proceeded to blow it through a lack of discipline. Don't let this occur, for you're a winner.

Let me give an example of how this can happen. Once again, our lovable, but deeply flawed little vegetable provides a real-life experience that educates us. Zarkoff Zucchini never fails to deliver. Every action he takes helps mankind and vegetablekind in some way or another.

In this particular example, we can learn some valuable lessons from the great Zucchini. I'm sure he would admit it wasn't one of his greatest moments. As a matter of fact, it can be added to his ever-growing list of embarrassing episodes.

That's the thing about legendary figures like Zarkoff Zucchini, they teach even as they err.

This particular series of incidents constituted an error in judgement. A couple of years ago, Zarkoff's wife had had enough. Zarkoff's constant philandering and out-in-the-open womanizing had pushed her to the brink of madness. His latest bimbo-chasing escapade had made the covers of every major tabloid, causing her great embarrassment.

Zarkoff had been caught drunk and naked at 3 a.m. in a Ritz-Carlton swimming pool. Tabloid photographs captured the lusty Zarkoff engaging in highly improper activities with three Los Angeles Laker fruit-cheerleaders. He publicly claimed he was lending emotional support to the girls after their team suffered a crushing defeat, but no one bought the story.

Zarkoff's wife finally could take no more and gave the great Zarkoff an ultimatum. "Stop your womanizing or I'm leaving," she was overheard screaming at him. The thought of the love of his life abandoning him put Zarkoff into a tailspin. He began drinking heavily and fell into a depressed state. A longtime carousing buddy offered some advice, seek treatment and receive some professional help.

That's exactly what Zarkoff decided to do. His wife reluctantly gave in and promised to give him one last chance to redeem himself. Couples therapy and marriage counseling were agreed upon and the two began consultation immediately.

It started out well. In front of the counselor, they candidly discussed their problems. Zarkoff even came clean on his affairs with their housekeeper, the housekeeper's cousin, and the cousin's friend. Honesty and openness seemed to be the therapeutic answer to all their issues. Zarkoff's lying past seemed to be done. His wife was actually considering allowing Zarkoff back into the house, as he had been sharing the doghouse with Rover, their beloved chihuahua.

After six weeks of therapy, it came to an abrupt halt. Late one evening, Zarkoff's wife heard Rover barking. This was highly unusual at this time of night. She went out to investigate thinking something may be wrong, possibly an intruder. What she discovered was far worse.

She was right in thinking maybe someone had breached their fence and entered the premises. However, this face was one she recognized. It was Lulu Ann, their marriage therapist. Her head was poking out of the doghouse, The pretty bell pepper was scantily clothed and her hair was a mussed mess. Without saying a word, she exited the doghouse and raced toward the gate. She was gone within a matter of seconds.

Zarkoff's wife was enraged. She knew her husband would be curled up in the back of the doghouse trying to hide. He was probably trying to come up with some outrageous lie as an excuse for having a near-naked female in his home. She called out to him, but received no response. Irate with madness, she lost all control. The nerve of her despicable husband, she was *their therapist*, for God's sake. She would show him!

Their barbeque grill was close by. She reached for the lighter fluid and began spraying the doghouse inside and out. After it was completely drenched in the flammable solution, she lit a match and threw it into the doghouse. It erupted in flames.

Zarkoff could hide no longer, for he was on fire. He desperately rolled out of the doghouse doorway, his pajamas ablaze and his hair completely burned off his handsome veggie head. He headed for his only means of survival, the swimming pool. The water sizzled as he plunged headfirst into the lifesaving water. The coolness helped to soothe his burns.

Zarkoff seemed to stay under forever. What awaited him on the surface was not going to be pleasant. That much he knew for sure. His wife was the angriest he had ever seen her. After a full minute, Zarkoff finally had to get a breath of oxygen. When his head rose out of the pool, he wished he would have just stayed under and drowned.

A bullet went through his ear. Another entered his shoulder. Yet another clipped his nose and it fell into the water. She paused to reload the pistol. This would be his chance to escape this crazed woman caught in a jealous rage. Zarkoff made a run for it.

Zarkoff was atop the gate when a succession of shots rang out. A bullet lodged in his buttocks. He fell to the other side as a bullet destroyed a testicle. Another obliterated his remaining testicle. Ball-less Zarkoff hobbled away as fast as he could. All he could hear in the background was his wife screaming obscenities.

Zarkoff made it to safety that horrifying evening, but it would be months before his wife would speak to him. He had blown it. Those weeks of marriage counseling had been working. They had made great progress until he messed it up. She even accepted the news about his triplet-ladies affair.

Now his marriage was crumbling before him. And now he needed two ball transplants. Ball doners were hard to find.

Once again, there's a lesson in this for all of us. Just because you've reached a plateau of success, that doesn't mean you can slip back into your bad habits. Just as Zarkoff fell off the wagon and began womanizing again, you can do the same if you're not extremely careful. One bite of the wrong food can send you down the same road as Zarkoff.

Females are to him what that crème-filled oatmeal cookie is to you. Don't let your guard down because you've experienced a taste of success. Zarkoff thought he had licked his addictive amorous tendencies, only to realize they had lured him back into a trap. It's the same for you. Bad foods will always be wagging their little fingers at you, lusciously temping you into sin.

Poor ole Zarkoff, he just can't seem to catch a break when it comes to the lovely ladies. You're different. Maybe you're not a world-famous veggie celebrity like Zarkoff Zucchini, but you have more willpower than him. It's up to you and you alone to make sure you don't slip up. Let's go back to the ways to avoid falling back into the fatty-food pit.

> *Zarkoff messed up,*
> *He's on fire.*
> *That's what he gets,*
> *For being a liar!*

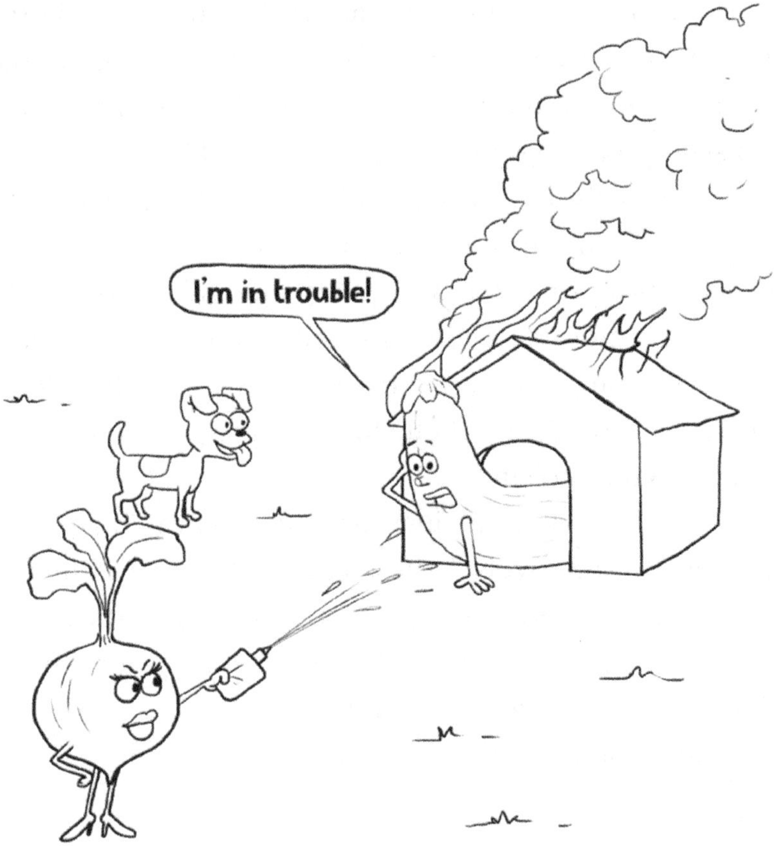
I'm in trouble!

Maintaining Tips II

The key to maintaining your weight is staying aware and never letting your guard down. You can never get cocky and celebrate your success by overindulging with the wrong foods. With that mentality you'll regain the weight and be right back where you started. You'll be just another statistic, another has-been. You'll be looked upon as someone who hasn't the discipline to close the deal.

Soon everyone will forget that you lost all that weight. The ones who do remember will now, subconsciously at least, view you as a loser. So what if you lost forty pounds? That will become old news once you regain it. No one will care that you did something remarkable in the past. They'll simply view you as who you are at the moment. Persevering through the ages and maintaining your weight is what gains their respect.

Remember that you're *never, ever* going back to your former eating habits. Testing the waters *lightly* is the way to go. Slow and easy is the proper approach. Every food that was previously on our hit-list is a potential spoiler. Every morsel of the bad stuff is like a grenade waiting to explode. At any moment you can be blown to bits and take the wrong fork in the road. Once you're navigating that path you're flirting with disaster.

Let's use steak as an example. Throughout your weight-loss battle, you probably didn't indulge in this treat. Now you can allow it back into your life, but you'd better be extremely careful. Have a lean one and thoroughly enjoy it. Then step back and regroup. *Don't get caught up in the trap.*

Every time you try another food, remember that you are still in a war. It may be a cold war, but it's war. Processed foods are relentlessly determined to control you. They never stop coming at you. They have no soul or compassion as they are forever trying to tempt you into failure. It's still the world verses you and you can never forget it. Every one of those salty, sweet, fatty villains is out to conquer you. They want you fat and miserable as that's their mission. Happiness is not part of their agenda.

Let's assume you love sweets, as so many of us do. Maybe you would like a dessert or a sweet snack. Great, go ahead and have a *small* piece of cake or candy and *slowly* enjoy every morsel. Now, stop and analyze the situation. You just consumed some sweets. *Can you handle it?* This is treacherous territory. You can fall hard from that high position you now occupy and it will damn sure hurt.

At any point, always remember that you can go back to the original stringent plan. If you sense danger, play it safe. Revert back to the personalized plan that worked so well and stay there for a few days. Then you can test the waters again.

Stalk that processed food item like a predator stalks its prey. Slow, deliberate, careful and cautious are the keywords. Think about that particular food item for days before you do battle with it. Get emotionally prepared to engage in warfare. If you learn to eat an item *occasionally* and in *moderation*, you'll be fine.

In this critical period, step on the scale at least once a week. The first time you see that you're a couple of pounds over your optimum weight, immediately go back to the program. Get back to where you want to be, then try again. This time you're more experienced and more aware.

Learn your body all over again because this is different than simply losing weight. In some ways it's more difficult. Maintenance is what places you in the winner's bracket. The streets are littered with remains of has-beens who couldn't survive the rocky road of temptation.

Winners never allow the enemy to creep up for an ambush. Show those nasty processed scoundrels who the real boss is. If they come snooping around your territory they're playing with fire. Send them packing down the road.

Go back to your weight-loss program fifty times if necessary. Use it as a faithful, dependable crutch. Eventually you'll figure out what foods are potential disasters for you. They'll be different for everyone. Eliminate them and mark them off as dangerous and totally restricted.

When it comes to fat, remember this fact. Your body needs a certain amount of fat, but not too much. Always get your fat from healthy choices. These include nuts, seeds, fish, and certain vegetable oils. Avocados are an excellent choice. Find the right combination for your unique body as you learn your personal maintenance requirements. Everyone's metabolism is different and you're on your own to discover what works for you.

A very fine line distinguishes necessary fat consumption from over-consumption. It's best to consume a small amount of fat on a daily basis, rather than over-indulge in a fit of bingeing. Experiment and find that perfect point where your body operates at optimum level. Go with your instincts and monitor yourself closely. Keep close tabs by using the scale during experimentation. This is a dangerous minefield that can rip you to shreds if you're not careful.

Let's assume you're where you want to be weight-wise. For a month everything has been running smoothly. A taste here and there of the bad stuff is all you're allowing yourself. Everything is going as planned. You're a star in your circle of friends and you're loving it.

Then you start to get a little cocky and make mistakes. You skip out on returning to the weight-loss program because you're overly confident. Your star will quickly become a falling star. Your lofty position among your peers will be no more. You'll come crashing down and nothing will remain but the crumbs of your success.

Do you think anyone will care that you lost weight only to regain it all back? No, they absolutely won't care. That's like a broke person bragging about how much money he had in the past. All that past money won't do a bit of good when the cashier at Walmart asks how you're going to pay for that merchandise.

People respect the here and now. Yesterday's star means nothing if it's lying on the ground all burned up. To stay in the game, you have to burn bright and stay bright. Maintaining is the hardest part for many people. Keep a close eye on your weight. You worked very hard to get to where you are, so don't blow it. Don't get fat again. Don't be like Zarkoff and give in to your weaknesses. Be a winner and stay a winner. You can do it!

Soaring high,
You're a Star.
You're on top,
Yes You Are!.

CHAPTER 8

The Exercise Plan

"The price of victory is high, but so are the rewards."
Bear Bryant

You Gotta Move

The body was meant to move. The evidence is all around us in the form of obesity. Take a good look at people the next time you go out. Fifty percent of the population are probably overweight, many of them vastly so. Sure, diet is a tremendous factor in this, but lack of exercise is just as much of a determinant. You have to make that machine move. It's that simple. The following story proves this.

"One calorie is one calorie." Zarkoff hesitated to let the kids absorb his words of wisdom. "Two calories are two calories," he continued. His audience of overweight teen tomatoes sat spellbound, glued to their honored guest speaker.

"Three calories are three calories!" a kid from the back row shouted in anticipation of Zarkoff's next intellect-barrier-bursting proclamation.

The Society for Overweight Tomato Tots was lucky enough to book an open date on Zarkoff Zucchini's busy schedule. Zarkoff immediately agreed to the event. Overweight tomatoes were especially dear to his heart, having had an ex-girlfriend who had been an obese tomato.

Zarkoff could never forget that day they met. Tammy Tomato was pretty and thin, with flaming red hair that flowed to the floor. Her eyes melted him on the spot. He fell for her immediately. Tammy and Zarkoff enjoyed a blissful year together as a couple. It came to an abrupt end when Zarkoff ran off with a pretty peach.

Tammy began eating as a way to cope with her loss. She gained 1,000 pounds over the course of a year. She became so big that she couldn't escape the doorway of the greenhouse that she called home. Zarkoff heard of this and guilt overtook him. It was because of him that she had gotten so large.

It just so happened that Tammy was sitting in the front row *and she was thin!* Tammy had lost every pound of the 1,000 pounds she had gained. She attributed it all to a daily exercise routine. The Society for Overweight Tomato Tots had made her an honorary member. She was living proof for the youngsters that any tomato could lose weight if they exercised.

Zarkoff was at a loss for words when he noticed her. He had always regretted running off with Peachy Peach, as that relationship didn't last long due to his affair with her sister. Now here was Tammy looking as good as ever. He wondered if she would take him back.

That thought didn't linger long as Tammy lunged at him. She was wielding a knife. The blade was long and sharp and headed right for his private area. Zarkoff stepped away just in time as the blade ripped into his designer jeans. His private area was exposed for all to see.

"It looks like one, only smaller," a kid cried out. Laughter filled the room. Zarkoff was completely embarrassed, but he didn't have time to worry about that. Tammy was coming at him again with fire in her eyes.

"I'll cut off that little troublemaker if it's the last thing I do!" she shouted. The knife's shiny blade gleamed as the sunlight bounced off it. She took another wide slice at him, barely missing Zarkoff's member. Security guards saw their opportunity and pounced on Tammy, subduing her as she lashed a verbal assault unfit for adolescence ears.

Tammy was taken away, but the damage had been done. Zarkoff was completely embarrassed. A tabloid reporter had been hiding in the crowd and had taken several pictures of his private parts. Now those pictures would be exposed to the world and everyone would know of his tallywacker size issues.

The real lesson to be learned by this story is Tammy Tomato's dedication to her exercise program. You too can lose 1,000 pounds if you exercise daily. I'm kidding, but you certainly will lose weight and tone up. Let's get on with the program and explore the world of exercise. It can be fun and change your life forever.

Lose a pound,
Lose a ton.
Keep it off,
You're never done!

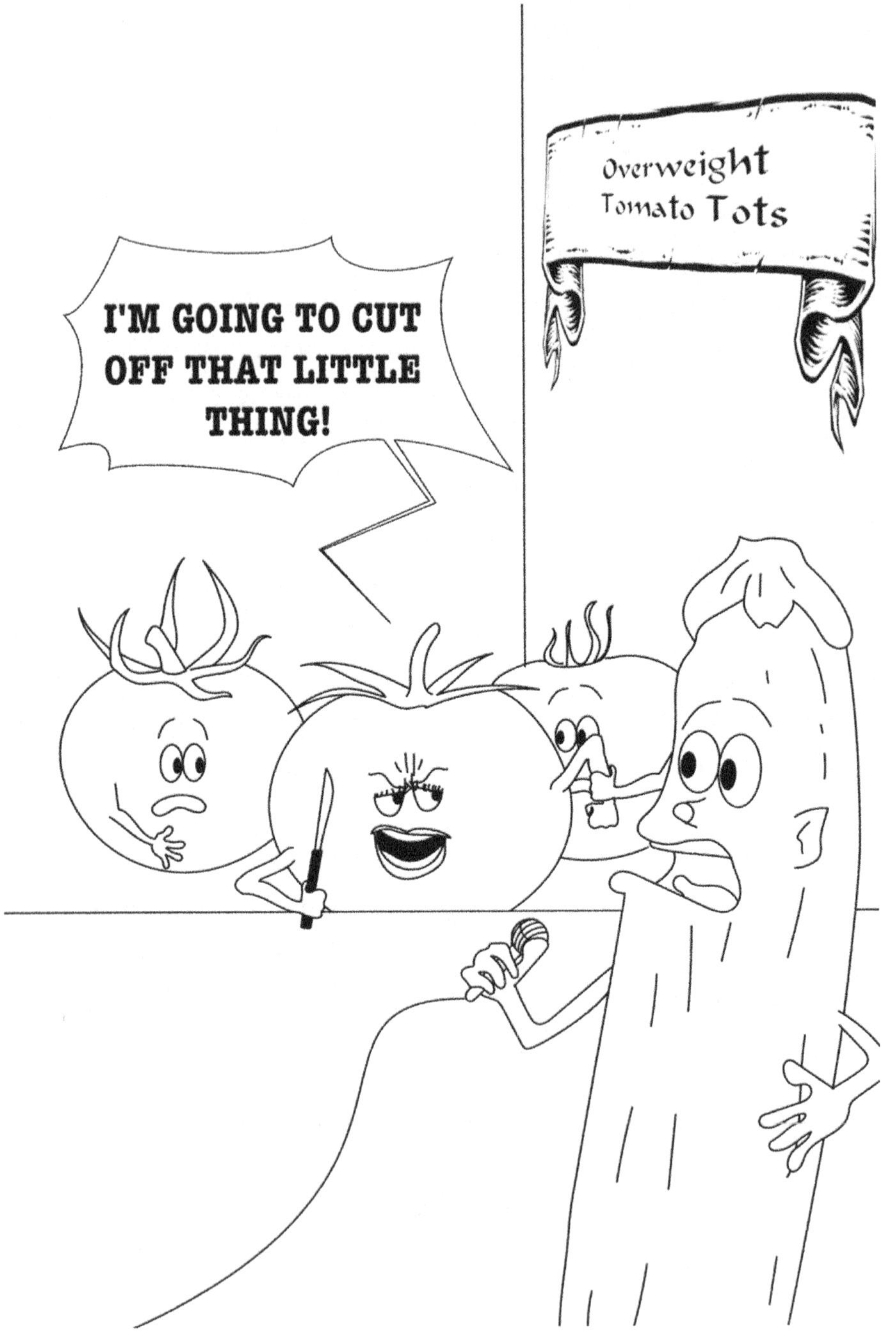

I'M GOING TO CUT OFF THAT LITTLE THING!
Overweight Tomato Tots

Clubs, Equipment & Clothes

There's one great thing about the game of getting fit. It's basically a fair contest where money won't give you an advantage. Money may allow more time for exercise, but other than that, it's pretty much a level playing field. If you possess plenty of money, don't think for a moment that you have an advantage over those less fortunate. The reverse is also true. If you're lacking in funds, don't think that you're at a disadvantage, for you're not.

There are a lot of fat, rich people and there are a lot of fit, poor people. All the money in the world isn't going to keep that cookie out of your mouth if you lack willpower. Just because you're not rich doesn't disqualify you from being the fittest, heathiest one in your circle. It's one of the few arenas on the planet where money takes a back seat to hard work and dedication.

Money may buy your way into a health club and that's fine. Health clubs can be a fantastic place to work out and can provide motivational support. However, that doesn't keep Joe Average from beating them at the fitness game if he so desires. If he wants it more, he'll win regardless of the exercise location.

The muscles in the body could care less if they're being worked in an expensive health club or the parking lot of a homeless shelter. They only respond to the action being issued upon them. Another analogy could be the stomach being filled in an expensive restaurant verses a free food bank.

It's what you eat, not where you eat. It's what you do at your workout, not where your workout is located.

Do you ever feel that lack of time is keeping you from exercising? A lot of people face this challenge. The day is filled with so many have-to-dos that it's sometimes hard to find time for exercise. If that is a real problem for you and you only exercise in a gym, then consider this.

How long is that round trip back and forth to the gym? Is it twenty minutes, thirty minutes, or maybe even more? With the time most people use to drive to and from the fitness club, they could have done their exercise routine in their home. Some people overlook the obvious and neglect this option.

If time and money are not factors, and you *enjoy* it, then by all means keep going to your health club. Some people really enjoy the social aspect of fitness clubs. There's nothing wrong with that, just remember you're there for a purpose. You're there to work, not turn it into a party.

There are some people who join these clubs simply to boast that they work out at such and such a club. They make an appearance and go through the motions of an exercise routine without really exercising. That's not going to get you very far. Do it for a reason, do it for yourself, for you'll be truly rewarded.

Many people choose to exercise in their home. It's actually very simple to do so. For the price of a couple of months dues on the health club, you can purchase some basic equipment for your home.

All you really need is a good pair of walking shoes and a set of used dumbbells. That will suffice, for what you're looking for is to get the heart rate up and to strengthen those muscles. There are numerous ways to do this. In actuality, you can get by without the dumbbells. Pushups, crunches, and other exercises where you're using your own body as weight resistance can be just as good.

Regarding exercise clothes, does anyone really care? I personally wear the street clothes which I wore the day before *if they're comfortable.* My exercise demonstration photos will attest to that. Yesterday's clothes can handle a final workout before they go into the wash. I'm a laundry efficiency fanatic, so I'm always cutting corners in that area.

As far as shoes, I've found a pair of basic work boots perform best for me. They're great for walking. They offer wonderful support for my geezed ankles and feet, as well as generating chuckles from surprised onlookers. Take care of your feet and they'll take care of you. The work boots also add a little extra weight to my leg lifts which I like. I don't really care if others snicker behind by back.

I actually enjoy seeing fashionable workout attire on others, so it's simply a matter of choice. Zarkoff was a sucker for tight-fitting spandex on his women. He said that was a very sexy look. Poor ole Zark had a one-track mind.

A treadmill or stationary bike might be a nice addition for some of you. They're especially good as an inclement-weather option when you have to stay inside. There are lots of quality ones out there on the used market.

Exercise equipment in general tends to retain value because in many cases it's rarely used. I'm sure you know someone who's purchased all the latest fitness gear only to hang clothes on it. They'll use it a couple of times and then it's back to their old habits. You may have even done this yourself.

A basic bicycle can be purchased for a minimal amount of money, even a new one. There's absolutely no need to go out and get a multi-geared fancy bike that the professionals use. So many people do this, mistakenly thinking that the more expensive the bike, the more fit you'll become. Really?

Sure, you can go further and faster with a fancy bike, but you would be missing the whole point. Aerobic exercise is the purpose for riding in the first place. I hate to break the news to you, but we old geezers aren't going to win any medals at the next Tour de France. Nobody really cares that you logged thirty miles of biking in one session, especially when your bike is designed to cover more distance with less effort. What they really notice are physical results. I'd rather work hard to go five miles myself.

I'm not trying to discourage you if you're really into that sort of biking. Go out and enjoy it. It looks like a great social activity along with exercise. What I'm saying is it's not going to make a difference in your aerobic value verses a regular cheap bike. It's all about getting that heart pumping and the heart doesn't give a hoot what brand of bicycle you're riding. The poor man can win at this game. All he needs is the desire to do so.

If daily mileage is important to you, then jump in a fast car and push the pedal to the floor. You'll get there in a hurry. Then you can tell everyone you knocked out 300 miles today. You'll get your mileage quota accomplished in a hurry. I have serious doubts that it's going to improve your fitness level though.

I've seen many people, in the heat of the *I'm going to get fit* moment, spontaneously go out and purchase an enormous, expensive, complicated, multi-purposed weight machine. Some of these things have more computer technology than a NASA rocket.

Once again, the poor man can hold his own here as well. A little set of dumbbells that gets used is a much better purchase than an expensive clothes-hanging device. I won't even mention how you'll stub your toe three times a day on those heavy protrusions sticking out at the bottom. Ouch!

Men seem to be the worst when it comes to bulking up the house with an ugly weight contraption. In a fit of action-hero delusion, we'll go out and spend the mortgage money on the latest weight machine being pushed by *Muscle Today* magazine. Its hideous presence and massive bulk will be used for a total of four hours before it transforms into its real purpose, toe-stubber.

Don't get me wrong, some people actually use these things. If you're doing so, keep up the good work. Just know there's no need to rush out and purchase a costly piece of fitness equipment. It could turn out to be the most expensive piece of furniture you own, and it certainly won't land you on the cover of *Better Homes and Gardens* for its aesthetic value.

Let me expand a bit on the subject of workout attire. I guess I'll have to emphasize again that the body doesn't care what clothing adorns it when it sweats. Does the woman wearing the name-brand workout suit get more fit than the woman working out in her underwear at home? No, because it doesn't work like that.

Just because you're making a fashion statement doesn't mean your body is going to respond accordingly. I've seen more than a few plump women strolling the gym showing off the latest clothing. I've also seen women wearing the most basic exercise clothes who have fantastic bodies.

Worry about that body underneath those clothes. The rest will take care of itself. Make sure your clothes are comfortable and don't rub you in the wrong places. Safe and comfortable, that's the key in this department. Let your body be your fashion statement.

The main point of this is that getting fit isn't related to money. If money could buy health and fitness, there wouldn't be any fat, rich people. However, if you look around, you'll see plenty of them. If you have money, then get out there and exercise and eat right. That's the only way that weight's coming off. If you don't have money, then your situation is the same. There are no excuses allowed related to money. We all have to work.

> ***Not much money,***
> ***But I am thin.***
> ***Who needs money,***
> ***I like to WIN!***

General Exercise Plan

The concept is simple. Make sure you do some cardio activity that gets the blood flowing and strengthen your muscles with some light resistance training. Many of you want to lose weight, so the aerobic sector of your routine is very important. That's what really speeds up your metabolism and eventually sheds those pounds.

Zarkoff Zucchini was a huge advocate of aerobic exercise. He claimed it helped with endurance and stamina. With his busy schedule and his numerous extracurricular activities, he certainly was one who needed an abundant supply of energy.

There was no doubt that Zarkoff was a man of incredible energy, having fathered numerous mixed-race fruits and vegetables. His DNA is spread across every continent. There is even a village in Antarctica populated by mostly Zarkoff descendants.

Zarkoff was once there as part of a fruit and vegetable delegation, spending a month at a seasonal research station. He did his research all right, researching pretty fruits and vegetables and how they respond sensually in a glacial-ice-covered environment. The response resulted in little Zarkoffs running around everywhere there today. His child-support bill is outrageous.

Let Zarkoff Zucchini be an example to us all. The fact that a vegetable of his caliber was a huge proponent of aerobic exercise says it all. If the father of half of Antarctica engaged in aerobic activity of all sorts, then we shall do the same. Hail to the greatest procreator ever of icy terrain-based fruits and veggies, the sperm-guidance instructor who provided a vast array of nutrient-rich foods to a veggie-deficient continent, the great Zarkoff.

Your aerobic exercise might not be quite as exciting as Zarkoff's heart-racing adventures, but you won't have jealous, weapon-wielding females chasing you down either. Drama sure seemed to follow poor ole Zarkoff, but somehow our esteemed leader managed to survive. We might not be so lucky, so let's keep our exercise safe and weapon-free.

Let's discuss our simple exercise plan. Losing weight is a major goal for many of you. I'll repeat once more, because it is *so* important, *be patient*. If you think you're going to lose decades of chub-chub in one week, you're setting yourself up for a *massive* psychological avalanche. Set your mind to the one-year theory and then watch as the weeks and months speed by. The year will pass and so will the chub-chub.

We're going to start with exercises that get the heart beating. Strength exercises will be brought in to your routine ever so gradually. Don't get me wrong, I certainly realize the value of strength training. However, a lot of you haven't exercised in a very long time. Look at the initial light aerobic exercise as a warmup for the strength buildup later. This is for two reasons. The first reason is that aerobics are major fat-burners and speed up the metabolism. After all, you are trying to lose weight.

The second reason is injuries. If you jump right into lifting heavy weights, you're apt to pull or strain something, or rip something out completely. Remember these muscles and connecting parts of ours are quickly becoming historical in nature. That means *we're old. We're geezers!*

That's why a simple walk around the neighborhood is how we'll begin our exercise program. We're going to ease into this, otherwise it's back to sitting in front of the TV watching nonsense and listening to canned laughter while our bodies try to recover from injuries.

What kind of shape are you currently in? What is your current fitness level? It matters not if you're already in great shape and simply trying to tune your body up, or if you haven't moved your body in decades. The concept is the same. Start at a level where you feel completely comfortable. Overdo day one and there won't be a day two.

For many of you that may be a five-minute walk or even less. That's okay, for no one is here to judge and punish. That slow five-minute walk today can be a jaunty hour-long walk a year from now. Walking, whether outside or on a treadmill, is an incredibly simplistic activity that works. It's easy to monitor and an exercise that rarely injures the body.

There you have lesson one of the overall exercise program. Walking is the primary component, particularly during the early stages. You can substitute a stationary bike or a regular bike if you prefer. Any low-stress aerobic activity will do the trick. The key is to make the heart beat faster for an extended period of time without risking injury. That's the only goal.

You'll start out very slowly and gradually build up your time and distance. How much time and distance are added and *when* they is added depends on your fitness level. If you're starting with a five-minute walk, then you may consider adding one minute per week. That doesn't sound like much, but that puts you at an hour in a year. An hour-long walk is a great feat for anyone of any age. Some of you may decide twenty minutes is your limit. That's fine, just do it regularly. That's the real key to success.

Please don't get discouraged if you're starting at the bottom fitness level. That only means your amazement-factor will be off the charts when you succeed. Others will respect you for what you've done, especially since you started from such a challenging position. If you're extremely overweight, then that's just the way it is *at the moment*. You're going to take charge and change the situation. You'll show them!

To all of you macho males out there, I know you're chomping at the bit to jump under those weights and transform yourself overnight. Leave those weights alone until your body gets used to some movement. You're not going to be Rocky Balboa in one week, especially if you're sitting in a wheelchair recovering from injuries.

When you instinctively feel your body can handle it, you'll incorporate some *light* weights into the program. You'll also include a couple of body-weight resistance exercises. This applies to men and women. Think of the weight training as a complete bonus. The walking or low-stress aerobic activity is still the bread-and-butter soul of your exercise program. Ingrain this into your psyche for it's a *forever* thing.

> *Look at me,*
> *In one year.*
> *I'll be fit,*
> *I have no fear!*

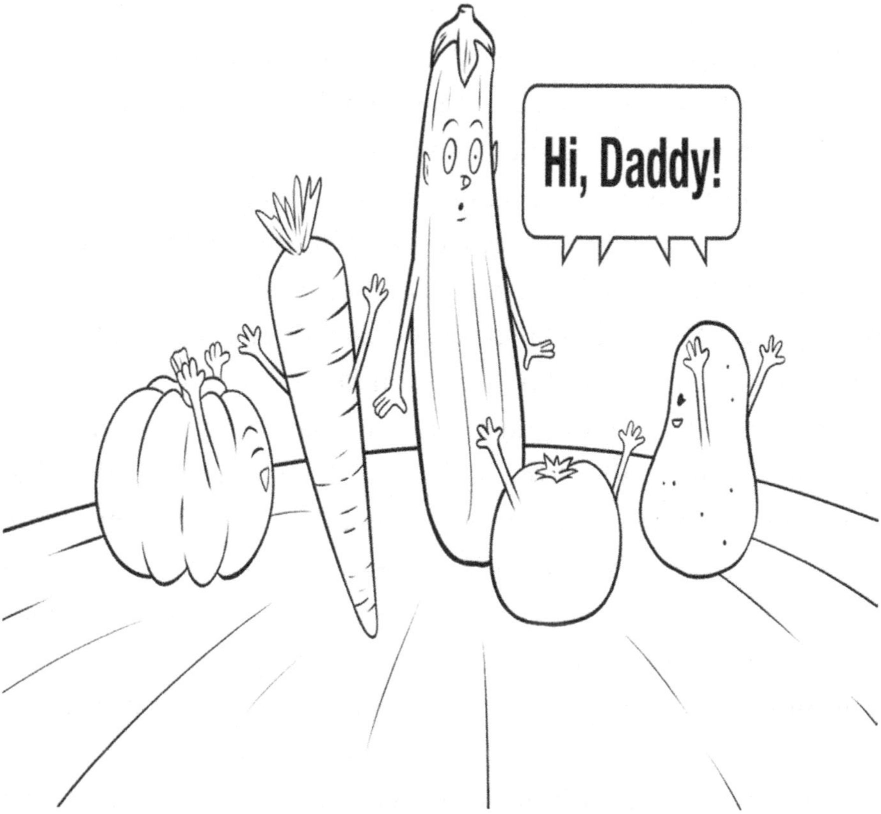
Hi, Daddy!

General Exercise Plan II

We'll delve into the details a little later, but for now here's the basic weight plan. The same principle applies here as the walking. You'll start with a weight so minimal you'll hardly notice it. You'll do two or three reps and put them away. Continue this for a week, then maybe consider adding a *minute* amount of weight or maybe an additional rep.

If you're looking a year ahead, and you should, you see that you'll be at a much heavier weight and many more reps by then. Patience is the key. Remember you're on the attack in the dietary department also. You'll definitely lose weight with this double-edged frontal assault on fat.

Try to get your simple startup workout in *every* day. The wonderful thing about the gradual incremental increase is the habit factor. You're developing a habit from the ground up. "Anyone can walk five minutes, right?" should be the way you'll view it. Take five minutes from your day and just do it.

That five turns into six and seven and eight while the habit continues to develop. You're at a lower risk of skipping your routine when it incrementally becomes a part of your daily life. Soon a twenty-minute walk will be as natural as that first cup of coffee in the morning.

At this stage I see no need for ever taking a day off from your routine. Definitely never plan a day off, for unexpected events affecting your schedule usually take care of your necessary rest periods. Simply plug yourself in like a robot and get it done. Try to keep the attitude of "never a day off."

Don't worry, uncontrollable events will take care of your rest requirements.

If you're one of those super-disciplined individuals, and I hope you are, you'll be able to plan an occasional day off. Try not to take more than one day off per week. Some individuals can go a month without a day off.

Length of exercises, intensity of workouts, sleep needs, and nutrition habits are among the many factors determining your body's rest requirements. Get to know your body and it will begin to communicate with you. It's truly amazing when that happens. When you're really tuned in, you'll know exactly what every little ache is telling you.

Sometimes the body is congratulating you on pushing it to just the right level. Other times it may be relaying important information that you're pushing too hard and it's time to take a day off, or at minimum, lower the intensity. Over time you'll learn the signals and what they mean.

Some days you may feel like skipping your exercise. Depression, time constraints, and daily worries are constantly working against you. Unless you're concerned about injuries or you absolutely know your body needs rest, *do not skip your exercise*. It's as much of a psychological backstep as a physical one.

Put yourself into a mindless zone and let all those deep thoughts melt into the background. Free your emotions and concerns and force yourself into an automatic gear. Begin stretching and then pick up your dumbbells, begin walking, or step onto the treadmill. You're still in stubborn mode at this point and raw determination is the guiding force. Make your body do it regardless of what your brain desires.

What happens next is amazing! After a few minutes you're into it, chugging along like a machine. Before you know it, the routine is complete and you're riding high psychologically. You'll look back and say, "What was I thinking? I feel great!" What began as a tremendous struggle turned out to a rewarding workout.

It's all in the mind. It starts with that winning mental attitude that rules everything. You are unstoppable if you believe in yourself. Your workout is done and you feel great about yourself. Your confidence is so high that others feel it. It's like an aura has enveloped you and shadows you everywhere you go. It all starts from within.

Compare this with a decision to skip your workout. All day long you would have walked around carrying that guilt in the back of your mind. You would be looking back and wishing you would have made the right decision to exercise. Once you've experienced these highs and lows, they'll motivate you.

The pedestal that you're perched upon after your workout is a feeling like none other. The low that goes with cancelling your workout is like a pain in your gut that won't go away. You live with it, at least subconsciously, all day long. Make that high your new drug, for it's a healthy drug.

All this is possible because you went robotic and started your routine. You put your body under automation and would not allow your brain to say *no*. All you needed was that little push and then you found yourself in a different world with a different mentality. One fork in the road can make such a difference, so follow the right path. You'll be rewarded for it.

Be determined to maintain your exercise schedule. You probably brush your teeth and shower every day, so exercise every day also. Make it a non-negotiable daily requirement that has to be done. Do something every day and tune up your body. Trust me, persistence and patience will eventually pay off. You'll see results and be so proud.

> *I'm a geezer,*
> *I'm so wise.*
> *I'm a geezer,*
> *I Exercise!*

Stretching & Injuries

Zarkoff Zucchini's rich heritage included two uncles who founded a prestigious law firm. Zucchini & Zucchini LLP specialized in sporting negligence injuries. Billions of dollars were awarded to their clients, most of them related to stretching. Corporations and individuals alike shuddered at the thought of being sued by Zucchini & Zucchini.

Their reputation in the field of stretching-injury litigation sent potential defendants cowering in fear. One high-profile case involved a well-known health club. They were accused of failure to provide ample stretching areas in their facilities. Veggie Health & Fitness provided no stretching areas whatsoever in their numerous locations. The results were preventable injuries by the club-goers who needed to be compensated.

One such club-goer who sought legal representation from Zucchini & Zucchini was a pretty little carrot who claimed a stretching-negligence-injury. Cooches Carrot was a regular visitor at Veggie Health & Fitness. She worked out to stay in shape for her job as a stripper. Cooches verses Veggie Health & Fitness would be a monumentally influential court decision.

Dancing at All Nude Veggies was physically demanding, so it was vital that naked girls stretch before engaging in gyrating activities. Veggie Health & Fitness had no such stretching facilities. Due to this negligence, Cooches strained her hamstring while simulating a pole climbing exercise. Now she was out for blood and compensation. Tips had dwindled down to a pittance. She could barely pay her narcotics dealer, much less her Louis Bourdon Exotics credit card.

Jurors sat spellbound as lead attorney Zavia Zucchini drilled witness after witness in an effort to prove stretching-negligence. It quickly became obvious that Cooches had a convincing case against the health club. Zucchini finally called Cooches to the stand to testify.

Jurors watched in horror as she was dramatically delivered to the stand on a stretcher. A couple of them openly wept at the young girl's misfortune. Zucchini & Zucchini knew just how to capture jurors' hearts. Although Cooches could walk just fine, the stunt obviously touched all who witnessed it.

Poor Cooches herself shed a few tears as a team of medics placed her in a wheelchair. Cooches then gave a very convincing testimonial of how she was wrongfully injured. She emphasized how hard it would be to continue nude stripping under these horrendous medical conditions.

It was finally time for the defense to call witnesses in their behalf. "Your Honor, we have a surprise witness we would like to call to the stand," stated their lead attorney. "I would like to call Zarkoff Zucchini to testify."

Zavia Zucchini watched in disbelief as nephew Zarkoff took the stand. How could his famous nephew be involved in this case? What could he have to do with a stripper's stretching injury? He watched intently as the defense team began grilling Zarkoff.

"Mr. Zucchini, were you present at All Nude Veggies strip club on the evening of August 11, the night before the alleged stretching incident at the gym?" asked the lead attorney.

"Yes, I was," answered Zarkoff.

"Did you have any encounter with the plaintiff, Cooches Carrot, on that particular evening?" the attorney asked. "Remember you are under oath, Mr. Zucchini."

"Yes, I did, sir," replied Zarkoff.

The attorney nodded. "And exactly what was that encounter, Mr. Zucchini?"

"Cooches gave me a lap dance that night, sir," quietly answered Zarkoff.

The attorney paused for a moment before he spoke. "And did anything out of the ordinary occur during that lap dance, Mr. Zarkoff?"

"Yes sir," answered Zarkoff.

"And exactly what was that out-of-the-ordinary occurrence, Mr. Zucchini?" asked the attorney. "Let me remind you again, you are under oath."

Zarkoff gave a quick glance toward his uncle. As he lowered his head in shame, he stated, "I was very intoxicated from drinking whisky. I got very aroused during the dance and accidently knocked Cooches on the floor. Then I fell on top of her, injuring her leg."

Everyone in the courtroom was stunned. Cooches had *not* injured her hamstring due to a lack of stretching facilities in the gym. Cooches had injured her leg in a lap dance incident involving Zarkoff Zucchini. The randy vegetable activist had once again let the wrong head do his thinking for him.

The case was quickly resolved by the jury. Veggie Health & Fitness was acquitted. Cooches would receive no monetary award for damages. It was a total disaster for everyone on the side of the plaintiff.

Zucchini & Zucchini had wasted time and energy pursuing a case that went nowhere. Family relations within the Zucchini clan would remain strained for months to come. Cooches would never again give Zarkoff a lap dance. The ensuing publicity did nothing to help Zarkoff's strained marriage. It was a dark moment for the young vegetable.

Let this be a lesson learned. Cooches admitted under oath that she had not stretched that evening of her infamous Zarkoff lap dance. Failure to stretch before a full night of gyrating on various laps had, at least indirectly, resulted in a strained hamstring.

The courtroom listened,
As Zarkoff said,
He was thinking,
With the wrong head.

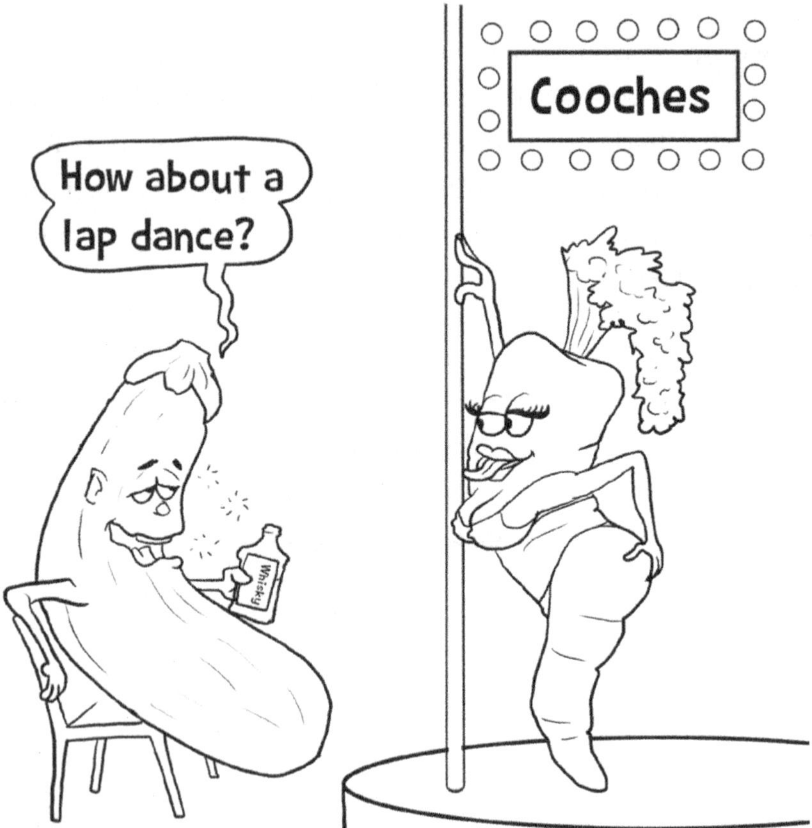
How about a lap dance?
Cooches
Whisky

Stretching & Injuries II

Let's move on from Cooches and get back to the subject at hand, the importance of stretching. Cooches forgot to stretch that evening and she paid the price. Don't let this happen to you. Never underestimate the value of loosening up those geezed muscles and joints before engaging in any physical activity, be it a crunch, pushup, or lap dance.

Regardless of whether you're a well-conditioned athlete or a *Matlock* expert who hasn't left the couch in thirty years, stretching is vital. The older we are, the more important stretching becomes. Young kids can awake from a deep sleep and immediately become loose, limber play machines. We're no longer kids.

Stretching is so important that if you have only ten minutes allotted for fitness, spend the entire ten minutes stretching. Make yourself flexible. Under no circumstances do you jump up and begin your routine without stretching. One major muscle strain or injury and you'll learn.

Most people in our age group will experience minor muscle strains even with proper stretching before their workouts. You are cordially inviting total disaster if you exercise without a full body stretch. As a general rule, always try to "think young."

In this case, however, always remember that you're a geezer. Old geezers need at least ten minutes of stretching before even changing a television channel on the remote. There have been incidents where geezers have been hospitalized with injuries related to changing from ESPN to ESPN2.

If you are going for a walk or a bike ride, it will primary be a lower body workout. That does *not* excuse you from loosening up your upper body and arms. Get your upper body as loose and limber as possible. Of course, your legs and midsection should be *very* loose.

Try to stretch every muscle in your legs. Gently limber up your lower back and stomach muscles. No muscle is too small to ignore. That could be the one that rips away from the connecting parts and puts you out of commission for a few weeks. You definitely don't want to be placed on *Matlock* watch and forego your routine.

If you're preparing for an upper body workout, ensure that your arms, chest, and ribcage areas are thoroughly loose. Roll your head around very slowly to loosen the neck muscles. Go both directions. This is *very* important at our geezer stage. Geezed necks are a major nerve center for overall geeziness. Don't neglect the lower body simply because it's an upper body workout. Spend a few minutes stretching your legs and midsection.

Everything's interconnected and when one geezer part decides to rebel against movement, it warns all other geezer allies to shut down along with it. The result is a total geezer freeze-up. Then you're back at the bar talking Little League glory days with other freeze-up buddies.

If stretching seems like a big hassle prior to exercising, you're right. You're so anxious to get started that it's only natural to want to get on with the program. The trick is to enjoy it. There's no way around this crucial step, so get used to it and embrace it. As you stretch, be imaginative. Let that geezy mind flow.

Think back to those pre-geezer days when you were a cretinous philistine, (that means being a dummy.) Think about being young and stupid and how good those days were. Being stupid was so much fun. As you stretch you can reminisce about your most foolish times. Come on, you know you did some naughty things. Geezers have so much material to pull out of that memory bank. Enjoy those memories before time steals them away. Stretching is an excellent time to let the mind wander.

Be patient as you stretch and don't rush it. Start very gently. It is possible to obtain a serious injury from stretching alone. Get to know your body and develop your personal style of stretching routine. Don't make it painful in the least, for that's a warning sign of a unified muscle freeze-up. You're doing something wrong if you have any pain.

In the winter, be especially careful and allow more time to warm up. Muscles take longer to loosen up in cold weather. Regardless of the weather, *never* underestimate the importance of your pre-workout stretching. It doesn't hurt to do a little post-exercise stretch also, or even mid-exercise. Make a point to stay limber at all times. Train those muscles and joints to bend and stretch at your will.

Develop the mindset *now* that stretching is *part* of your program, a *huge* part. If you don't exhibit the patience required to perform this critical step, you're going to pay in a big way. Major, or even minor injuries, can discourage you to the point of completely abandoning your exercise program. Then you'll become just another freeze-up victim telling white lies at the bar as your body continues to deteriorate. *Do not let injuries occur. Always stretch!*

Despite what every fitness expert advises about stretching and starting out slowly, most people eventually suffer an injury. I'm as guilty as anyone here. I think it's human nature to want to push yourself to the limit. Determination to succeed sometimes pushes you to the edge. When you exceed your physical limits, injuries occur.

I know many of you will be dummies like me, and sure enough you'll push yourself too hard. The result will be an injury of some sort. Let's stop the madness right here. Ninety percent of all injuries can be avoided by some simple stretching and starting your fitness program incrementally. By this, I mean adding to it very slowly.

I don't have to tell you that as we age our bodies lose flexibility. Over the years we've become well aware of that fact. Stiff and rigid joints remind us every day. Although we can overcome that somewhat by stretching, exercising, and eating right, we're probably going to have to accept this condition. You can only fight aging to a point.

Our bodies now break instead of bending, so we have to know exactly where that breaking point is. Learn your body and its limits. Find that breaking point *without breaking*. Stay well under that point as you begin your exercise program.

You can eventually raise the bar somewhat and get a little closer to the edge. Go with the flow and use your intuitive senses to read your body. This will start to make sense as you progress through your program.

Most of you will be starting your nutrition program at the same time you begin exercising. The change in diet alone will be a monumental undertaking, so don't add additional stress by overemphasizing the exercise program. Pace yourself like the turtle, not the hare. This will avoid those painful injuries. You'll get to the finish line and it will be a smooth process, not one full of braces, bandages and pain pills.

Th first segment of your exercise plan should be getting the body used to some movement. You can't expect an old body to just decide one day that it's now sixteen again. You have to negotiate a deal with your body. Both parties have to give and take and meet in the middle.

You agree not to push the body too fast and the body agrees not to break. Both of you end up winning with this agreement. The body becomes stronger and healthier and you're feeling good about yourself. Stubbornness on the part of either party and the whole thing falls apart. Everyone becomes a loser in that scenario.

You took forty years or so to work on getting out of shape, so take a few years to get back in shape. Trying to get in shape in one week is asking for big trouble. Shock and awe won't cut it in the fitness arena. The body doesn't react well to suddenly being punished.

It wasn't the body's fault all those oatmeal cookies and ice cream were stuffed inside it for decades. It didn't ask for a dozen soft drinks a day for thirty years. It didn't ask to be stored away like a junk car in front of a TV for decades when it should have been driven. Things get rusty when they're not used.

The body didn't ask for this. These were all intellectual decisions made by its manager. Now the manager has to deal with the current situation in a reasonable manner. Revolt by the body isn't a pleasant thing and injuries are the grim reminder.

Here's the bottom line on injuries. Avoid them at all costs by stretching and starting slowly. Did you get that? *Start your exercise plan slowly!* Do something every day, but that something doesn't have to destroy ligaments and tendons. Time is now your friend, not your enemy. Be the turtle and survive the marathon.

If you do have an injury, you have to deal with it. You cannot get discouraged and quit the game. Learn all the signals and try to distinguish between a slight muscle strain and something worse. Often you can continue your normal workout even with a minor injury. Other times you cannot.

If it's a borderline case in your opinion, play it safe. Possibly choose an easier exercise and approach it slowly with less intensity. Maybe you could take a day or two off with nothing but a stretching routine. Maintenance of injuries is an acquired art that requires a touch of common sense.

One or two injuries and you'll be highly motivated to *avoid* them entirely. It's frustrating to be chomping at the bit to exercise when your body is broken. Do not fall to pieces if you have a major injury. Work other muscle groups and *really* watch what you eat. Your metabolism will slow as you slow. Fight it out and you will eventually heal. Avoid the next injury because now you know the penalty. Good luck!

Always stretch,
Make it a rule.
Don't get hurt,
Don't be a FOOL!

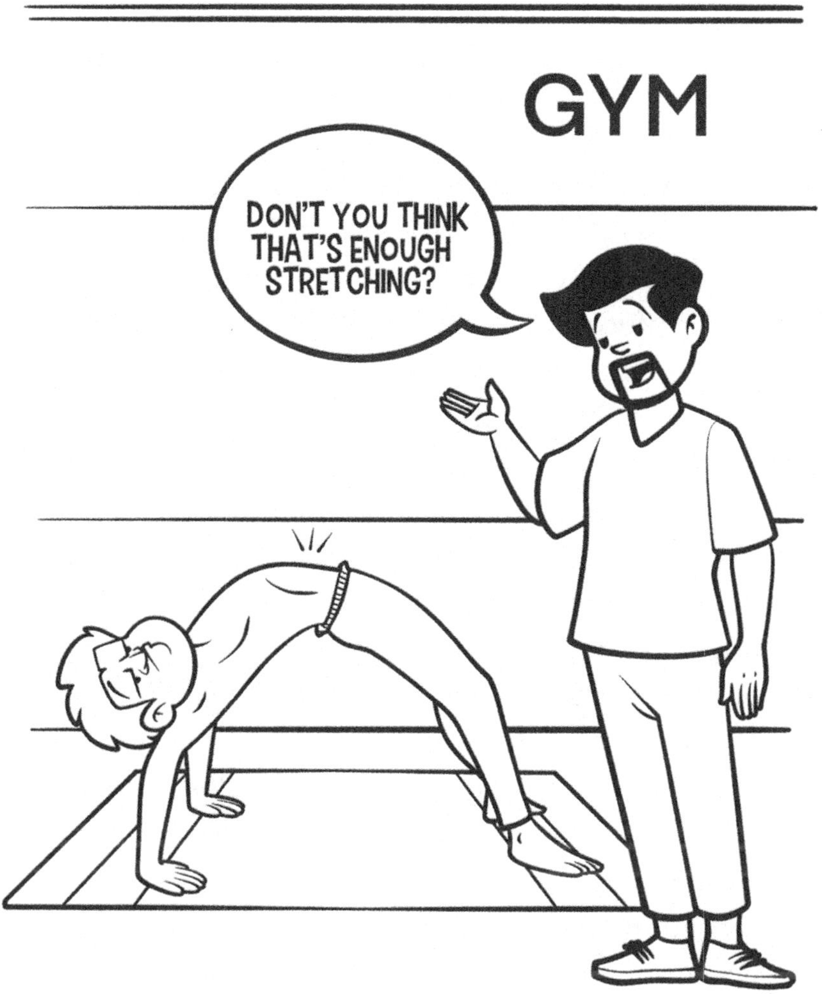
GYM
DON'T YOU THINK THAT'S ENOUGH STRETCHING?

The Joy of Walking

Walking should be the heart and soul of your exercise program. You *must* engage in some aerobic activity. If you can't walk outside, I suggest a treadmill, stationary bike or regular bike. Any exercise machine that gets that geezed heart beating will suffice.

Walking with friends can be gratifying, but make sure it's all about the walking. The focus must stay on the walk and not transform into a gossip session. One case of a walking group that went awry involved our amorous friend, Zarkoff Zucchini.

It started innocently, a group of female office workers who decided to walk during their lunch hour. They were doing so in an attempt to lose weight. They performed administrative duties at the Global Center for Vegetable Equality. The three workers included a grapefruit, a watermelon, and an eggplant. All the girls were pretty, but somewhat overweight, and the watermelon especially so.

One beautiful autumn afternoon they were doing their usual laps around the parking lot when a big, black limousine pulled up. Who could be so important that a limousine was required for their transportation? The girls slowed a bit and watched as two occupants climbed out from the back seat.

"Look!" exclaimed Eleanor Eggplant, "that's Omar Onion, the head of Gardens for the World Foundation."

"Oh my," cried Gabriella Grapefruit. "That's Zarkoff Zucchini with him. He's the famous vegetable activist."

"Oh, that Zarkoff is so handsome," Melanie Melon said in her sultry voice. "I would love to meet him."

"Maybe you'll get the chance," said Eleanor Eggplant. "I think they're here for two days. There's a veggie awareness event going on until Friday."

As fate would have it, Zarkoff would encounter the three girls separately later that morning. Zarkoff being Zarkoff, innocently or maybe not so innocently, invited each of the girls to join him and Omar later that evening. They would be going to Veggie Tiki, a poolside restaurant and bar that had become a local institution.

Zarkoff got an early start when he arrived at Veggie Tiki. He began downing shots of tequila and liters of beer. Before he knew it his head was spinning. He called his office and had all afternoon meetings cancelled because he had a stomach virus. Zarkoff was an accomplished liar when he had to be.

His secretary reminded him that today was his wedding anniversary and his wife would be expecting to hear from him. Zarkoff downed another shot and quickly forgot about that trivial task. He never thought wedding anniversaries were of much importance anyway.

Around his eighth shot of the fiery alcohol, an old friend just happened to sit down beside him at the bar. It was Kiki Kale, an adult film star Zarkoff had befriended a few years back. They had quickly bonded back then because they shared the same strain of herpes virus. Kiki was soon retiring and was actually looking for a serious mate. Zarkoff would be a great catch.

A few shots later Zarkoff and Kiki were smooching away at the bar. A drunken Zarkoff told her he would gladly be her long-term mate. They would begin their committed relationship immediately. Kiki was overjoyed at the news, but she had to go back to the studio to finish filming her last movie. Cameras were waiting.

Kiki left and Zarkoff continued throwing back shots of tequila. Soon he noticed a familiar face in the seat that Kiki had just relinquished. It was Gabriella Grapefruit, one of the young ladies he had met earlier. She was looking pretty at the moment, very pretty.

Zarkoff may have been drunk, but that didn't interfere with his natural charm. As a matter of fact, alcohol seemed to make him more lovable. It wasn't long before he and Gabriella were kissing where he and Kiki were doing the same earlier. Gabriella fell under Zarkoff's spell and they agreed to begin dating. An ecstatic Gabriella soon left the bar due to prior obligations, but she was looking forward to their planned dinner date the next day.

No sooner than Gabriella walked out the door, Eleanor Eggplant strolled in. Zarkoff had never seen such a more gorgeous eggplant in his entire life. She had shed her office attire and replaced it with a low-cut blouse and the shortest shorts he had ever seen. She was hot and voluptuous and she had her sights dead set on the famous veggie activist.

The two quickly established a chemistry that exploded right there in the bar. Charlie Cucumber, the longtime bartender, had to warn them about their public display of affections. Children were present in the restaurant area and had begun to take notice. Eleanor was only present for an hour. She too had to leave due to prior obligations.

It had been a successful hour. Zarkoff was meeting her for dinner the following evening. An enraptured Eleanor left the bar riding high on cloud nine. She couldn't believe her good fortune. Zarkoff Zucchini was her new man.

As Zarkoff turned up another shot, he noticed the most beautiful watermelon he had ever laid eyes upon. She was walking right towards him. It was Melanie Melon! She too had changed into different attire, a skimpy dress that barely covered her dark green body. She looked so much better than she did at the office building. She was hot!

Zarkoff had always been attracted to large women. Melanie was the biggest watermelon he had ever seen and he could barely control himself. He had to get to know this lovely sexpot better.

Melanie took an immediate liking to the smooth-talking, famous zucchini. Zarkoff soon had her under his magnetic spell and they began planning a future together. Melanie became extremely amorous over this news. An intoxicated Zarkoff meant every word he said at the time. They even discussed marriage plans. They both wanted a future together and maybe have some kids.

The evening ended with a long kiss in the parking lot as they went their separate ways. An elated Melanie Melon couldn't wait until their planned dinner date the following evening. She would be having dinner with Zarkoff Zucchini! She was already planning what she would wear for the big night. She would dress to impress.

The following day a hungover Zarkoff barely made it to his morning meeting. His head hurt so much that all he wanted to do was go back to sleep. What did he do yesterday? He had no memory of anything after Kiki Kale left the bar.

He did have a faint memory of making a date with Kiki, but it was too hazy to register completely. Charlie Cucumber had politely told him to leave the bar because he was too drunk. He did remember that much. Everything in between was a total blackout.

As the morning progressed Zarkoff began to feel a little better. Maybe he would go out and get a little fresh air on his lunch break. As he exited the front door, he noticed three girls who appeared to be extremely disturbed. He recognized them as the girls he had met separately yesterday morning in the building. Maybe he could console them as they were becoming increasingly distressed. A few assuring words from a famous veggie like himself surely couldn't hurt the situation.

As he approached them, he started getting a weird feeling. These girls seemed more familiar than he previously thought. Was something playing tricks with his mind or was it just his hungover state of mind? Anyway, he proceeded to walk over to them.

Zarkoff smiled as he spoke. "Hi girls. It's me, Zarkoff from yesterday. Do you remember me?"

At the sound of his voice their heads turned. At that moment all the memories flooded into Zarkoff's horrified brain. "Oh my God! I'm in big trouble!" he muttered to himself.

Six eyes gleamed at him, infused with anger. Gabriella made the first move. She gave him a devasting right to the side of his head that knocked him to the ground. Zarkoff saw stars as he awaited further punishment that would undoubtedly be coming.

Zarkoff was correct in his thinking. Eleanor grabbed a jagged rock that was lying nearby and side-armed his face. Zarkoff's nose went flying into the air. Gabriella joined back in as she began kicking his brand-new testicles. The pain was unbearable.

A crowd gathered as the melee ensued. "Watch out, she's going to sit on him!" Zarkoff heard someone shout.

At that moment Zarkoff thought his chest would be completely crushed. Melanie, the large watermelon had jumped and her enormous bulk fell upon him. The girthy gal was bouncing on his midsection in an obvious attempt to kill him.

"You said you would marry me, you piece of rotten veggie garbage!" Melanie shouted as she lifted herself up and landed back on him with brutalizing force. "You said we would have children together, you triple-timing, silver-tongued, liar gourd-face."

Zarkoff couldn't breathe as the blows to his head were quickly sending him into another coma. The pain being inflicted upon his newly-transplanted testicles by Gabriella's violent kicks was unbearable.

"Don't worry, Melanie," screamed Gabriella as she issued one last blast to his swollen testicles. "He won't be making kids any time soon."

Zarkoff wanted to die as he writhed in agony. As he slipped out of consciousness, he saw one last face. It was that of Kiki Kale. His old actress friend had made a surprise visit to see her newly-acquired boyfriend. After being told of the situation, she too wanted Zarkoff dead. She was consumed with the same fiery anger as the other three.

"You didn't miss anything, girls," shouted Kiki as she wrapped her hands around Zarkoff's neck in an attempt to strangle him. "All you would have gotten from this lousy parasitic louse would be a bad case of herpes."

At that moment a security team arrived and tore the girls away from Zarkoff. One of them shouted, "I think he's dead!"

They immediately began to administer CPR on the motionless Zarkoff. A medical team arrived and shocked Zarkoff with a heart defibrillator. His heart began beating again just as Eleanor Eggplant broke away and issued one more kick to his blood-soaked body.

Zarkoff fell into yet another coma. He spent eight months in the hospital, but he did survive. Extra security was placed in his room due to death threats from assorted females. It was another episode of misery for the flawed zucchini. His wife heard of the incident on the national news. To do this on their wedding anniversary was unforgivable. She packed her bags and headed to cousin Lillie's. It would be six months before she would speak to him again.

Zarkoff's reputation sunk even lower in the public arena. How could such a brilliant man make such dumb decisions? Only Zarkoff Zucchini knew the answer to that one. He would never escape the stigma of the so-called Four-Girl-Attack.

Zarkoff vowed to become celibate the rest of his life. Unfortunately, that didn't last long. An affair with a sweet little nurse named Olive ensued shortly after his heart transplant. Zarkoff was pronounced a hopeless case by many as his reputation continued to wane.

As usual, there's a lesson in this tale. Be careful when you see a group of girls walking together. They could be conspiring to commit murder. Always be on guard for homicidal walkers. Be especially aware of your surroundings if you are a womanizer, and always remember to carry protective weaponry.

Try to be a walker with ethics and don't plot to kill people while you walk. Now that you know that, let's get back to the true business of walking. It's a very important ingredient in your fitness routine.

> *Two, three, four,*
> *Women or more.*
> *Cause problems,*
> *That's for sure!*

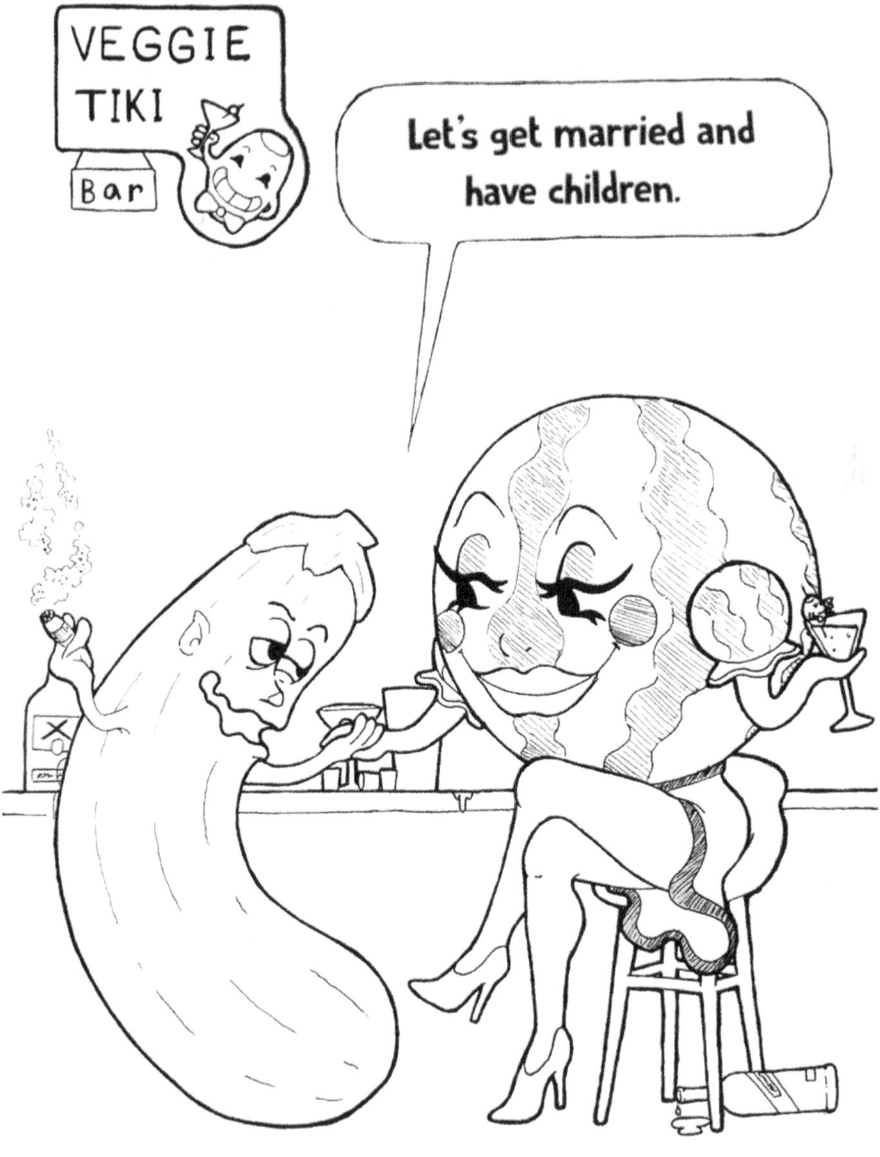
VEGGIE
TIKI
Bar
Let's get married and have children.

The Joy of Walking II

Walking is convenient, easy, and free. It is one of the first motions the body learns as a child. It's a coordinated movement of muscles, all working together in unison to move a human from point A to point B. Walking is genius simplicity from the creator of our species. It's the most natural exercise we can do. I use it for most of my lower body workout, as I rarely supplement it with weight exercises or squats.

You need not be an athlete to walk. You can be the clumsiest person around and still perform this activity. Even the most uncoordinated can easily pull it off. So many people overlook this type of activity. Sometimes the most obvious solution gets lost in a haze of an overwhelming array of choices. When that occurs, it's best to take a moment and back off. Take a look at the big picture and reanalyze everything from a distance. The answer may be staring you in the face.

Many people start an exercise program with the wrong mindset. They falsely believe that exercise *has* to be tedious and boring. They picture it as work verses fun, something that is not enjoyable. That's the wrong way to look at it. Instead of capturing exercise inside a frown, picture it as a big happy smile. Maybe even plaster those happy faces around your workout area to remind you.

Don't get trapped in the "boring" mentality when it comes to walking. Walking is lots of fun. Breathe the fresh air, enjoy the scenery, and watch all the interesting people that you'll encounter as you walk. Just remember that you're not there to engage in conversations, pet someone's dog, or set up a Zarkoff-style encounter. You are there to walk!

Let your mind wander. Tap into the deep, meditative part of your soul that needs to escape technological imprisonment. One of the greatest benefits of walking is temporary extrication from the electromagnetic dome that practically enslaves us.

If you must, carry your little music box with you on your walks. However, I urge you to try a few walks with nothing but your mind and soul to entertain you. Many of you will find that you never needed that distractive device. There's so much locked up inside your subconscious that needs to be freed. It's the same as a dog when it goes out to walk and play. It's sheer joy and happiness.

Let your mind run recklessly through the past, present and future. *Take time to think.* It's truly amazing how the body and mind synchronize when you're in this state. It's possible to finally snap out of this trancelike condition to realize you're done with your entire walk. You've exercised and weren't even conscious of it. How easy is that?

There's something about walking that is soul-soothing, a sort of medicine for all that ails you internally. It's an incredibly healthy way to deal with the pressures of life that relentlessly attack us. Not only are you treating your body to one of the greatest forms of exercise, but you're also releasing mental stress in a positive manner.

The next time you are anxiously awaiting a potentially stressful encounter, try taking a short walk beforehand. You will find yourself better equipped to handle it. You're more relaxed physically and mentally. You'll be sharper and more likely to deal with situations in a calm and cool manner. This prepares you to make better decisions in a delicate situation. You'll have the edge on your competition. They probably sat around and let worry consume them while you tuned up the soul for battle.

Many of you may be dependent on some sort of sleeping aids, anti-depressants, anti-anxiety medication, or pain-killers. It's probably been an incremental process and undoubtedly tough to lick. However, with the proper attitude and your walking routine, you'll stand a real chance of eliminating some of these nuisances that have taken control. Clear this with your physician before dropping any medications.

You may possibly be able to replace those pharmaceutical remedies with exercise. Walking is the first place to start. You never know, you may find you never needed those crutches in the first place. The solution may have been within you the entire time. Try it.

Walk for fun,
Walk to unwind.
Walking is good,
Good for the mind.

The Joy of Walking III

Regardless of your physical condition, walking is a great workout. Of course, there are conditions that can render us incapable of walking. I urge you to be creative and find an exercise that works for your particular disability. The rest of us really have no excuse not to walk.

As we discussed earlier, it's all about incremental advancement. Adding a minute to your time every week or so is the secret. Never forget this a one-year-project at the bare minimum. Look into the mirror and see the future.

Many of you guys will want to switch into macho-man mode at this point. Walking is for the weak who can't run and sprint. Walking is for women. That will be the mentality for many of you as you sprint off at jet-speed to break a long-standing Olympic record. You will be wrong. One month from now those women will still be smiling and walking as you nurse your hamstring pulls and shin splints.

Let's face it, as if I have to repeat it, we're too damn old to be racing twenty-year-olds competitively in the physical arena. Start using some of that wisdom you've accumulated and drop that conditioning-media mass of malarkey that consumes you. Release that *Terminator*-hero wannabe fantasy that's tortured you your entire life. No one really gives a hoot if you're walking or running. They've got their own problems to address. Just get out there and walk and see all those pretty ladies that are already doing it.

There's nothing wrong with a jog if it doesn't injure you and you enjoy it. My personal experience was pain in my knees after several months of jogging. I was younger and was afflicted with Macho Disease along with an extreme case of Peanut-Brain. These two ailments together caused me to continue running until my joints continuously ached day and night.

Macho Disease had completely engulfed me and Peanut-Brain had a chokehold on me. I was doomed to an eternal future of idiotism. At this point I visited a physical therapist who happened to be my ninety-year-old, uneducated, rural, deep-south grandmother. I explained how running was killing my knees and I was completely lost as to what to do. She calmly said "Stop running."

I immediately saw the light with her Zarkoffish simplistic answer and began walking. My extreme degree of mental deficiency had me locked away in ignorance. My grandmother showed me a way to break free from my idiotism that enslaved me. I'm now a role model for my fellow unfortunates. Ever since I graced the cover of *Peanut-Brain Quarterly,* I've helped others conquer that once-thought-to-be-incurable malady.

Okay, that's enough bragging on my accomplishments. Although walking is still my mainstay form of aerobic activity, I still run in occasional short bursts just to get the heart rate up a bit. If you runners out there are doing so problem-free, then by all means continue onward. Always remember that you can convert over to a fast-paced walk at any time if you so desire. You won't really lose anything in the aerobic department.

Learn to walk with your entire body. By this, I mean don't be afraid to engage your midsection, upper body and arms during your walks. Also focus on your posture. This burns extra calories per stride and that's our primary goal. Fat is our enemy and we're on a mission to burn it off.

You'll find that the more you focus on your complete body, the *slower* you'll go. Yes, you'll be walking at a slightly reduced pace. Thirty minutes of entire-body-focus walking will register *less* distance than your normal walking pace. You may rightfully ask why that is considered a positive thing. How can *slower* and *less* be a good thing when you're trying to lose weight and get in shape?

The answer is that your caloric burn-off rate stays the same, or more likely shows a slight increase. Here's the proof. Try this experiment on your next walk. Walk a few laps using your normal stride and focus. Most likely, you're of the mindset to get that next mile in as fast as you can.

Then do a few laps engaging the entire-body-focus approach, focusing all your concentration on standing erect. Keep your head held high looking straight ahead, chest poked out, upper body parts and abs straight and slightly tensed, and add a swinging motion to your arms.

Continue forward with a smooth and steady stride, which is now a slightly shorter stride. Your mind is still dead-set on getting that next mile done as quickly as possible, but you'll find your pace actually slows somewhat.

Take a moment to analyze this aerobic experiment. You're probably more out-of-breath than you were using your normal walking form. That's a good thing because it means you're chewing up those calories, and you're using your full body to do it. When your concentration is focused solely on distance goals, your body is *efficiently* accomplishing this by neglecting any muscles deemed unnecessary to achieve this goal.

That's a wonderful outcome if you're a competitive runner, but is that your thing? Do you want to have mileage-bragging rights at your upcoming luncheon with the other girls, or do you simply want to lose weight and get in shape? The same principle applies here as with the slightly Macho-Diseased bicyclist whose only ambition is to ride more miles than the next guy. I briefly addressed this earlier, but let's touch on it again.

I have many friends who are avid bicyclists and I truly understand the competitive spirit. If the competition is what drives you, then the following few paragraphs won't apply to you. If that's the force that keeps you in shape, then absolutely continue down that path. I truly admire it. This only applies to the lost soul who got caught up in the whirlwind and lost track of his primary goal, to lose weight and get in shape.

Do you want to burn calories, tone up, and get lean and strong? Or would you rather pay an extra ten thousand dollars for that bike that registers more mileage? Sure, you'll get in shape riding that bike, but it has nothing to do with counting miles. It's all about burning calories regardless of how fast you're going.

Jumping-jacks for thirty minutes will really sizzle those calories away, but did you accomplish many miles? As I stated earlier, if mileage is your primary concern, choose a faster instrument of motion. Maybe a Ferrari, a Porsche, or possibly a space rocket will get it done.

Walk every day, *And you will see.* *Great you'll feel,* *Thin you'll be!*

The Joy of Walking IV

Sometimes the big picture gets lost in the haziness of the details. Sometimes we lose sight of our original goal when we get bogged down with the particulars. We forget the spark that started the fire as extracurriculars flood our senses. Don't overcomplicate matters by allowing others to steer you down an alternative path. Sometimes that path leads to frustration and disillusion. Then you quit and resign yourself to season seven of that TV series you love. Don't let that happen.

The bottom line, as it applies to walking, is to burn those calories as we tone our bodies. Most of you reading this book are chiefly concerned about feeling good and looking good. The means and methods really don't matter as long as they're safe and practical. You want to look in the mirror and see a lean, healthy body.

Walking is a great time to focus on improving your posture. As all of us geezed time-travelers know, posture declines as you age. What was once tall and straight is now a little stooped or hunched, and not quite as firm as the good ole days. It doesn't have to be that way forever.

What's great about the entire-body-focus approach is that you're constantly aware, at least subconsciously, of maintaining correct posture. You're keeping your head upright, your chest is projected forward, and your abs and lower back are tight and straight. Over a period of time, this along with your essential stretching can do wonders for your posture. Like everything else with his program, don't expect overnight miracles. Simply plug along and enjoy the ride, and good things will follow.

The next walking-related subject we'll address will be interruptions. As you may already know, once you halt your walk for any reason, it's difficult to start back again. The mind and body go into *I'm-finished* mode. Then it's like a computer restart. Aren't those updating interruptions annoying?

The absolute biggest obstacle to a steady, uninterrupted walk is a neighbor. Many of you walk around your neighborhood because it's so convenient. You know everyone and everyone knows you. As you're enjoying your brisk walk and your mind is going back to a pleasant memory from the past, you hear that familiar voice. It's Jane Neighbor!

You know who Jane Neighbor is. She's the one who first learned of retired Dr. Sillick's affair with Rosetta Sanchez. Within two hours the entire community knew when and where they met and the erection-issues they overcame. Jane Neighbor may be the nerve center of the neighborhood, but she's also a walk-destruction expert.

Jane Neighbor will expect you to immediately stop what you're doing and engage in conversation with her. Your past history is to cave-in to her demands and talk to her because you're of a loving, polite nature. You understand the entirety of her self-esteem is based upon being the gossip queen. She's had underlying issues ever since she snitched out her twelve-year-old sister for kissing the next-door neighborhood kid. What a wonderful feeling that was.

As Jane approaches you, do not panic! Remain calm and remember the statement you've prepared for this moment you knew would occur. This is the critical phase of the encounter that you cannot blow. It's the moment of truth hitting the gossip queen and shattering her ego into a thousand bits, but you have to do it for your own survival.

It's an emotional disaster that will probably send her straight to the psych ward. There she'll quickly become the indisputable knower-of-all-meaningless-things, the go-to girl for the mentally disturbed, the psychotherapist's nightmare of nightmares. Her life will continue, but don't worry, you're still a part of her life. You can bet that she's telling her fellow roomies about your particular peculiarities, and how she once saw you pee behind your house that day you accidently locked yourself out.

As you hear Jane's screechy voice, turn towards her as you slow your pace. *Do not completely stop walking.* She wants to talk because that is her sole purpose for living. She wants to approach you and engage in conversation. *Don't do it!* Look her in the eyes with a smile and politely say, "Jane, I'm so sorry, but I just started a serious exercise program and I can't stop. Can we talk later?"

Then turn away and *really* pick up the pace. Walk the fastest you've ever walked in your life. *Get away from her now!* Every second counts. Put much distance between you and this obsessed dominatrix of useless information collecting. Your message to her must be loud and clear. *You are very serious about your walk.* You can't allow yourself to be weak. If you give in for even a millisecond, she'll pounce on you and devour you.

Most likely Jane Neighbor won't give up after one attempt at ruining your walk. The next day when you go by her house, she'll be waiting for an ambush. As you walk past her front yard, she'll leap from the bushes and attack. She'll be armed with some new information concerning Dr. Sillick and Rosetta's rendezvous. She'll be out for blood.

There's a way out of this. As you approach her house, approximately a block before, begin a fast-paced jog. Pull your hat down over your face as much as possible. Pretend you're so focused on your jog that you don't even hear her as she assaults you verbally with juicy gossip. She'll immediately spread the news of your madness to her gossip-underling staff that she has strategically placed around the neighborhood, but you will have survived.

Another area of danger involves pets. So many of us love those furry animals that are so adorable. The problem is you *can't* pet them on your walks. Many of your neighbors, friends, or strangers that you pass on your walks are walking their dogs. If you're a true animal lover, you may be tempted to stop and show your affection towards them.

You have to be tough and pass them by. They're a booby-trap that can destroy your walk. We know how that works, miss a chunk of one walk, and that leads to two, then to three, and you're traveling down the road towards total abandonment. If you're a true dog lover, you'll figure out a way to pet dogs *and* get your walk done. Don't let Rover destroy your walks!

Walk nonstop, *Do not chat.* *If you do,* *You'll be fat!*

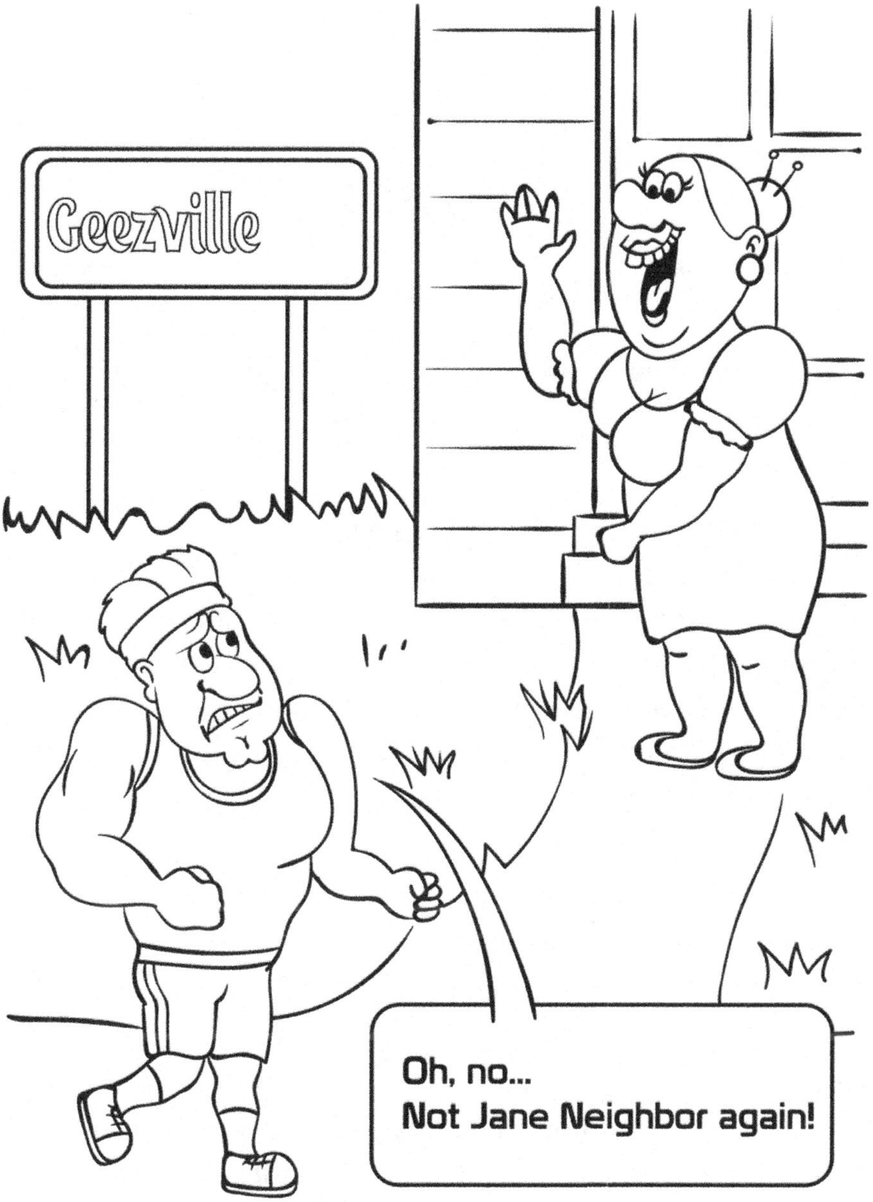
Geezville
Oh, no...
Not Jane Neighbor again!

CHAPTER 9

The Exercise Plan II

"Blow their minds and do something remarkable."
B.B. Dixon

Walk This Way

The waves gently rolled in as the warm ocean breeze stirred the umbrella in Zarkoff's sweet rum drink. He watched the island palm trees dance to the rhythm of the Bob Marley song playing in the background. Oh, how he loved the beach life, such a relaxing time away from all the madness of his other world thousands of miles away.

Zarkoff had always wanted to visit Thailand. For years he had heard about its beauty and the friendliness of its people. They didn't call it "The Land of Smiles," for nothing. It had been over two years since he had a vacation, and it was finally real.

Here he was, amongst sandy white beaches, warm ocean breezes and wonderful people. It was wintertime back home, but here the weather was as beautiful as could be. There wasn't a cloud in the sky and the temperature was perfect. There was nothing more he could ask for, or so he thought.

"*Sawatdee kha*," a voice called out. It was the sweetest voice he had ever heard. "Can I get you another drink, Mr. Zucchini?"

Zarkoff looked up to see the most beautiful coconut he had ever seen in his life. She was absolutely stunning, with her dark hair, beautiful skin, and a smile as big as the sun shining above. It was true what he had heard, the coconuts over here *were* the most beautiful in the world. Wow!

Zarkoff was a loss for words. He was in a dreamlike state, a blissful blessing from above. He finally regained his senses to reply. "Well, yes, sweetie, I'll have another drink. What is your name?"

"My name is Chintana," she answered back, flashing a smile that melted him. "It means 'good thought.' The world can always use more good thoughts, don't you think?" She smiled again as her sweet voice echoed across the water.

"Yes, it sure can," answered Zarkoff. "Would you like to join me for a drink?"

"Sure, that sounds great," Chintana cheerfully replied. "As a matter of fact, I'm just getting off work. Would you like to join me and my friends at the bar?" She pointed towards the open-air bar a few feet away.

Zarkoff could not believe his eyes. There must have been ten or twelve Thai coconuts gathered around the bar. Every single one of them was as beautiful as Chintana. They all could have been cover girls for *Fruit & Veggie Fashionista Magazine*. Never had he seen such a collection of stunning women in a single location.

"Yes, I would love to," answered Zarkoff, trying to contain his excitement.

They strolled to the bar and Zarkoff was introduced to all the girls. They immediately recognized him for being a famous vegetable activist. He quickly became the star attraction as they clamored for his attention. They had never met a famous veggie before. They peppered him with questions and showered him with attention.

So here he was, surrounded by eleven of the most gorgeous coconuts in the entire world, all of them worshipping him as if he were a god. Zarkoff pinched himself just to make sure it wasn't a dream. How fortunate could one zucchini be!

Unfortunately for Zarkoff, one of the lovelies was aware of Zarkoff's somewhat stained reputation. Years ago, Connie Coconut's cousin had visited America and fell in love with a wonderful, charming zucchini. The zucchini proceeded to break her heart when she caught him running around with a mango actress. She never recovered from this emotional devastation. That cheating zucchini was Zarkoff.

Connie came up with a plan. Payback would be coming Zarkoff's way and it wouldn't be a pretty sight. Connie covertly let everyone know of her intentions. Connie would have revenge for what Zarkoff did to her cousin. Upon learning of the situation, all of the girls were fuming with anger. They too wanted Zarkoff to pay for his evil deed.

The plan was put into operation. The girls first plied Zarkoff with free drinks, so much so that he could barely stand. All the while they were constantly touching him, whispering in his ear, and promising all kinds of fun. Eleven beautiful coconuts were united with one goal. Zarkoff didn't stand a chance.

Connie suggested they all go for a walk on the beach. Sunset would be coming soon and it was exceptionally beautiful on this particular island. Zarkoff was in full agreement, especially after Connie suggested everyone go skinny-dipping.

The girls walked down to a private beach that only the locals knew about. Now they could really set their plan into action. Zarkoff was all smiles as five of the girls disrobed before him. As his attention was diverted the other six girls rushed towards Zarkoff and knocked him to the ground.

The girls quickly bonded as a team, binding him with thick rope and gagging him by plowing a prearranged bag of smelly elephant doo down his throat. They blindfolded him and dragged him over towards the wasps' nest that buzzed with activity.

"That's close enough, girls," ordered Connie. "No one wants to get stung."

The girls then walked over to the rockpile and each grabbed a large rock. "Okay, girls," said Connie. "Make sure you hit the middle of the nest and then run like hell. Are you ready?"

They all shook their heads in agreement and each launched perfect shots into the huge nest. Then they raced to safety, never looking back. Their part of the mission was complete. Now it was the angry wasps' turn.

Zarkoff had never felt such pain in his life. All the drinks in the world couldn't ease the agony of several thousand angry wasps all stinging him at the same time. After a couple of thousand stings the poison began acting on his system and he began convulsing. His eyes rolled back into his head. His face turned blue. His arms and legs jerked as more wasps gained revenge for the rock attack.

Suddenly he stopped breathing and his whole body stiffened like a board. He was quickly losing consciousness. Death was once again eminent and again it was related to angry women. He promised God that if could just survive this he would never talk to another female again. Then he passed out.

Ten months later he awoke from his coma. As he opened his eyes, he saw Connie Coconut and her cousin Coolie standing by his bedside. "How do you feel now, Mister Mango Lover?" calmly asked Coolie. "Are you happy you cheated on me?"

And just like that, they both left the room. Zarkoff slipped back into the comfort of his coma. Six months later he awoke for good. He left the lovely country of Thailand and all its beautiful residents behind. He learned a valuable lesson and you should learn a lesson from this also. *Never go walking if eleven people want you dead.*

Make this an important rule for your walking program. Before every walk I ask myself, "Do eleven people want me dead?" If the answer is no, then I begin my walk. If the answer is yes, I choose not to walk for safety reasons. You should do the same.

> Zarkoff did bad,
> He paid the price.
> Mean ole wasps,
> Don't feel nice.

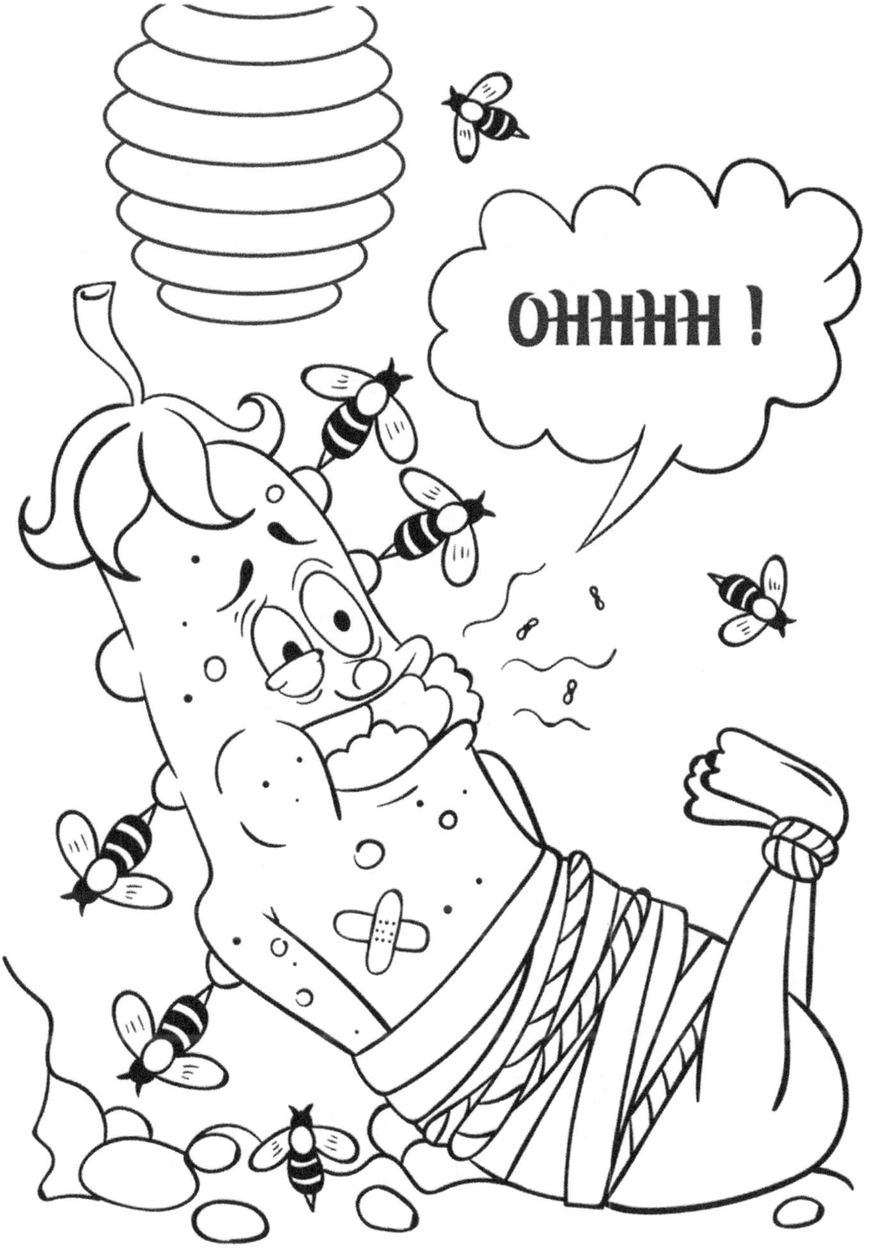
OHHHH !

Walk This Way II

Now we must go forward and not dwell on our unfortunate hero. He survived and we will too. Walking will be a big factor in our survival, as it will keep us fit and healthy. Let's progress on to some more walking-related topics. We'll start with a subject briefly mentioned earlier, the sun and all its power.

Many of you live in areas where there is lots of sunlight. The sun is a powerful entity. It's no wonder it was treated as a god over the ages. It demands respect and rightfully so, for without it our planet is doomed. We need small doses of it to receive vitamin D. If we're not aware of its power and take it lightly, it can come back with a vengeance in the form of skin cancer.

When you're outside walking or engaging in other outdoor activities, try to shield yourself from the sun. I know many of you think a dark tan is attractive, but is it really worth the risk? Look up some pictures of skin cancer and that should change your mind, not to mention those awful bandages that grace your body after the surgery. We all know that geezed-up bodies are especially at risk, so be careful.

I'm amazed at the young girls I see walking or jogging without a hat of some sort. Sometimes I want to stop and tell them that pretty face of theirs isn't going to be so pretty in twenty years if they continue. The sun can do a number on the skin in the form of premature aging. Even if you're lucky enough to avoid skin cancer, it will still make your skin leathery and unattractive.

I think it's a good idea to cover as much of your body as possible from sunlight. Be especially aware of your face and wear a hat that serves a purpose. Find one that really does the job and covers the entire face. Try to cover your neck by pulling up your collar or other means. I've seen some pretty rough looking necks on some otherwise very beautiful women. Protect your pretty self.

Put fashion on the back burner when it comes to sun protection. Being lax in the protection department is risky business. You may think that fancy little hat is a sign of your fashion sense, but unless it provides protection it's worthless. Keep up that mentality and you'll be seeking some fashionable bandages to wear on your face. It may not be tomorrow, or maybe it won't happen at all, but do you really want to risk it?

The primary concern is shielding yourself from those dangerous rays that slowly but surely damage the skin. Respect the sun and it will respect you. Make a habit of wearing a hat outside. Try to cover your arms and legs as well. Once you get used to it, you'll be fine. It's not as hot as you think.

Don't fret ladies, you'll still get male attention. Burnt skin isn't a requirement. There are lots of men out there who prefer a woman with soft and sexy skin. If you still can't get a date, look up Zarkoff. He'll find you attractive.

Here's a subject few people take seriously, the surface upon which you walk. Hard surfaces can really put a strain on geezy joints. Although walking is a low impact form of exercise, you have to take a long-term view of it. There's still a constant pounding that can slowly wear down those ancient joints and moving parts. Two miles a day is over 700 miles per year. That's a lot of grinding on geezed knees and joints. Geezers don't need any more aches and pains, so take this subject seriously.

Search out some softer surfaces for your walks. Maybe there are some trails nearby that you can use. Perhaps there's a park nearby with a grass or dirt surface. Dirt and grass are usually great choices. You'll cover more distance per minute on the harder surfaces, so don't get caught up in the mileage-bragging-rights trap.

As mentioned before, don't worry about the miles you're covering as much as the effort that goes into those miles. Maybe the grass you're walking on hasn't been mowed in a few weeks and it's a little more difficult to navigate through it. Embrace the challenge and don't worry about the distance you're covering. Your body is applying more energy per step, so it all works out in the long run.

It's really all about a general awareness of the possible surfaces and making the best choice. You may decide to walk alongside a concrete or asphalt path instead of walking directly on it. When given a limited choice between asphalt and concrete, go with the slightly softer asphalt option. Seek out the best places around you.

Is your favorite place to walk a track, field, or another location where you're constantly going around in a circle? If so, change directions occasionally. I know it may seem a little strange, but I think it's healthier on the joints, especially the knees. Imagine the long-term effects of a constant left or right turn, especially on our battle-scarred working parts.

Wear those creaky joints out in a fair manner and don't discriminate against one or the other. At our age, we're trying to let our bodies wear evenly. I personally want every organ in my body to start a downhill slide simultaneously. After that my exit will probably be quick and relatively painless. Then I can relocate to that big happy hour in the sky.

Don't stray too far from home. This makes it easy for you to just say no to your walk. Try to keep your walking area close by. Keep things practical and convenient because you can't risk abandoning your exercise program. I don't have to tell you to choose safe areas in which to walk. You're old and wise enough to know to avoid large venomous snakes and murderers on the loose.

Try to avoid walking in smoggy or crowded areas. Sometimes it's your only option, but don't make a habit of it. All that grimy pollution won't be doing your lungs any favors. Heavily traveled roads certainly take away from the joy of walking. The more cars you encounter, the more you risk being involved in some of sort of vehicle verses pedestrian incident. Take a guess at which one gets the worse end of that deal. Geezer down!

Try to find a peaceful area in which to walk, one that's quiet and safe. If it's impossible, then invest in a stationary bike or a treadmill and get it done at home. Jumping-jacks and other calisthenics are another option.

I really haven't mentioned enough about the treadmill/stationary bike options. They are both excellent devices to get a geezed heart beating faster. I possess sort of an old school mentality, so I'm always leaning towards the outdoor option. However, in many ways the treadmill and bike options make more sense.

The biggest advantage they offer is the opportunity to escape inclement weather. You certainly don't want to walk in a fierce thunderstorm, dangerous heat, or frigid cold, although I've experienced all of this. Some of my decisions bordered on downright stupidity, so I offer no defense. Mom dropped me on my head as a baby, or at least that's the story I'm sticking to.

Many of you don't have room in your home for a treadmill or bike. If that's the case, and you're facing weather conditions, then simply innovate. Do some jumping-jacks or run in place. Throw on one of those old rock and roll CDs and get funky. Relive the disco days of yesteryear. It really doesn't matter as long as you're creating an aerobic workout.

Just open up your mind and move that body. Get that workout done and you'll be feeling proud the rest of the day. Happy hour will be so much more fun because you deserve it. Whatever you do, don't go sit on the sofa and mindlessly turn on that remote. You'll be doomed for sure.

Another alternative exercise is swimming. I highly recommend this well-rounded form of exercise. It offers a great combination of aerobic and strength benefits along with being very easy on the joints. I love swimming! If you have a pool available, then by all means utilize it. Analyze the water before you jump in. If the water is colored urinary yellow, opt for another form of exercise. Super geezers and babies tend to be aqua polluters.

Exercise videos are another great aerobic option. Even if you only add it into your rotating mix of exercises, it's a wonderful choice. Choose an easy-to-learn one that doesn't require a technology degree to figure it out. Keep it simple. Make *sure* you go the low-impact route so those geezed-up joints can handle it. I also don't have to remind you to stretch! We're well aware that we're brittle and ancient and on the verge of breaking in half. Go easy and try to stay in one piece.

Perhaps one day you've accomplished your exercise routine, but you're still feeling overly energetic. You're ready for a little bonus exercise. One of the simplest is something we described in detail earlier. Park along the outer edge of the parking lot the next time you go shopping. You'll get in a little walk and your car is safer from the door-bangers who orgasm from denting others' vehicles.

The next time you're waiting on an elevator, consider taking the stairs. It's a wonderful bonus exercise. If it's only a flight or two, it's nothing more than a little exciting, aerobic adventure. You never know what or who you may discover as you trek up the stairs. Maybe Zarkoff's up there with a street hooker. You'll also avoid those sometimes-awkward moments in a crowded elevator where everyone's analyzing strange body odors.

Other bonus exercises include lawn work, cleaning the house, washing your car or trimming hedges. Try walking or biking to any short destinations that constitute your regular errands. The choices are only as limited as your imagination. If nothing else, bonus exercises provide a psychological lift. It's part of a healthy mentality towards your fitness program. Think back to the days before you committed yourself to becoming fit. You likely would never have considered *walking* or *biking* to the store around the block.

You're a geezer,
That's okay.
You can walk,
Every day!

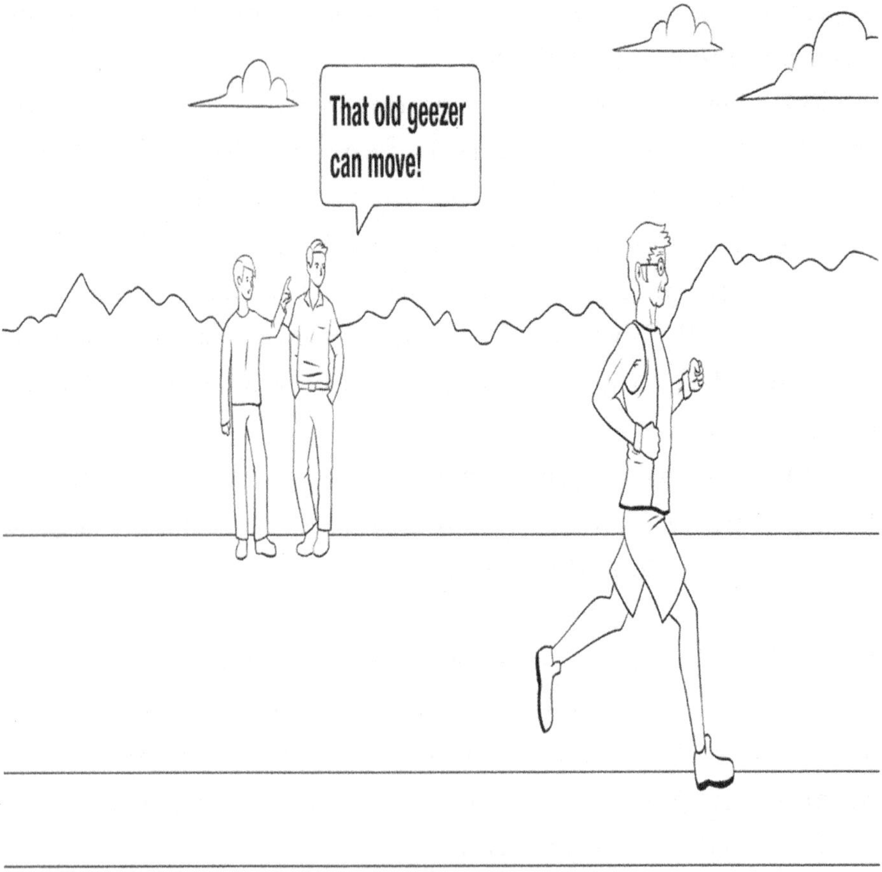
That old geezer can move!

Get It Done

Over and over, I've emphasized the warrior mentality you have to acquire and master if you want to become fit. You have to believe in yourself and stay focused on the end goal. Every day is just another cog in the machine, another brick in the wall, another tiny step forward. However, when you put all those hard-fought victories together, you've got something of substance.

When you fight through a particularly challenging day and squeeze in your exercise routine you're building confidence for the next day, and the next, and the next. It's a foundation that's built to last and not crumble with the first big wind that howls by. You're proving something to *yourself* and you're going to make damn sure you do it. Congratulate yourself for making it through the day and move on.

Nobody else is really going to care, but they'll sure take notice when that day finally comes and they realize you did it! You lost that weight you so desired to lose, or you're toned and cut to the point they could only dream about. The point here is to keep plugging along like a machine and everything will fall into place. Keep at it and don't take no for an answer. The old saying, "Where there's a will, there's a way," is more applicable here than anywhere. Get it done!

Many of you may enjoy traveling, or possibly your job requirements involve extensive travel. We all know how difficult it is to do certain things when you're away from your home environment. Exercise is no exception. Your treadmill is not awaiting you, the weather is vastly different with possible extreme conditions, your bed isn't so comfortable, the late-night dinner with your boss left you with a cloudy head, and so on.

Traveling is one of those situations that really separates the true winners from those who think they're winners, but can't cut it when the going gets tough. It sometimes takes a will of steel to persevere and survive. The following story illustrates this point.

A great zucchini once proclaimed, "See the future and the future will see you." What this means exactly, I have no idea, but it won Zarkoff Zucchini a Nobel Veggie Prize. The award ceremony was held in Stockholm, one of Zarkoff's favorite cities. Although Zarkoff always claimed it was the cultural museums that drew him to this historic city, in actuality it was the hidden red-light district that kept luring him back.

Zarkoff was so proud of his award. It was personally handed to him by the King of Sweden. The committee tried to revoke it shortly afterwards due to a venereal disclosure by the king's wife where she blamed Zarkoff Zucchini. Zarkoff denied any venereal wrongdoing and with limited evidence, the embarrassing episode was quickly dropped.

Zarkoff had put on a few pounds and had recently begun an exercise program. Stockholm was his first travel challenge since he decided to lose some weight. Keeping up a fitness program while traveling had always been difficult for Zarkoff.

This time Zarkoff pledged to himself he would truly commit to his exercise program. One of his longtime girlfriends back home had commented that he had a little pudge around the middle. That was a major turning point. When the ladies took notice, it was time for action. That was the only motivation he needed.

Zarkoff was halfway through his hour on the treadmill when she walked in. It was 6 a.m. and he wasn't expecting anyone else to work out so early. The fitness room seemed to light up with energy the moment she walked in. Wow! She was a knockout rutabaga if there ever was one. Her Nordic features were of the classic beauty that drove Zarkoff crazy. Her sparkling blue eyes reminded him of the heroines of ancient fairy tales. Her gait was one of self-confidence and charm.

She quickly introduced herself. "Hi, I'm Roskva Rutabaga. I know who you are. I saw you receive your award yesterday on TV. Congratulations, Mr. Zucchini."

Zarkoff was at a loss for words. The last thing he expected this morning was a gorgeous rutabaga to join him in the fitness room. He had always had a weakness for rutabagas. His wife was a rutabaga. As a matter of fact, she was a descendant of a Swedish rutabaga clan. It was too bad all of his affairs had put their marriage in such a bad state. What difference would one more make? Their marriage was so shattered as it was. Zarkoff finally spoke.

"Thank you," he stuttered. "Yes, I'm very proud of it."

"See the future and the future will see you," said Roskva with a smile. "That's the quote that won you the prize. Am I correct?"

"You certainly are, sweetie. I'm impressed. May I ask if you're single? I hope I'm not being too direct so early in the morning."

"Oh, you're not, Mr. Zucchini," The room lit with brilliance as she flashed her blue eyes. "And yes, I am single."

Zarkoff proceeded to pile on his considerable charm and within ten minutes had arranged a date. Roskva was an outdoor enthusiast and the two of them would go kayaking the next morning. Sweden's wild rivers would provide the perfect romantic setting for a girl such as Roskva.

Zarkoff was excited beyond belief at his good fortune. A knockout rutabaga was joining him on a romantic kayaking expedition. He could get a little exercise and enjoy the company of this stunningly-beautiful girl at the same time. Wow!

The morning arrived and Zarkoff stood by the kayak anticipating the presence of Roskva. Zarkoff strained his eyes as he saw a figure in the misty morning fog. It was Roskva! He could barely control himself. Then another figure suddenly appeared in the distance. It looked to be another female and she was carrying a rather large bag. Who was this other individual joining her? And why? He thought it would be just the two of them.

They greeted him at the kayak. "Mr. Zucchini," said Roskva, "I'd like for you to meet my mother. Her name is Ritta."

Zarkoff was completely caught off guard. Her mother! Ritta looked somewhat familiar, but maybe it was just his imagination. He sure wasn't expecting this, but he had no choice. He had to go through with the kayaking trip. The three of them, along with Ritta's large bag, piled into the cramped kayak. They launched into the water.

The excursion started off pleasant enough. Small talk dominated the early stages of the conversation. Without warning,

Ritta latched onto Zarkoff's arm and stared into his eyes. "How's sister Ria these days?" she calmly asked. "I haven't seen her in years."

Zarkoff felt his heart skip a beat. Now he remembered who this lady was. She was his wife's sister! He had only seen pictures of her, but there was no doubt this was her. Oh, no! How did he get into this mess! Once again, Zarkoff was in big trouble. Really big trouble!

"So, you're interested in my daughter, are you Mr. Zucchini?" Ritta said, quickly becoming more emotional. "Well, I guess my sister would love that, huh, Zarkie?"

Before Zarkoff could reply he was punched in the stomach so hard he couldn't breathe. He never saw Roskva's strong arm undercut into his gut. He felt nauseous. As he doubled over in pain, he got a glimpse of Ritta pulling something from her bag. It was thick rope and heavy-duty tape. The situation was looking very bleak.

Within seconds Ritta expertly had him tied and bound. She must have been practicing this forever, for he couldn't move one inch of his body. He watched in horror as she pulled out a rather large concrete block, then another, then a third. She quickly attached the heavy blocks to Zarkoff's helpless body.

The situation had become even more bleak. She was going to push him into the frigid waters for him to drown. Zarkoff began wondering what creatures would eat his decaying body at the bottom of the river. How he wished he had never cheated on his wife! He was going to die for sure this time.

The shock of the icy water awakened all his senses. His life flashed before him. All his do-good activism would probably never be remembered. All they would focus on would be his sensationalistic death at the hands of a revengeful woman, a crazed maniac intent on retribution for her sister's constant suffering and embarrassment. He slowly sunk down until he landed on the bottom. He hoped he would die quickly.

Zarkoff held his breath for as long as he could. He would finally exhale and it would all be over. His little zucchini lungs would fill with icy water and he would die. The bottom of a Swedish river would be his eternal resting place. This would be the punishment for all his years of infidelity. Why did he have to chase women? Why did he have to die because of it? Zarkoff began exhaling his final breath. It was "goodbye world."

Just as the last bit of air left his lungs, he spotted something out of the corner of his eye. Was it …could it be …yes, it was! It was a cheaterfish, the first one he had ever seen. Cheaterfish were one of the rarest species of fish in the world. There weren't many of them because they weren't capable of raising families. The reason was because they spent all their time cheating on their aquatic spouses instead of being responsible. Males and females alike did nothing but cheat. Oh my, did they love to cheat. The STD rate of cheaterfish was six times that of a normal fish.

Zarkoff couldn't believe what he witnessed next. The cheaterfish swam by him analyzing the situation. This was a large male cheaterfish, over six feet long, and he seemed genuinely alarmed that a fellow cheater was in such distress. Cheaters needed to support each other in times of need.

The cheaterfish stared into Zarkoff's eyes. For a moment they seemed to communicate telepathically. The cheaterfish reassured Zarkoff that he would be ok. There was a cheater bond between them that only cheaters could understand. Zarkoff would live to cheat again! The cheaterfish was determined to rescue Zarkoff from what seemed an eminent death.

He tore into the outer binding of tape and rope with his huge teeth. He shook his head violently while gripping the binding. The first layer ripped away and fell to the bottom. Again, he latched onto the binding that imprisoned his fellow cheater. Another large chunk fell to the bottom. Zarkoff could now move his arms and began helping the cheaterfish. The last bit of binding ripped away and Zarkoff was free.

Zarkoff didn't have a chance to celebrate, not yet. He knew that if he popped his head out of the water, the two murderous avengers would quickly grab him. He would certainly die a horrible death. The cheaterfish seemed to be thinking those exact thoughts. He once nearly died at the hands of his ex when she caught him in a fish-bed with a pair of pretty salmon.

She had strung him up and was ready to castrate him when a fellow cheaterfish rescued him. Cheaterfish never abandoned their compatriots. It was commandment number three of the Cheater Ten Commandments. *Thou shalt always help a cheater in need.* The cheaterfish came up with a plan.

He swam alongside Zarkoff and motioned for him to straddle him and hold tight. They were going for a ride! Cheaterfish were known for exceptional quickness due to much practice running from their irate mates. Zarkoff mounted the large fish and held on for dear life. Immediately the large fish zoomed into high gear, leaving the scene like a dragster car. Within seconds they had safely distanced themselves from the enemy.

Zarkoff popped his head out of the water and took in a precious breath of fresh air. Another few seconds without oxygen and he would have likely died. He glanced towards the cheaterfish with a look of gratitude. The cheaterfish acknowledged him with a flip of his tail.

Zarkoff had to thank his new friend. He removed the Nobel Prize that dangled from his neck. He placed it around the cheaterfish. The cheaterfish then raced off into the distance towards a school of pretty female trout. There was cheating to be done!

Zarkoff looked off in the distance. He could see two girls still in the kayak. They had opened a bottle of champagne and were obviously celebrating his demise. They were dancing, playing music, and laughing hysterically at his presumed death. One of them lit a flame.

Zarkoff strained his eyes to see what was going on. The other girl pulled out a paper, no it was a picture, a picture of him! They placed the flame underneath Zarkoff's picture and it erupted in flames. Screams of joy echoed across the river. Zarkoff was dead and gone and good riddance! "Long die Zarkoff!" he heard them shout.

Zarkoff eventually made his way to a nearby village. He quickly arranged the next flight out of Sweden. He covertly left the country and took some time to lick his emotional wounds. This would be one of the most difficult periods of the little zucchini's life. His wife left him and this time she claimed it was for good. He was a confused little veggie and was desperately seeking direction.

Zarkoff tried everything, religion, hard drugs, gardening, more hard drugs, but nothing seemed to work. It would be a full year before Zarkoff recovered emotionally and resumed doing what he did best, philandering. He stayed friends with the cheaterfish that had saved his life. The two exchanged emails frequently.

Never cheat, *On your wife.* *You just might,* *Lose your life!*

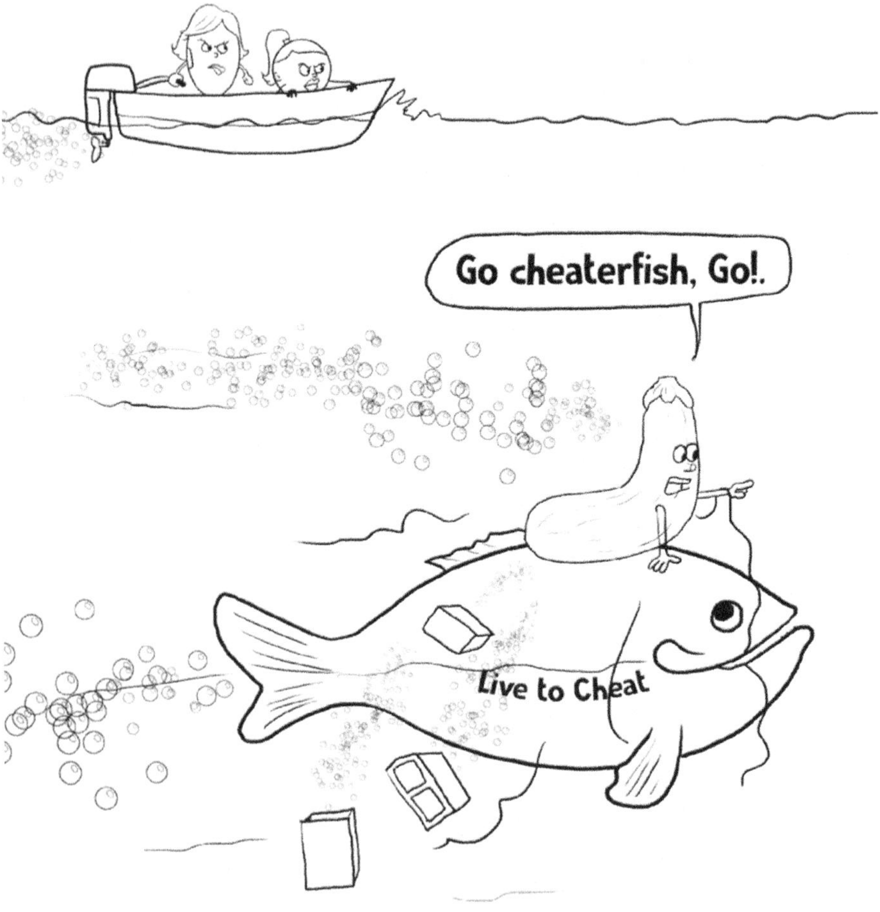
Go cheaterfish, Go!.
Live to Cheat

Get It Done II

As usual, there's a lesson to be learned from this tale of both sorrow and cheer. That lesson is to always screen a potential date when exercising on a business trip. You never know if that person is a murderer intent on taking your life. Always ask, "Do you want to kill me?" If they say no, continue exercising. If they say yes, leave the premises immediately and fly as far away as possible.

Zarkoff had a brilliant mind, but he really didn't have what it took to survive the brutal world of maintaining a traveler's exercise regimen. You have to do better than that. You may not have the underlying issues that distract poor Zarkoff, but absolutely there will be challenges that await when you travel. Just remember, there are no excuses in this brutal game we're playing. Miss a few days of your routine and you're going to pay. Cry all you want about how difficult it is to maintain your fitness regime while away, but it's only going to fall upon deaf ears.

Nobody really cares to hear it. All anyone responds to is success, results and actual physical transformation. That's what will make you amazing, the fact that you took a vision and brought it to fruition. You attained something you *really* desired. It's you against the world and the sooner you realize it, the better. Exercising on the road is not easy. Find a way to get it done.

Never forget the humor in all this and use it as an ally. Others may snicker at your creative little ways to make it work. They won't be laughing when you leave them in the dust. They'll be watching as you gallop towards the finish line and that gold medal. Make yourself and your fitness obsession into a running joke, but deep inside keep that intense fire burning. As Zarkoff stated, "See the future and the future will see you."

Many of you will be in hotels or unfamiliar homes as you travel. This adds an extra layer of inconvenience that shatters many well-laid plans. It simply becomes too much effort to make it worth it. Then there are changes in routines and schedules that can throw you for a loop.

Mix it all together and it's a formidable opponent. It's a ton of adversity that stands tall in front of you, daring you to cross that line inside their territory. This is no time to be timid and shy. Don't just step a foot over that line, blast through it like a wild animal and attack it head on.

As with most of this fitness and nutrition program, it gets easier as you continue practicing good habits. Every time you travel you gain more experience. You learn to defend yourself against the onslaught of never-ending challenges of life away from home.

Make that first time work, no matter what stands in your way, and the second time will be easier. It's a little psychological game you're playing with yourself. Do it once and you can do it again. Confidence is a powerful force that's hard to contain once it's unleashed.

Whether you're with family, friends, or business associates, let nothing interfere with your passion to succeed. Don't be hesitant to tell them you need time for your workout. Most will respect you for it and will probably be jealous of your determination to stay fit. There may be the occasional fool that belittles you and tries to embarrass you. Let him speak, for every word he's saying he's going to regret. That old saying, "You're going to eat your words," rings true here.

They are only displaying their own insecurities because they secretly admire your unwavering dedication. The ones who put up the most resistance can provide ammunition to you in the form of motivation. When the alarm clock rings and you're hesitant to get of bed and exercise, think of that puffball airhead who gets a juvenile kick out of antagonizing you.

Revenge will be coming your way and you won't have to say a single word. You're going to be fit and puffball will still be a bottom-dweller thriving on carcasses of the weak. Leave that poor unfortunate behind and move on.

Do what it takes when you're on the road. If you have to skip a breakfast, lunch, or dinner out, then so be it. Sacrifice where you will lose the least. Triage out your obligations and slice away a borderline commitment to make room for your workout. If you really want it, you *will* find time to exercise while traveling. Get ruthless and make it happen.

A simple solution is one that keeps coming up, go to bed earlier and get up earlier. What keeps us up at night? You know what it is. We're well aware of the triaged victim that we have to sacrifice and leave to die. It's an old enemy that has to be dealt with harshly. It's that television that can so easily suck an extra hour out of your evening. That hour could be your exercise hour. Deliver a knockout blow as you kiss the grandkids goodnight and go to bed an hour before everyone else.

Staying out of the hotel bar for that last drink and heading to bed is another option. There's your invaluable hour right there. You just made a decision that will allow you to survive the next day in the brutal world of fitness discipline. Only the weak use the excuse, "I don't have the time." Travelers have to work harder.

Don't worry if you're stuck in a hotel, you can make it work. Hotel rooms are an excellent place to sneak in a workout. Stretch that geezed-up body thoroughly and get to work. Throw a towel down on the floor and do your crunches, push-ups and dumbbell routine. Did you remember to bring those dumbbells?

Do you need a little cardio time? Run in place, do some jumping-jacks, dance around like your genitalia is being nibbled on by a thousand ants, anything that gets your body moving and that geezy heart beating. Get the sweat pouring from your body and clean out that worn and wise container where we shelve our soul.

It's over before you know it. You knocked it out and you're feeling good about yourself. When it's done, you're feeling like you can conquer the world as you walk out into the wild jungle that is another day. Don't forget the hotel fitness room if that's your thing. Just be on alert for pretty murderers who want to kill you.

Let's run through a few more tips on surviving those trying times of traveling while in the midst of a workout program. Remember that you're playing a psychological game with yourself. You have to hang on to the program at least enough to survive. You can jump back full force into it when you're back home. The trick is to arrive back home feeling good about yourself and your dedication. Make that effort while on the road and you'll survive.

GEEZER ALERT!

Come On Ole Geezer, Keep Reading. No Nappie Yet!

How about the days you're actually engaging in the act of travel? These days can be especially trying. Airports, security, and ground transportation can make for a long, agonizing day. However, there's one thing that's always in abundance. That's downtime and waiting for something to happen.

Before we delve into this, there's one very important note that shouldn't even have to be mentioned. *Bring your own healthy snacks to the airport*. If you happen to be driving to your destination, do the same. Don't get caught in that nasty food trap. Eat before you're actually hungry, because temptation of those over-priced fat-bombs can overwhelm you in a moment of weakness.

Waiting and airports go hand-in-hand together. That allows for quick naps and lots of opportunities to rest your body. If you do the following, you'll be glad to get that rest. Here's an example. Let's say that you need to leave your home for the airport by 6 a.m.

Wake up *super* early and complete your entire workout. Yes, you'll be extremely tired, especially if this is not your normal schedule. That's okay, because you did what you had to do to keep your program alive. You're a winner. Nap and rest as much as you can during your travel ordeal.

Another version of this is to double your routine the day before traveling, then take the following day off. A word of caution, be *very* careful anytime you push yourself beyond what you normally do. As you know, there's always a lurking possibility of injuries hiding in the shadows. They're just aching to jump out and grab a geezer.

Never push yourself beyond your comfort level. Possibly add fifty percent more to your routine if that's more comfortable. You could also reduce the intensity of the workout slightly. When you're adding to your routine, extra walking is a safer option than the weight-lifting department. It's the geeze factor, so play it safe, my fellow old coot. We don't want to break down at the airport like an old car in the desert.

The next tip was briefly mentioned earlier, exercising *at* the airport. I admit watching a geezed coot doing crunches, push-ups and jumping jacks could provide some comical entertainment for bored travelers. You can at least somewhat hide behind some chairs as you're doing the floor-based portion of the routine.

Never expect to totally get away with it though, because it's always some two-year-old that will discover you. In all their innocence, they'll point and exclaim to the crowd around them, "Look at that old person doing funny things on the floor." You've got be tough and endure it.

Remember that you'll likely never see those people again and you provided a bit of entertainment in an otherwise drab environment. Who knows, maybe you'll get famous on some sort of social media. The two-year-old probably has his three-year-old buddy acting as his video guy and filming everything that moves.

Staying in hotels,
Flying on planes.
An exercise program,
You must sustain!

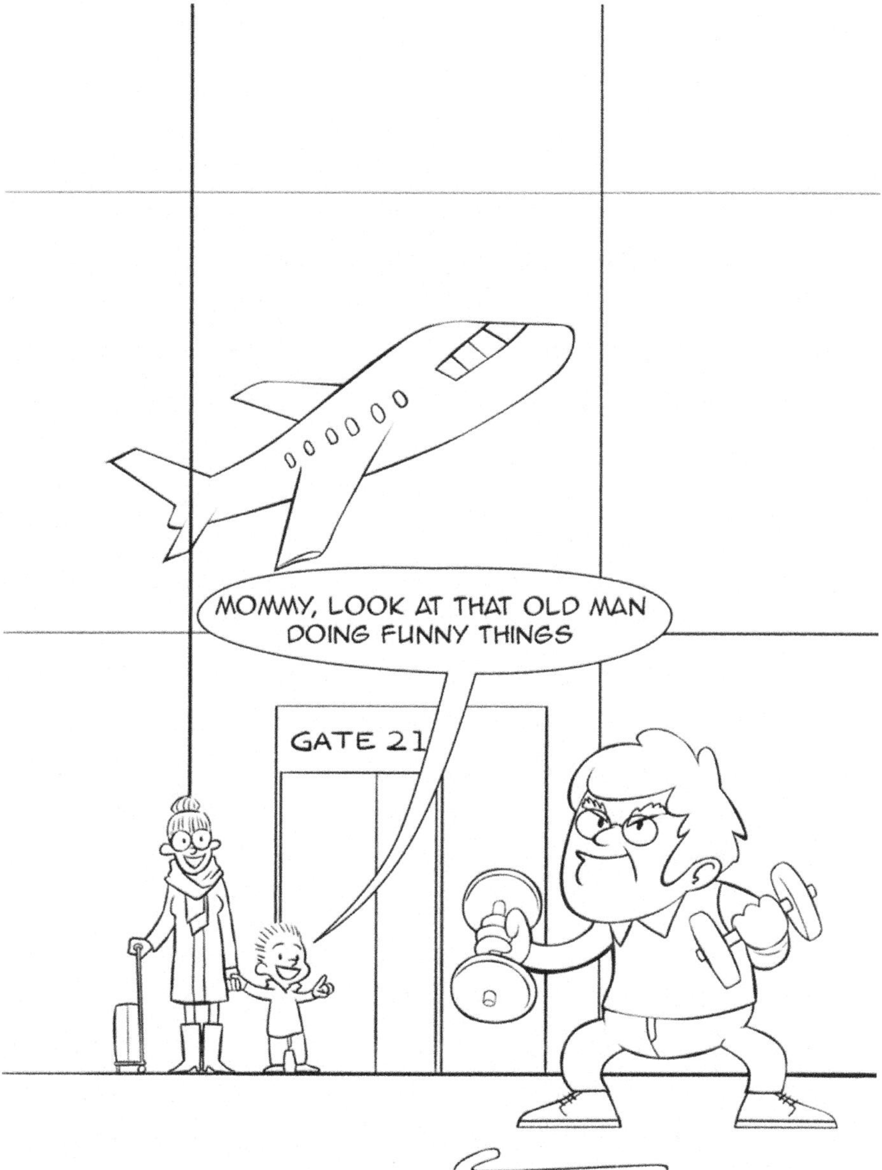
MOMMY, LOOK AT THAT OLD MAN DOING FUNNY THINGS
GATE 21

Get It Done III

When you finally arrive at your destination, things will become a little easier. Settle in and arrange your battle plans for getting through it. Additional exercise tips include utilizing a chair or some other item as a dumbbell, walking the unfamiliar area scouting out potential happy hour locations, or swimming in the hopefully pee-free hotel pool. You can substitute water aerobics for any exercises that are difficult to fit in. Another substitution example would be doing calisthenics in the room instead of outdoor walking on a rainy day.

The next subject somewhat coincides with the traveling issues. It concerns short-term exercise planning. This will happen naturally as you progress through your exercise program and become more professional. Don't overanalyze it. It's really just common sense and we geezers have a wealth of it stored up.

I'll run through a few examples. Suppose you're golfing tomorrow and you expect to be doing a lot of walking. Today's schedule is tight and you're worried about missing your workout. A possible solution would be to sacrifice a portion of today's aerobic workout and really concentrate on the other exercises.

Try to keep all of those muscles moving in a balanced nature. If one group is worn and tired, then work something else. The key is to keep moving, for our old bodies could go into permanent freeze-mode at any time. Reincarnation is right around the corner for us, or possibly a long rest in Heaven. I trust that none of you are going to the firepit below where my mean ole Uncle Thomas resides.

Suppose you are flying out of town in three days. You will also be away for three days. I admit it's a certain hassle to check in those dumbbells with the airlines. Since you'll only be gone for three days, there's a way around it. For the next three days, concentrate heavily on your dumbbell/abdominal workout. Add a little more than usual, especially the dumbbells. By the third day, your upper body will be ready for a long rest.

Fly away and while you're out of town, concentrate on your walking/aerobic routine. This gives your upper body a deserved rest while you work your lower body extra hard. Maybe you could slip in some crunches and push-ups if possible. Once you arrive back home, you slide back into your normal exercise sequence.

Once you get into a regular workout schedule, you'll find yourself doing *anything* to accomplish your exercise routine. You will juggle work, social commitments, and domestic duties to accommodate that important workout. When you've reached this point, you'll probably never turn back. You'll be as hooked on exercise as much as you were to that bowl of ice cream that used to rule you. You are committed.

Try to always think ahead without worrying about it. Stress isn't what we're looking for as it speeds up our already geezed-up bodies. It's really simple. If something is coming up in the near future that could possibly interfere with your exercise, plan for it now. With proper short-term planning, you won't skip a beat. Be aware of the immediate future and relate it to your fitness program.

The next subject we'll discuss will be how to avoid workout interruptions. *This is very important.* An interrupted workout is a huge problem. You run a great risk of never resuming it. From the very beginning, you need to set some *hard* rules regarding your workout.

Rule number one involves that thing that stays attached to you night and day. Put away that addictive phone and let voicemail handle it. Remember those pre-geezer decades when we lived without a mobile phone? You survived many years without one of those devices, so you can certainly go an hour without it. Don't worry, you won't miss anything. The world will still be as messed up in one hour as it is now.

Exercise is top priority. Make peace with those who live with you and work a deal. Tell everyone of importance that you're not to be disturbed during exercise. Work with your partner to protect each other's time. Fiercely guard that workout time like it's the most important thing in the world.

If your house is on fire, stay there doing curls until the flames completely engulf you and char you to the ground. Finish that workout no matter what the situation. That's the dedication I'm looking for. Just kidding, but do try to develop that mentality towards interrupted workouts.

Let's proceed to the next chapter. Here's the plan itself and how to manage it. It's simple and easy and designed especially for a geezed-up body.

To stay fit,
Have a plan.
You can do it,
Yes, you CAN!

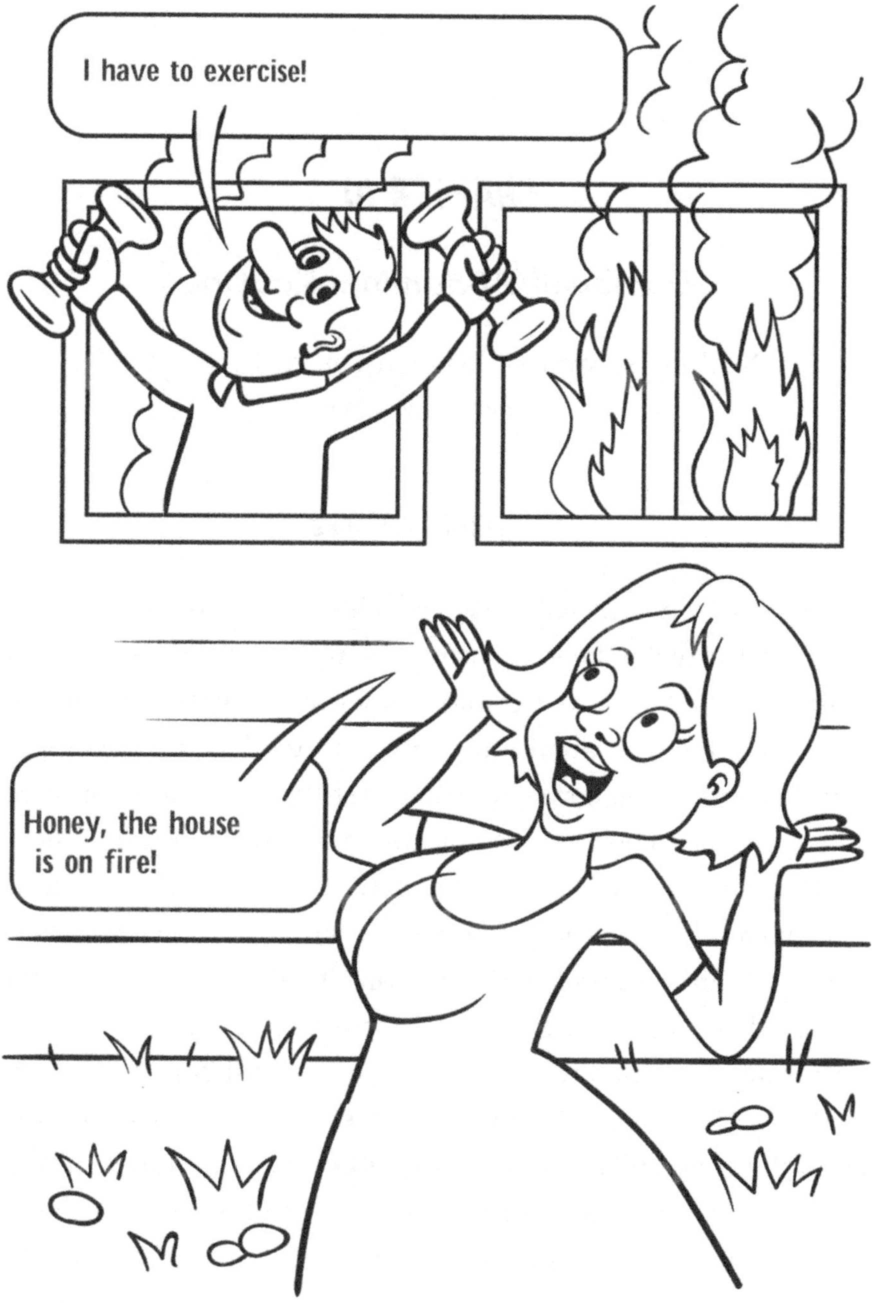
I have to exercise!
Honey, the house is on fire!

CHAPTER 10

Dumbbell/Abdominal Routine

"Nothing's impossible when you really want it."
Robert A. Walker

Simplicity Works

Longevity and survivability are vital if you're to make it. That's why we're keeping things simple here. Complicating matters only leads to trouble, sometimes big trouble in the form of complete abandonment. Our goal is to develop a simple exercise program that will last through the long-term. We want this to become an automatic part of your daily life.

Walking or another aerobic activity will be the staple of your basic exercise plan. You should attempt to do this every day, with only an occasional day off. It's the calorie killer that we need to keep those fat cells from taking over. The other important part of the program is our dumbbell/abdominal routine. This keeps us toned and strong and balances our overall fitness. Five or six days per week of these simple exercises should keep those muscles in good working order.

Combine this simple approach with a sensible, healthy diet and you're destined for success. It won't happen overnight, but you didn't gain that excess weight overnight either.

Plug along methodically with your daily exercises and you will be rewarded. That excess weight will try to trick you at first by refusing to budge. Don't let that discourage you, for it will eventually come off one pound at a time. At some point, your metabolism caves in to your persistence and rewards you by slicing pounds off at a *much* faster rate.

The dumbbell/abdominal routine has only seven exercises. They are geared equally for women and men. Only three of these require dumbbells, and you can use the same dumbbells for each one. Our goal isn't to fill a room with expensive, bulky equipment to impress others. We're not interested in that. What we are interested in is losing weight, getting toned and maintaining it for life.

The seven exercises are abdominal crunches, leg-lifts, dumbbell presses, dumbbell flies, dumbbell curls, push-ups and squats. These exercises have been placed in a certain strategic order for maximum efficiency. As you are doing one exercise, certain muscles will be resting up for their turn. Then you use those muscles while the others rest. This enables you to go as fast or as slow as you like. The pace should be one that you feel comfortable with and can keep up day after day without burning out.

Remember that we're discarding all that hype from the past that never worked. That advice was probably geared to the twenty-something kid who desires the perfect body just like their celebrity fashion hero. Their heads are spinning in circles at their precarious age, one where they know it all, but know nothing. At that age they're desperately seeking a mate to marry, have 2.2 kids, and get divorced as soon as possible. You know the routine.

We're not out for that perfect body. If it happens, then it's a wonderful thing. It's just that it's not our end game. Ours is more simple and much more realistic in its approach. Wipe out all that silly clutter from the past and settle in to something that *works*. This has been tested and is guaranteed to work, with one critical qualification. *You have to work.*

Please pause now for an important message

Early cavewoman did these ***exact*** *exercises that I'm promoting. Ancient stone ledgers have been recovered at Paleolithic archaeological sites, containing records of seven* ***miracle*** *exercises that guaranteed cavewoman would lose ten pounds per week, week after week. These are the seven exercises I'm promoting and* ***only I possess the secret*** *behind them. For a small fee I will share my knowledge with you. These prehistoric artifacts have been analyzed by expert archaeologists and were found to be actual* ***miracle*** *exercises. To find out more, go to my website and sign up with your credit card. For a mere $599 per month, you too can lose ten pounds every week. Don't worry, we'll put you on autopay. You will be paying forever!* ***Sign up now*** *and lose weight!*

I hope you all know **that was a total joke**. Just buy me a beer if you ever meet me and I'll be forever appreciative. Drifting back into reality, there is a very good reason why the exercises are limited to seven. As I'm writing this, I'm looking at a popular fitness book that sells well, but offers no practicality whatsoever. It serves as an excellent cocktail coaster though.

Why is it not practical? It tells us to become fit we have to execute certain exercises on certain days during certain weeks, switching between intermediate low volume, intermediate medium volume, intermediate high volume, advanced low volume, advanced medium volume, advanced high volume, all the while rotating each exercise on specific odd days and even days, then reverse the exercises and work backwards. *What the ....!*

Even Euclid, the ancient Greek mathematical whiz wouldn't be able to figure this one out. Take a guess at how many *mandatory* exercises are described within it. *42!* That's right, you'll get fit if you learn these 42 exercises and call upon Einstein's ghost to guide you through the intellectual haze.

Your brain may become fit trying to analyze it, but your body probably isn't going to make any progress. It's headed back to the safety of a *Gunsmoke* rerun, something nice, simple and soothing. "Screw this fitness stuff," it says, as it clicks down upon the remote.

Now you see the reason for limiting the number of exercises. It's better to actually perform seven exercises daily than to attempt 42 exercises, quickly become discouraged, and quit entirely. It's overwhelming to try to learn new exercises and keep track of them, especially when you're just starting out. The dedication and discipline requirements alone drain your mental energy. Simplicity is the answer to longevity. Accept it, geezer.

Another advantage to keeping things simple is the freeing up of the mind. Once you've mastered the basics of this simple plan, you need not stress over your next exercise. It will become nearly automatic. After you've practiced it for a few months, you can almost place yourself into a meditative state.

The crunches, curls and such will just happen as your mind wanders anywhere you choose. What sounds better, having to concentrate on what variation of which exercise is coming up and stressing over it, or picturing yourself on a sandy, white beach with the gentle waves rolling in? I prefer the easy, peaceful route.

The less you have to think about something, the easier it is to just plug into the system and get it done on a daily basis. Sure, it's probably true that there are a couple of muscle groups that don't get worked to perfection using this program. If you want that, get on the internet and order that book with 42 exercises, each with 6 variations, for a total of 252 different tasks to complete.

One other thing, factor in the geezer quotient and does anybody really care? You're old and no one expects you to bring home the gold in body building competitions. And who the hell is going to do an inspection of your body to make sure your tiny stapedius muscle is receiving the proper workout? It's one of approximately 600 muscles and I think you'll be okay if it's not toned to perfection. Zarkoff may be inspecting some of you ladies out there, but I'm pretty sure you'll pass with flying colors regardless of your fitness status. Being female is the only requirement with him.

These seven exercises mainly concern the middle and upper body, with the exception of the squats. There is absolutely no need to get fancy with these exercises. They are all very basic. They work as well for women as they do for men. These aren't overnight-body-beautiful gimmickry pieces of magic promised by the con-men. These are real exercises that deliver results over time.

Gradually, you will feel and see improvement in your body. These same seven exercises are listed in hundreds of fitness books, usually alongside a host of other complicating exertions. The trick with these particular seven is they're a perfect combination to achieve a generally fit body. Perhaps one day I'll improve on them, but for now I'm completely satisfied. Hopefully, you will be too.

Seven exercises, Nothing to it. Easy to learn, Easy to *do* it!

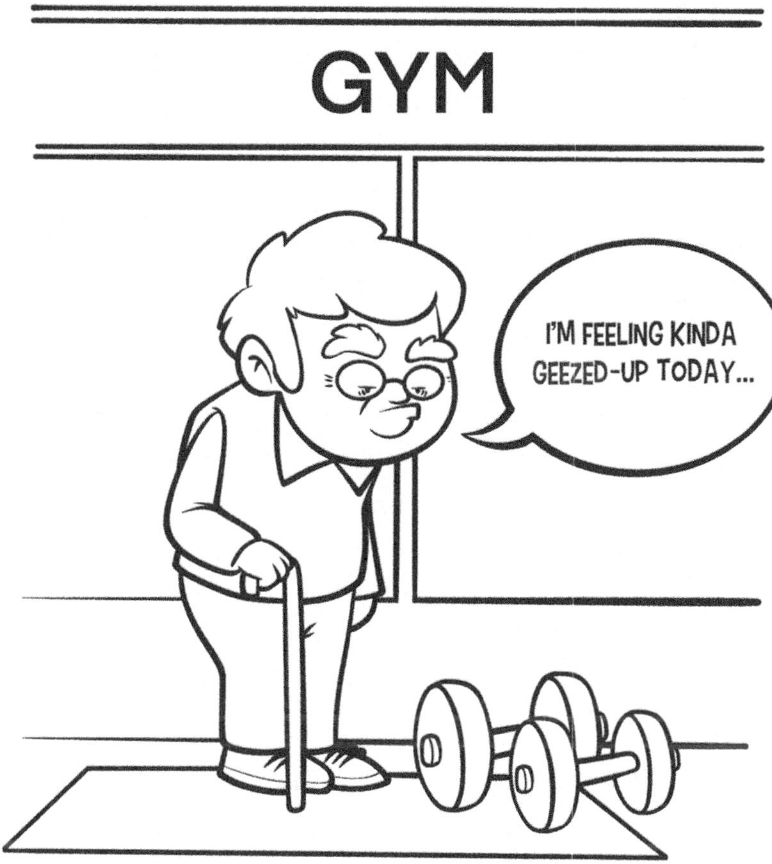
GYM
I'M FEELING KINDA GEEZED-UP TODAY...

The Seven Exercises

Here are the exercises described *in the order* that I prefer to do them. I like to perform the first set of *each* exercise in a very loose manner, with no focus on intensity. Look at the first set as *more of a stretching exercise* rather than the exercise itself. It's like a car building up speed as it enters a freeway. It's the most natural way to flow into each exercise and helps to prevent injuries. It's the geezer factor as you may guess.

You did stretch, right?

LEG-LIFTS: These strengthen the upper and lower abdominal muscles. I'm sure you know the importance of your core muscles. You will *no*t see immediate results from working these muscles. You will, however, feel it relatively quickly. Do not get discouraged because the mirror you're staring into doesn't show a ripped midsection. This part of the body requires time for visible results. Keep up the routine as if it were your job. *Don't quit.* Be very careful and don't strain a muscle, for it's quite easy to do. To *see* results in the abdominal area, you have to eat right. Never skip these important exercises. Here's how to do them.

Lie flat on your back on an exercise mat, blanket or adjustable abdominal bench. Lower your legs just to the point where you feel your back lifting off the floor. This is for optimal abdominal benefit. Keep your legs fairly close together and your feet several inches apart. Change the position periodically if you like. I like to mix it up during my routine. Now *slowly* lift your legs up while mentally focusing on your core. Try to create that little core burn that lets you know you're working the right muscles. Don't make the mistake of arching your lower back, which lets your abdominal muscles relax. Inhale on the way down and exhale on the way up.

After a few months of mastering this exercise, some of you may want to do what I mentioned earlier. I actually wear heavy work boots to add a little weight. I guess you could add weight by any method you like. The key here, if you choose to do this, is to experiment and progress *slowly* with any additional weight. You know why. It's the geezed-up potential injury factor.

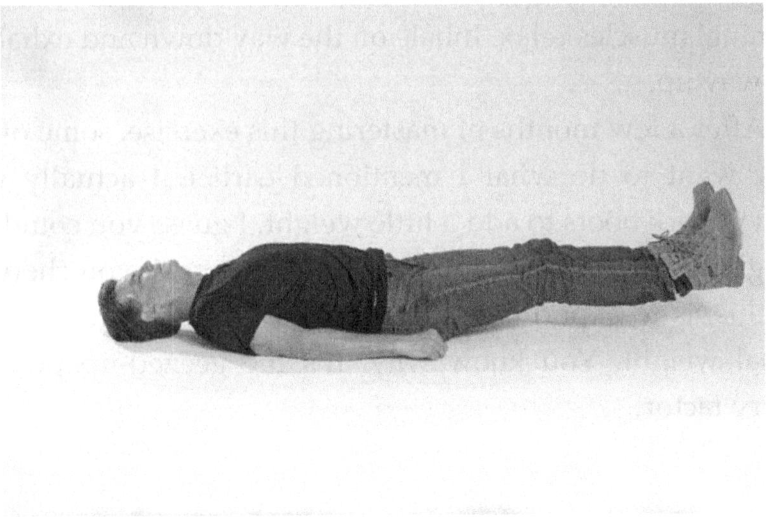

LEG-LIFT

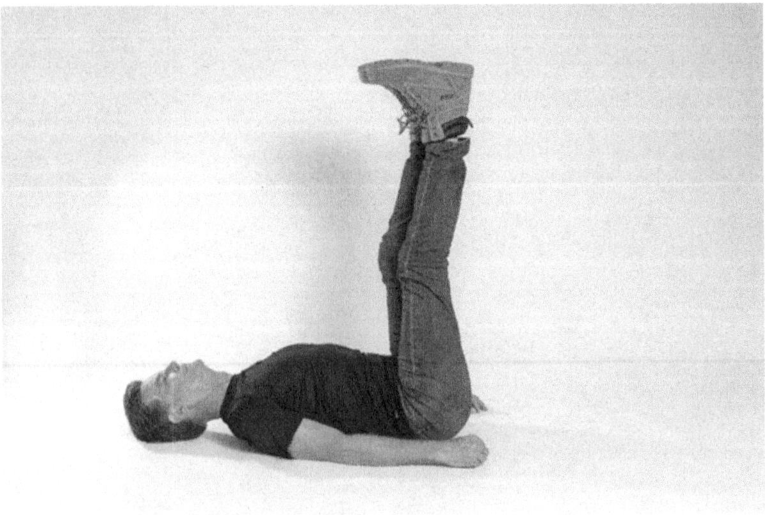

CRUNCHES: These are similar to the leg-lifts in that we're concentrating on the core. Once again, don't expect to be Superman or Wonder Woman after doing a few sets of crunches. It's not going to happen. The core exercises are extremely important whether they're visibly showing results or not. Keep them up no matter what. Here's how to do them.

Lie flat on your back on an exercise mat, blanket or adjustable abdominal bench. Have your knees bent. You can keep your feet flat on the floor or you can be slightly on your heels. I mix the two for no particular reason. Lift your hands up to a comfortable position. There are several different thoughts as to where to place your arms and hands. Many suggest placing your hands behind your head, while others suggest holding your arms and hands a little further to the front. The latter is the method I prefer, but choose whatever feels comfortable. The bottom line is to work that core and stay injury-free.

Contract your core as your lower back presses against the floor. Exhale as you *slowly* lift the head and shoulders upward a few inches. Be very aware of this movement and don't strain your neck or pull it forward with your hands. Hold this position for a moment and try to create that little burn we crave that lets us know we're succeeding. At this point I sometimes slowly lift my feet upward a couple of inches. It seems to engage the lower core a bit more. Inhale as you slowly lower your back to the starting position. Try to master this simple exercise and make it part of your life.

I sometimes like to do a knee-in version of this exercise. As you know, I thrive on simplicity and try to stay away from multiple variations as much as possible. However, this is one that I feel is beneficial. The only real change is that you raise your knees upward to the point where you can nearly touch them with your elbows. I would consider this a slightly more advanced version of a crunch. By mixing the two versions you'll probably reach a little more of the core area. The goal is to create that tiny burn and *not hurt yourself.*

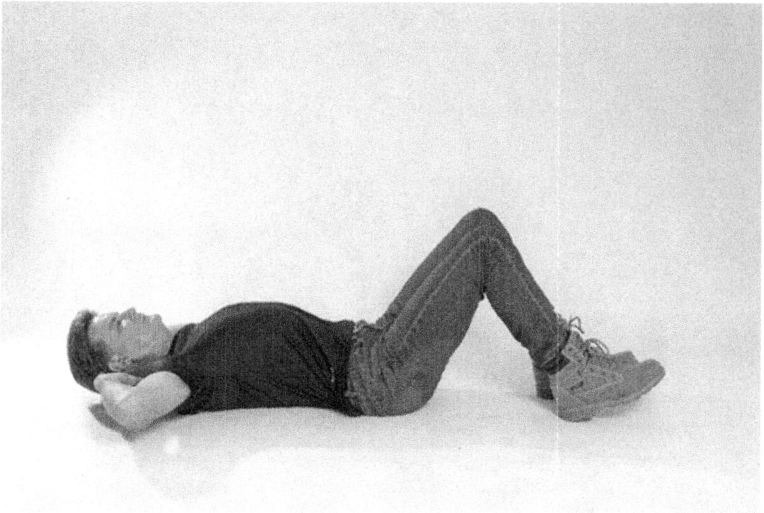

CRUNCH

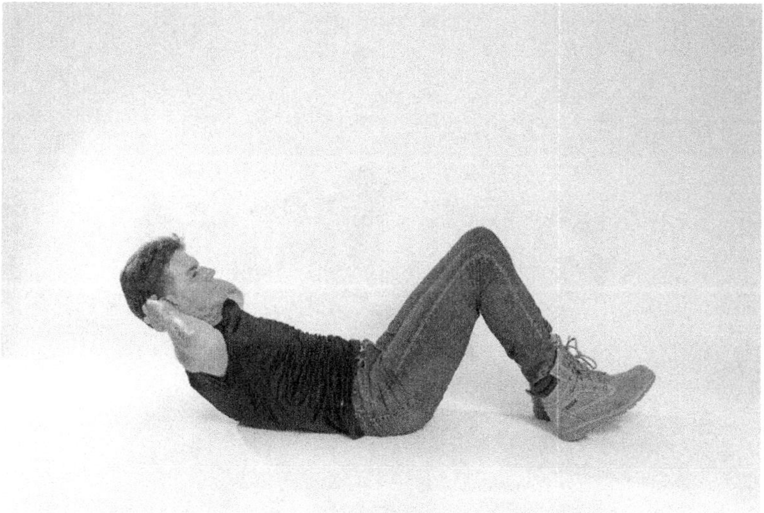

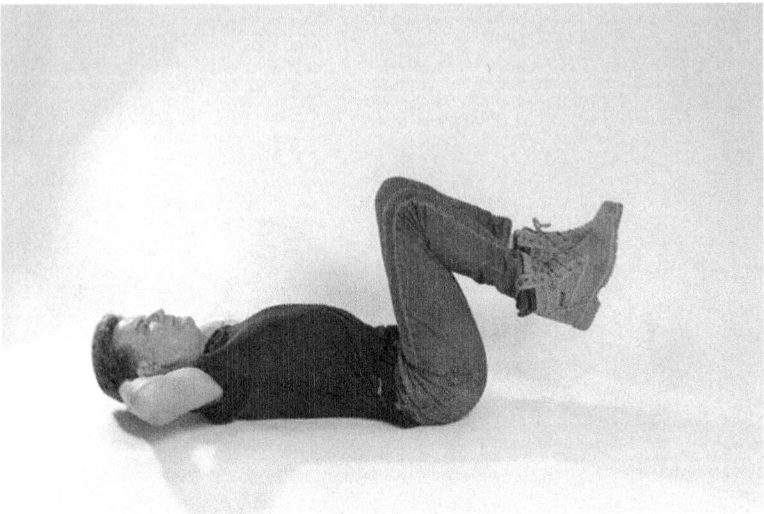

KNEE-IN CRUNCH

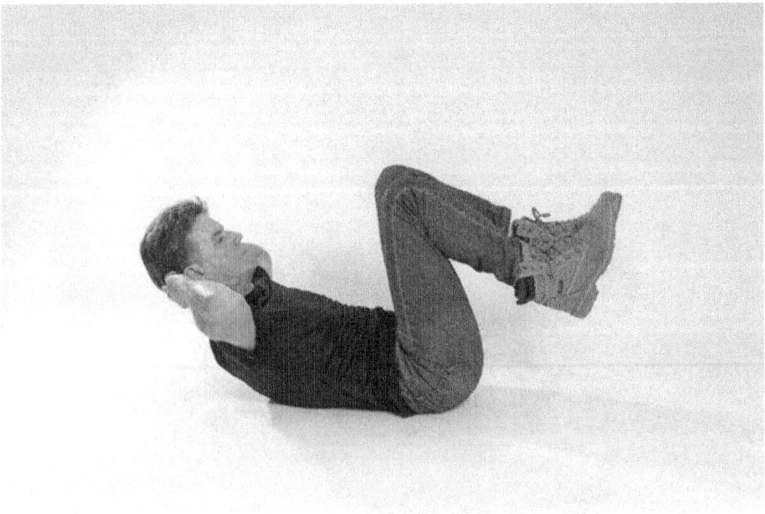

DUMBBELL PRESS: The dumbbell press is a great exercise for the chest and upper body. The weight of the dumbbells is of great concern. There will be a section later in the chapter regarding weight amounts and number of repetitions. You must put a lot of thought and slow experimentation into this before you begin the routine. Whatever you do, don't just go pick up the closest dumbbells you can find and start plugging away at this exercise. Your geezed-up body will resist and you will pay. Here's how to do them.

Lie on an exercise bench with a dumbbell in each hand and your feet flat on the floor. You can also lie on an exercise mat or a blanket on the floor. You may lose a tiny bit of the benefits this way because you're missing a couple of inches of the total exercise. There is one advantage to this though. You're somewhat reducing your chance of injury. Those inches I'm talking about are actually the prime potential injury zone, especially for geezers.

The bottom line is to not concern yourself with an exercise bench if you don't currently have one. They cost money and take up room, and I've never heard anyone comment positively on their aesthetics. "Oh, what a beautiful workout bench that is! It matches your expensive European furniture so well. I just adore the beautiful sweat stain in the middle!"

There is another reason I avoid a bench. I actually like using it, but I travel a lot and can't afford to get used to it. It's a psychological thing. You get used to something, it's temporarily taken away, and the mind shifts into the "all or nothing" mode. The result can be a devastating abandonment of the program while under the psychological loss of the bench.

Therefore, I don't allow myself to get connected to a bench. It's funny how the mind works sometimes. Most of you probably possess normal brains, so maybe this doesn't apply to you. If so, carry on and be very grateful you're not cursed with quirky mental afflictions. I'll now continue.

To prepare for the dumbbell press, push the dumbbells up to the point where your arms are directly over your shoulders and your palms are up. Tighten your abdominals and tilt your chin toward your chest. Lower the dumbbells down and to the side until your elbows are slightly below your shoulders, or level with them if you're on the floor. Focus on your chest as you roll your shoulder blades back and down. *Slowly* push the dumbbells back up without locking your elbows or raising your shoulder blades. Exhale as you're doing this. Hold for a brief moment and then repeat the downward movement.

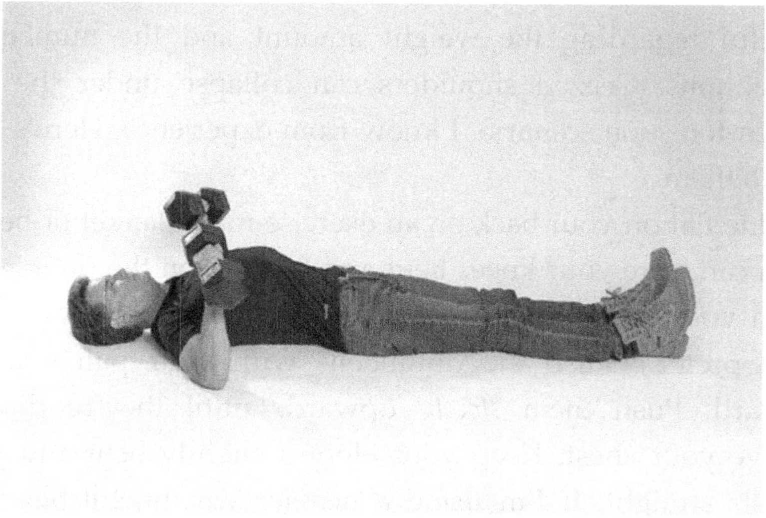

DUMBBELL PRESS

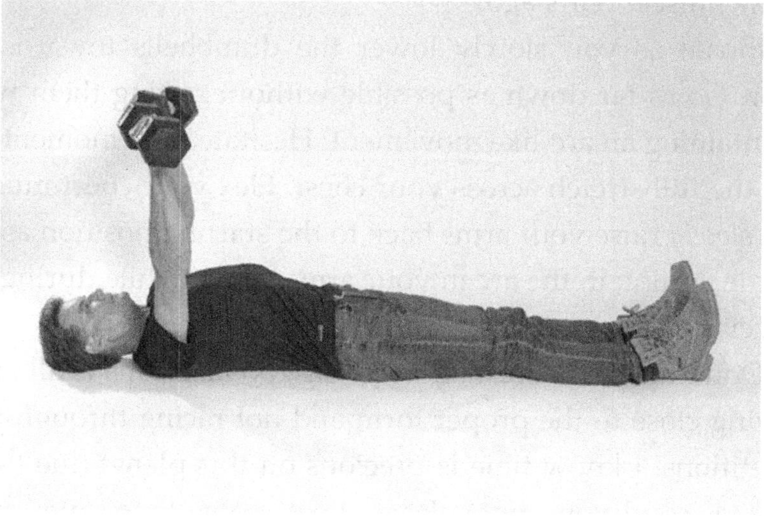

DUMBBELL FLY: The dumbbell fly engages some of the same muscles as the press, as well as others. Sometimes I'll mix the two exercises in one set. As with the press, be very careful regarding the weight amount and the number of repetitions. Geezed shoulders can collapse under the too-much-too-soon scenario. I know from experience. Here's how to do them.

Lie flat on your back on an exercise mat, blanket or bench. You can have your knees bent and feet flat on the floor, or lie with your legs stretched out. You can mix both positions if you prefer. Grasp the dumbbells with your palms facing inward. Push them *slowly* upwards until they're directly above your chest. Keep your elbows slightly bent and your wrists straight. If I'm using a heavier weight, I'll bend the elbows a bit more to accommodate it, at least for the first set. It's an old geezer warmup trick I learned after straining a geezy muscle years ago.

Inhale as you slowly lower the dumbbells towards the floor. Go as far down as possible without resting them while maintaining an arc-like movement. Hesitate for a moment and feel the full stretch across your chest. Flex your chest muscles and *slowly* raise your arms back to the starting position as you exhale. Maintain the arc in your arms all the while during this exercise.

Don't make the mistake of going too fast. This is all about staying close to the proper form and not racing through your repetitions. I know time is precious on this planet due to our geezed condition, but please take your time and avoid injuries. You've got another couple of good years left in you, you old geezer.

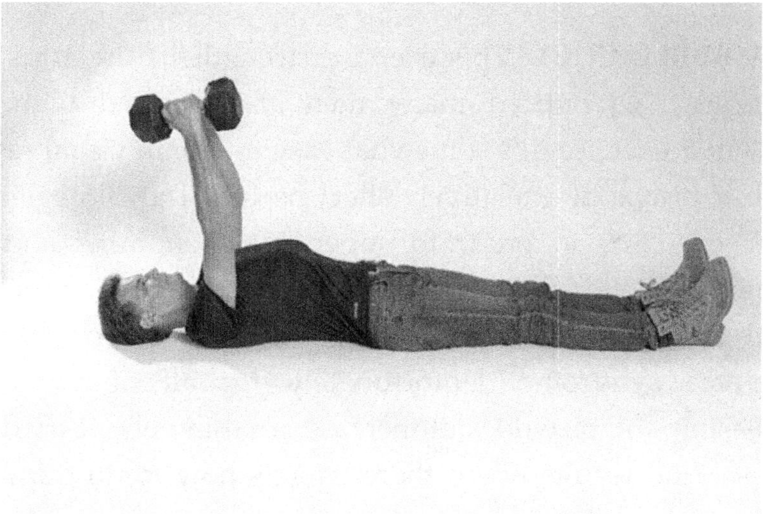

DUMBBELL FLY

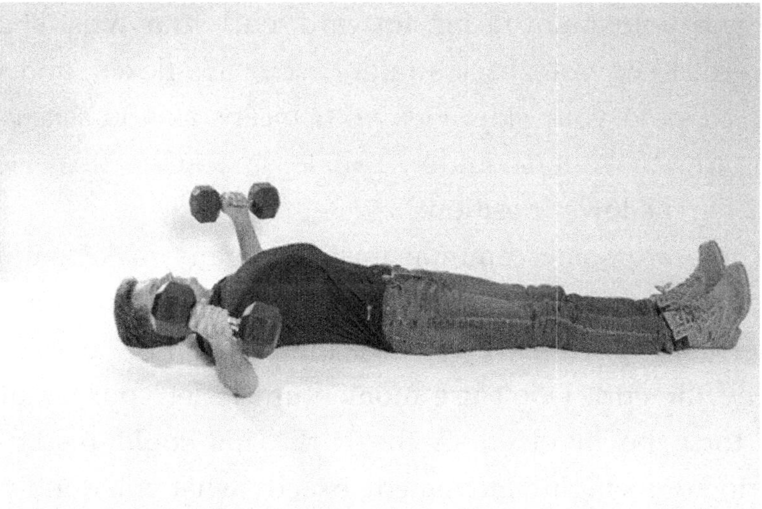

DUMBBELL CURL: This exercise strengthens the arms and forearms. I've noticed many men are obsessed with this particular exercise. It's somewhat easy to obtain visual results in your biceps in a relatively short period. They'll neglect all other exercises in order to super-size their arms and get women to notice them. This is probably due to some childhood psychological disorder of a sexual nature, or possibly little-wee syndrome. Unfortunately for all of us males, increasing arm size doesn't increase anything else. I tried this and saw no results down there. Here's how to do dumbbell curls.

Stand with your feet about hip-width apart holding a dumbbell in one hand. With your arm straight down at your side and your palm facing forward, curl your wrist slightly forward. Keep your back straight, your abs flexed, and your arms close to your side. Flex your biceps as you *slowly* curl your arm to your shoulder. Exhale as you do this. Slowly return to the lower position.

There are some common mistakes many make with this simple exercise. Make sure that you concentrate on form rather than speed. Don't change the position of your elbows during the curl. Don't use momentum to let your shoulders and torso be involved in the curl. This could result in a heaving or swinging movement, exactly what you don't want. Do these the correct way and your arm size will increase. If you want to increase male genitalia stuff a large sock inside your underwear.

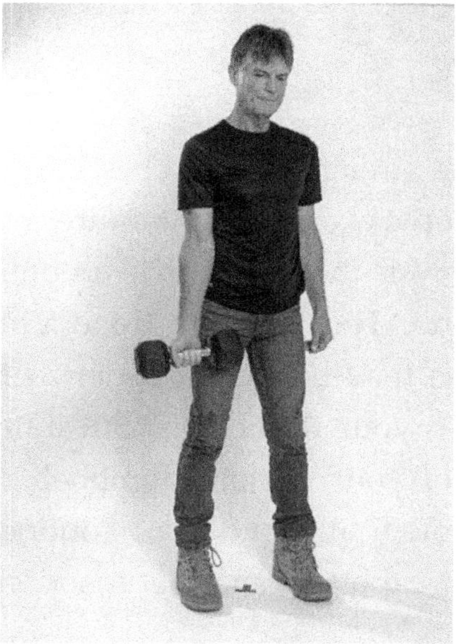

CURL

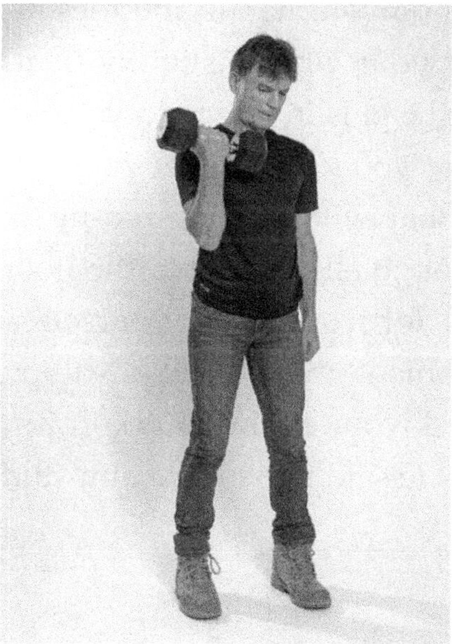

PUSH-UP: These strengthen the chest, arms, shoulders and core. This is a simple exercise that requires no weights and not a lot of space. That is the biggest reason push-ups are included in the routine. They can be done virtually anywhere. Occasionally, you may be caught somewhere for a few days without access to your dumbbells. Substitute a push-up for each repetition of your normal dumbbell routine. This will keep you psychologically into your routine. Push-ups are a valuable secret weapon in an emergency. Here's how to do them.

Get on the floor on all fours, positioning your hands slightly wider than your shoulders. Extend your legs back so that you are balanced on your hands and toes. Keep your feet hip-width apart and your elbows slightly bent. Make sure your back is flat, your head is in line with your spine, and your abs are tight. Inhale as you *slowly* lower yourself to the floor.

I've noticed that with our geezed-up bodies, it is sometimes better to not go all the way to the floor. Experiment and see what works for you. Hold yourself at the downward position for a moment, then *slowly* push up. Exhale as you do this and don't lock your elbows. Zarkoff Zucchini was a huge fan of push-ups. He said they made him stud-like.

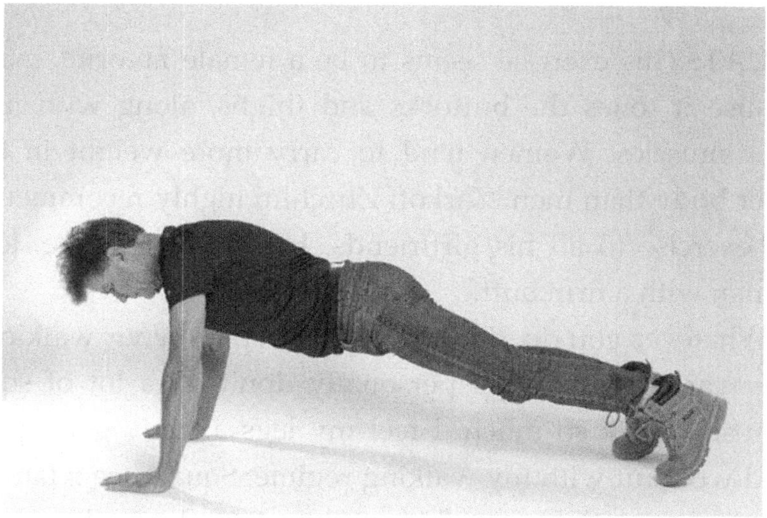

PUSH-UP

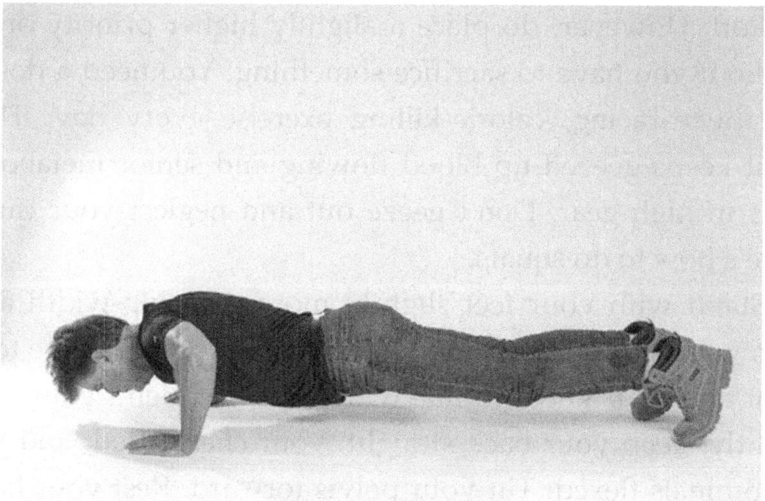

SQUAT: This exercise seems to be a female favorite, mainly because it tones the buttocks and thighs, along with many other muscles. Women tend to carry more weight in their lower body than men. Zarkoff Zucchini highly recommended this exercise to all his girlfriends. He loved a strong, leggy woman with a firm butt.

Whatever you do, don't let squats replace your walking or other cardio workout. I personally don't do a lot of squats because I walk so much. I feel my legs already get a pretty good workout with my walking regime. Squats are a fantastic exercise and can show visible results relatively quickly.

Squats and a cardio workout together can really do a nice number on your legs. It will definitely make you desirable to Zarkoff. However, do place a slightly higher priority on the cardio if you have to sacrifice something. You need a dose of that heart-racing, calorie-killing exercise every day. That's what keeps geezed-up blood flowing and senior metabolism rates in high gear. Don't geeze out and neglect your cardio. Here's how to do squats.

Stand with your feet slightly more than hip-width apart with your toes pointing forward. Keep your hips square to the front and your knees in line with your feet. Bend your knees slightly, keep your back straight, your chest lifted, and your abdominals flexed. Tilt your pelvis forward. Rest your hands on your hips or by your side and keep your heels on the floor. I also sometimes hold my hands in front of me to start. It's just a geezer habit.

Breathe in as you bend at your knees and hips. Now *slowly* squat down as if you were sitting in a chair. Keep your weight over your ankles, your back flat, and chest lifted. Check that your knees are in line with your feet. Don't allow the squat to go below seat height. Aim to keep your thighs parallel to the floor.

As you squat, extend your arms straight out in front of you. Exhale as you slowly stand up, keeping your heels on the floor, and bring your arms to your sides. Flex those buttock muscles as you keep your back flat, your pelvis tilted, and your knees slightly bent. Do these daily and make Zarkoff proud.

Those are the seven simple exercises that will work if you methodically perform them regularly. Make them a part of your daily routine along with your cardio program, and you're on your way towards becoming fit. Be patient and you'll see results.

Geezers we are,
But that's okay.
We can exercise,
Every day!

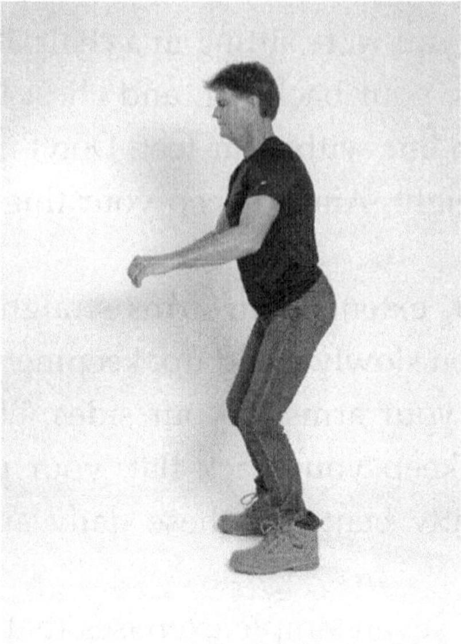

SQUAT

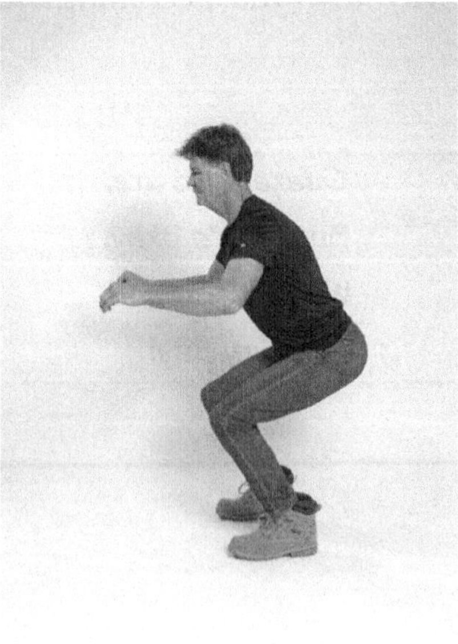

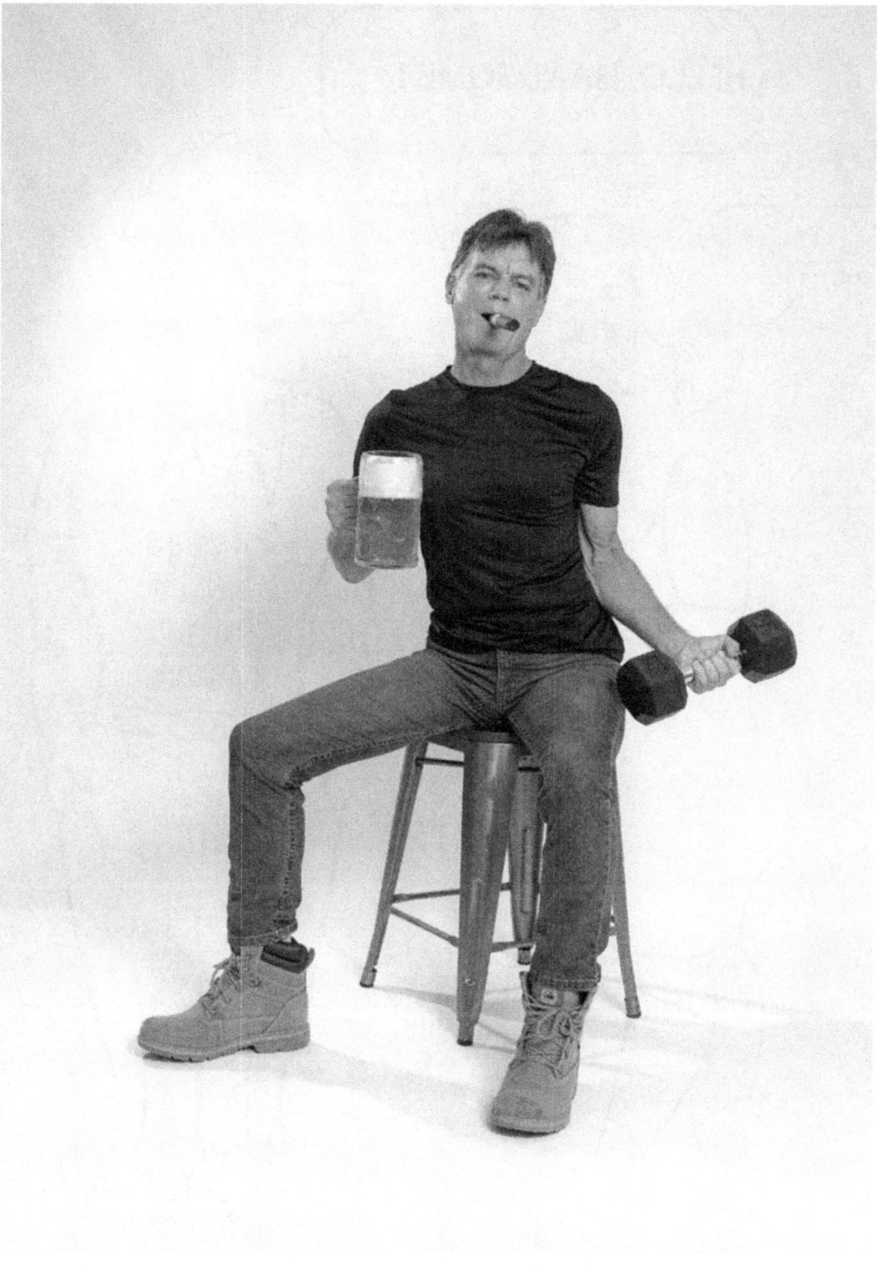

IMPROPER EXERCISE TECHNIQUE

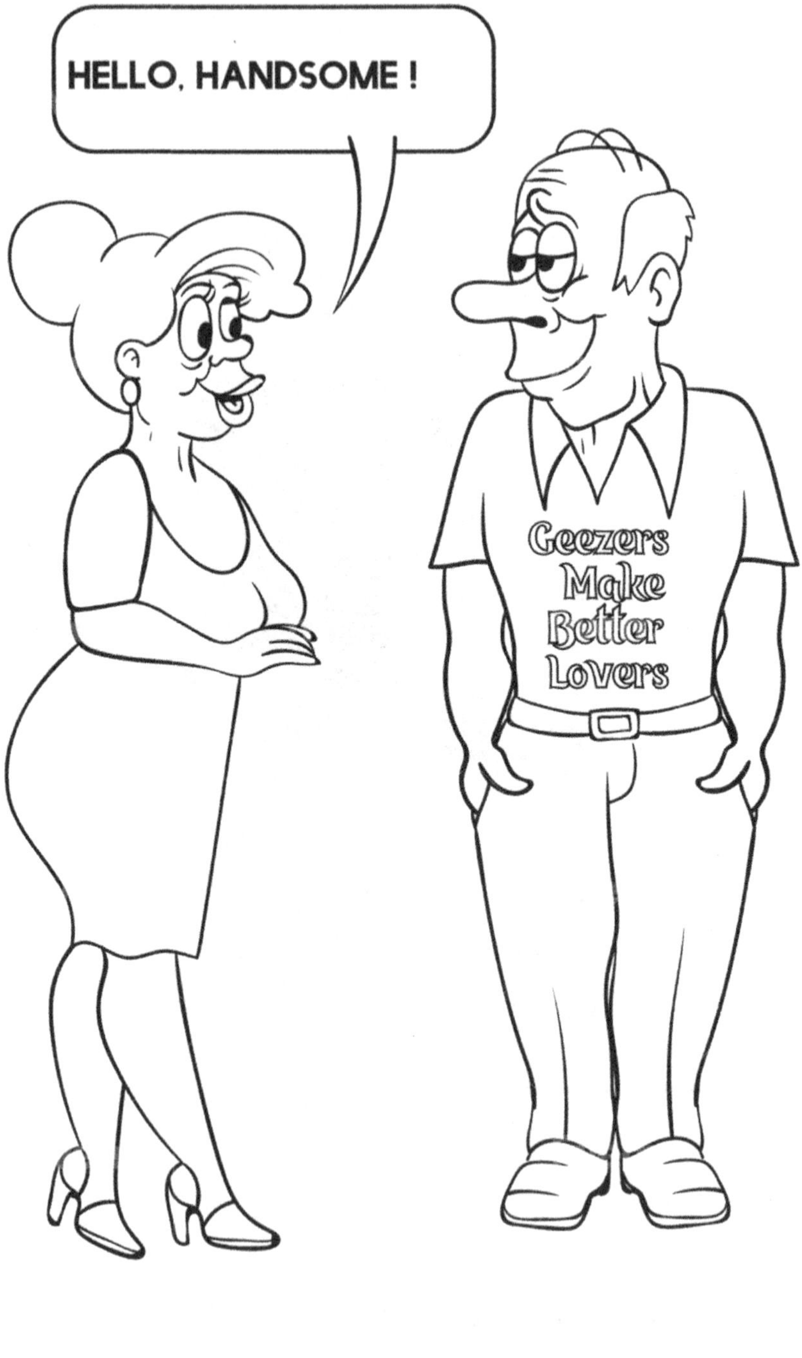
HELLO, HANDSOME !
Geezers Make Better Lovers

Exercise Tips

Now let's address some important questions. How much weight and how many repetitions are questions that need to be taken seriously. It is critical that you choose the proper weight for your particular situation. It is also important that you discover that fine line on the number of repetitions that works best for you. Too little, and especially too much, are not where you want to be.

I'm not trying to be repetitious, but this has to be repeated over and over. Injuries are a real threat, especially when you are starting out. Those of you laughing at me for continuously drilling you on this will be the first to suffer. The Karma God will get you. Go too fast and try to be Mr. America in three days and you will pay the price. Too much weight, too many repetitions, and going too fast will knock you out of the race early on. *Start slowly and carefully and avoid injuries.*

Start out with a weight that you can perform several repetitions consecutively with very little strain. Don't be in a hurry to add more weight. Always play this safe. Even if you were a twenty-year-old this would apply. The fact that we're all at Heaven's gate really reinforces this rule. It doesn't take a lot to tear something in these worn bodies. We're not made of elastic anymore.

When you are absolutely sure you can handle a heavier weight, you may want to consider this method. Do three quarters of your workout with your normal weight, then perform the last quarter with the heavier weight. Do not start your workout with the heavier weight, for your body needs to ease into this as naturally as possible. You have to be loose and limber when you're introducing anything new to a geezed-up body.

Never add more than a few pounds at any one stage. This is treacherous territory as far as injuries are concerned. After a week or two, or twelve weeks if that's what it takes, move up to one half of your workout with the heavier weight. Once again, make sure it's the *last* half of your workout. If you have *any* doubt about being able to handle the weight upgrade, *stop immediately*. Put the weights and your ego aside and use common sense. If you continue to bull your way through it, you're taking a huge risk.

After a few weeks of this, move up to three quarters of your workout with the heavier weight. Continue this for an extended period of time. Repeat the process and jump up to a full workout with the heavier weight when you feel comfortable. When you're finally performing your entire workout with the heavier weight, don't even consider adding more weight anytime soon. Let your body become accustomed to the routine.

Geezed bodies need movement more than bulk-style training. We're looking for a toned, lean, strong body rather than the shirt-ripping comic-book-hero approach. I hate to once again remind my fellow geezed macho guys, but those days have passed us by. Just go with the lean and healthy look. Don't worry, the ladies at the weekly bingo game will still pay attention to us.

When the time comes to upgrade your weights again, you will instinctively know it. Be in no hurry to do this. Let it be totally natural, smooth and easy. Repeat the one-quarter incremental plan again, being just as careful as before. You have the rest of your life. The dumbbells are your friends, not your enemies. Treat them as such and grow to love them.

How many repetitions will you do of each exercise? The short answer is to never stray from your comfort level. Never risk an injury by doing something your gut tells you not to do. Starting an exercise routine is always the most difficult part, but once you're plugged into your particular system, you'll be locked in like a machine. *So don't panic in the beginning.*

Start out very slowly. If you have not exercised regularly in years, proceed as follows. Stretch like you've never stretched before, for you are venturing off into the front lines of battle. Get as loose as you possibly can without injuring yourself. Yes, you *can* injure yourself by simply stretching. Geezers never get a break in this business.

Start out with two curls for each arm, four squats, two push-ups, two presses, two flies, five crunches, and five leg-lifts. Don't be afraid to do *less* if that's what you're comfortable with. I know there will be macho-man resistance here, because men hate to admit they can only do two push-ups, or two curls, and so on. Hey guys, we're not the "studly" characters we used to be. I know you used to be a high-school star linebacker, but that was a long time ago. Used-to-be doesn't mean anything in geezer-land. Our ladies want the here-and-now.

Take a hard, honest look at yourself before you jump. If you're truly in reasonable shape at this moment, then go for it! The message I'm trying to get across is that a lot of you are mis-perceiving yourself to be in better shape than you really are. Don't let the ego rule over common sense. Start as slow as you need to and don't be embarrassed. You'll win in the long run.

Do this simple routine for a couple of weeks, along with your cardio workout every day. If you're injury-free, try doubling the repetitions. Go another two, three, or four weeks and double it again. If doubling down seems a bit too much, then just add fifty percent at a time. The main goal is to add in small increments and avoid injuries.

Do you see how fast you can move up? Remember that we're looking at this as a minimum one-year project. The quantity of repetitions will creep higher and higher, and before you know it, you'll be where you want to be. It doesn't take long to work your way up to a twenty-minute workout. That's nothing to be ashamed of, for you'll see results for sure. Just be patient.

In the beginning and continuing throughout the first year, it will be a constant balancing act. You'll be juggling weight-amounts and repetitions to always be improving, yet always being careful to avoid injuries. Don't worry, it will become intuitive and instinctive as you move along. Listen to your body as it slowly gets used to being worked again.

Always try to keep the exercises balanced as well. These seven exercises are designed to complement each other. Always be proportionate as you increase. For example, don't sacrifice crunches to focus on more curls, or vice versa. All of our muscles rely on each other for help, so never neglect any particular group. Be completely fit, a lean, mean senior machine.

Here are a few final tips regarding these exercises, particularly the ones that require dumbbells. Geezed bodies can snap at any time, even with the weight you're accustomed to lifting. I once saw an aged geezer break into two pieces after he picked up a spoon. I glued him back together. Here's a trick that really helps. Let's assume you're preparing for your first set of a dumbbell exercise.

Instead of immediately reaching for the dumbbells, run through three simulations of the exercise without the dumbbells in hand. This somehow warns the muscles as to what is coming. I guess it's a final stretching procedure that thoroughly prepares them for battle. You can also apply this practice to the first repetition with the dumbbell, but in a different way.

Let's use a curl as an example. On the very first repetition, don't be concerned about using proper form. Think of it as a final stretch. Engage your entire body as you slowly progress through it, making sure there are no jerky movements. The stress of the exercise is divided amongst other muscles that otherwise wouldn't be engaged. It's as if they're all working as a team to help each other. This way no particular geezer muscle is caught off guard and strained. The targeted muscles are now ready for action.

Here's one final note worth mentioning. When you pick up your dumbbells always lift with your legs, and not your back. People sometimes get careless because dumbbells are relatively lightweight. They're anxious to carry on with their routine and move too fast. It's even more critical for us geezed-up exercisers. We always have to be extra careful. We want to survive to be able to work out tomorrow.

Here is an example routine of a client of mine. She's 65 and fit. She has been very successful because she applied herself, started slowly, and methodically kept at it. She hadn't exercised in thirty years when she started and she had a horrible diet. However, she had the drive, dedication and discipline to pull it off.

After eighteen months she's feeling great about herself and her whole demeanor has changed. She's forty pounds lighter and there's more to come. She considers the following as the optimum regime for her along with her daily walk. Note the emphasis on the core exercises. Yours will probably differ from hers, but you too can be just as successful. Even if you progress and ***stop*** at one-quarter of her workout you're a success. Just keep at it day after day. ***Remember, this took eighteen months!***

Stretch *thoroughly* for a ***minimum*** of ten minutes!

Lie with your back on a blanket and stretch your core for one minute. Place your arms behind your head to loosen your rib cage area. Slowly progress through the exercises focusing on proper form.

3 leg-lifts, 3 crunches, 3 knee-in crunches. Repeat again. Repeat again. Repeat again.

3 dumbbell presses, 3 leg-lifts, 3 crunches. Repeat again. Repeat again. Repeat again.

3 dumbbell flies, 3 leg-lifts, 3 knee-in crunches. Repeat again. Repeat again. Repeat again.

3 curls each arm, 3 push-ups, 3 squats. Repeat again. Repeat again. Repeat again.

Stretch again!

Walk uninterrupted for 20 minutes, 30 minutes, or …

START VERY SLOW! THIS IS AN ADVANCED WORKOUT!

Don't underestimate,
A geezer's heart.
All those years,
Made us smart!

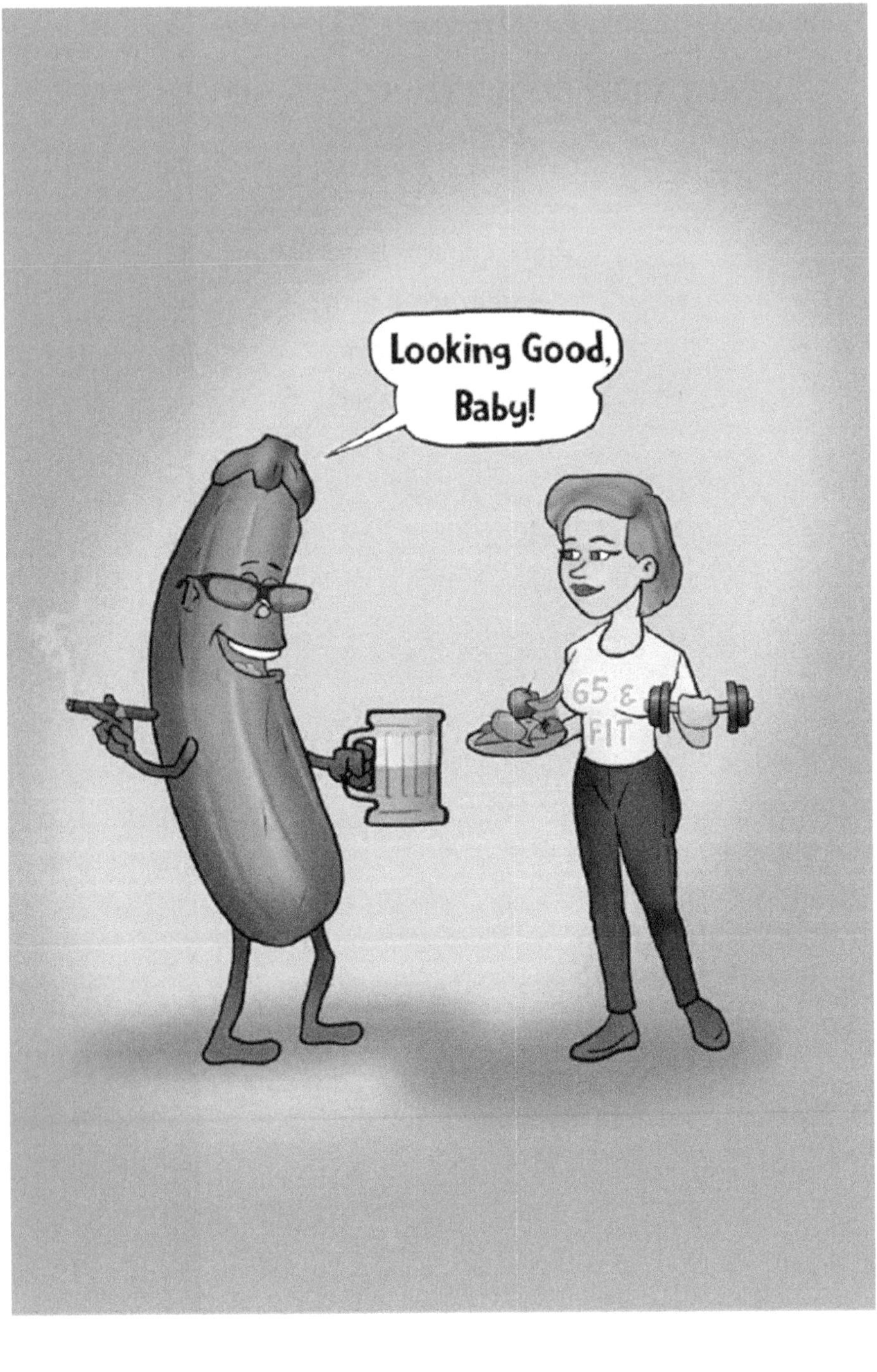
Looking Good, Baby!
65 & FIT

CHAPTER 11

You Can Do It III

"Grab your dream and make it come true."
Patra Koonkarnkhai

Determination & Desire

The driving force behind your success will be your determination and desire. Do you really want it, or are you just playing a little game with yourself? Are you going to stick through it, or are you going to cave in and give up at the first obstacle that challenges you? Are you willing to sacrifice the time and effort to make it work, or will you revert to your old habits and take the easy way out?

Zarkoff Zucchini was a vegetable who possessed an abundance of drive and ambition. He represented the little guy, the working-class vegetable who got no respect. Zarkoff was a genuine hero, a legendary figure that will be eternally remembered. The following story illustrates the character of this great vegetable.

It was a hot summer day in Phoenix, Arizona. Zarkoff Zucchini was attending a fund-raising event for disabled jalapeno war veterans. A foundation was being set up to assist those who had sacrificed so much in the Great Pepper War of

2010. Thousands of peppers gave their lives and countless others were wounded or psychologically traumatized from the horrible conflict.

As usual, Zarkoff Zucchini was the guest of honor. His presence alone had brought in the elite of high-vegetable society. Millions of dollars were expected to be pledged towards helping disabled pepper veterans. Zarkoff would be the keynote speaker at the event. He was the figurehead, the main event, the headline act.

He would be going on stage in five minutes. Zarkoff peeked through the curtain that separated him from his audience. It was a black-tie affair with all the trimmings. There were veggie-world leaders, heads of major veggie-corporations, and a splattering of veggie-entertainment icons in the crowd.

Placed in the front-center seat was Jaime Jacinto Jesus Javier Jalapeno, nicknamed Five-J for obvious reasons. Five-J was the most honored and distinguished war veteran in jalapeno history. He found fame and eternal honor after leading the charge in the Battle of Burning Butt.

Five-J courageously led his fellow pepper soldiers behind enemy lines to rescue a group of jalapeno schoolchildren. They had been kidnapped by Jalapenos Out for Blood, a band of bloodthirsty, renegade, jalapeno terrorists. They had been known to kill young hostages just for sport. Five-J was incensed as he stormed into battle.

Five-J's exocarp was shot 64 times and he nearly bled to death. His pericarp was completely destroyed as his seeds littered the battleground. He courageously continued to fight and inspire his soldiers. He was near death when the last small capsicum was lifted to safety by a helicopter. There could never be a bigger jalapeno hero than Five-J.

Zarkoff was closing the curtain when something familiar caught his eye. Sitting two seats down from Five-J was...could it be...was it her...no way...yes, it was! It was Jellano Jalapeno, the famous singer! Zarkoff had a brief affair with the fiery Latina a couple of years ago. It was short, but intense, and ended when Zarkoff began dating her backup singers.

At one point he was seeing all four of the Jalapenettes. None of them was aware he was seeing the others. They were all very spicy ladies, even hotter than his habanero girlfriend.

"Ladies and gentlemen," called a voice from the podium, "I now hand it over to the one and only, the true force behind vegetable rights, Zarkoff Zucchini!"

Zarkoff walked out onto the stage. The crowd stood and went into a thunderous applause that seemed to go on forever. At one point it felt like the building would collapse from the vibration. Zarkoff had never felt more appreciated.

It finally subsided and Zarkoff spoke. "I am here today to honor the courageous jalapeno veterans that fought for justice and liberty and freedom. They have sacrificed so much and we..."

"You're not here to honor anyone, you pig!" shouted a female voice from the crowd. "You're a rotten scoundrel," cried another voice. "You're a shameful disgrace," yelled a third voice. "You deserve your wee to be chopped up and fed to the fish," a fourth voice called out.

Zarkoff was in shock. How could this be happening? Four pretty jalapenos were standing in front of him and they were displaying their fiery character. It was Jellano and her Jalapenettes. How was he going to resolve this without being completely embarrassed?

Suddenly the four peppers simultaneously charged the stage. They were enraged beyond description, boiling with anger. Five-J rose from his wheelchair to follow them. Zarkoff knew he was in deep trouble.

They executed their plan exactly as they had practiced it. Jolie Jalapenette blindsided Zarkoff on the side of the head with a cast-iron frying pan. A stunned Zarkoff fell to the floor. Julie Jalapenette bound him with rope and tape. Janie Jalapenette pulled out her industrial scissors, sliced up Zarkoffs trousers, and ripped them from his body. Zarkoff's exposed wee was there for all to see. The crowd snickered at how small it was.

Five-J took the camera from the podium and focused it on Zarkoff's privy parts. It was now being viewed on the big-screen TV for all to see. The crowd erupted in laughter at his miniaturized member. Jellano Jalapeno then approached Zarkoff carrying a large bucket. Zarkoff opened his eyes just as Jellano poured the contents of the bucket onto his privy area.

The burn was immediate. It was a bucket of sliced jalapenos, habaneros, and the feared Carolina Reaper, the hottest known pepper on earth. His little wee was on fire! The pain was unbelievable! A more horrible death he could never imagine. How did this happen? Why did he anger these fiery girls so?

Suddenly another bucket appeared on the scene. Jolie Jalpenette kicked at the pile of peppers that rested on Zarkoff's wee. Then she poured out the contents of the latest bucket. Zarkoff screamed so loud that even the attendees in the back seats heard him. It was a batch of nothing but Carolina Reaper peppers, all sliced to produce maximum heat. His wee was now scorched to the point it had become one big blister. Even if the girls stopped now, he feared it would never again operate properly. This pain was like none he had ever experienced.

However, the girls didn't stop there. Julie Jalapenette appeared with a gallon-jug filled with a liquid substance. "Let's see how this feels, wee man!" she said as she chuckled. "It's pure, concentrated Carolina Reaper extract, the hottest substance known to the planet. One drop can send a man into a coma. Let's see how a whole bucketful feels on your roaming wee!"

She poured it onto Zarkoff and it seeped through the pile of peppers onto his privates. Julie was correct in her analysis as the pain became so intense that Zarkoff fell into a coma. Just before he lost consciousness, he saw Janie Jalapenette approaching with yet another jug filled with the powerful extract. She gleefully poured it over his seemingly lifeless body.

The girls joined hands and lifted their arms in glorious victory. Zarkoff's wee would never stray again. It was done forever. "A bad wee is no longer!" they all cried in unison. "No bad wees! No bad wees!" they began chanting. Soon every female in the audience was chanting along with them.

Zarkoff awoke from his coma six months later. A nurse informed him of the bad news. His wee had been amputated. Doctors had to do it to save his life. They feared infection might spread into his bloodstream. His wee was surgically detached and thrown into a dumpster. A hungry possum ate it as a mini-appetizer.

Zarkoff was devastated. His entire identity had been taken from him. His whole existence revolved around impressing the female gender. Even though his wee had been a small one, he had been very proud of it. Now his life was shattered beyond repair. There would be no more wee activity ever again. His world had ended.

This is where Zarkoff's true character actually revealed itself. It took a full year, but he finally rose above his depression. Zarkoff's leadership skills once again prevailed as he overcame his devastating loss.

Zarkoff founded a group for others who suffered devastating wee injuries. Burned & Gone Wees International quickly became the premiere wee rehabilitation center in the western world. Dismembered male fruits and vegetables flocked in for group therapy. A satellite group called Wees Gone Forever sprouted up in Asia, and it too quickly grew into prominence.

Zarkoff Zucchini will be remembered for his contribution to wee victims as much as his vegetable activism. His enduring legacy will never fade as wee survivors around the world pay tribute to him every day. A wee enlargement research center was founded in his honor.

One day small wees will be a thing of the past, and it will all be due to the hard work and dedication of our valiant hero.

The entire male population, and many frustrated females, owe a great deal of debt to Zarkoff Zucchini. What a legend.

> Zark's little wee,
> Sure did burn.
> Now it's gone,
> He never learned.

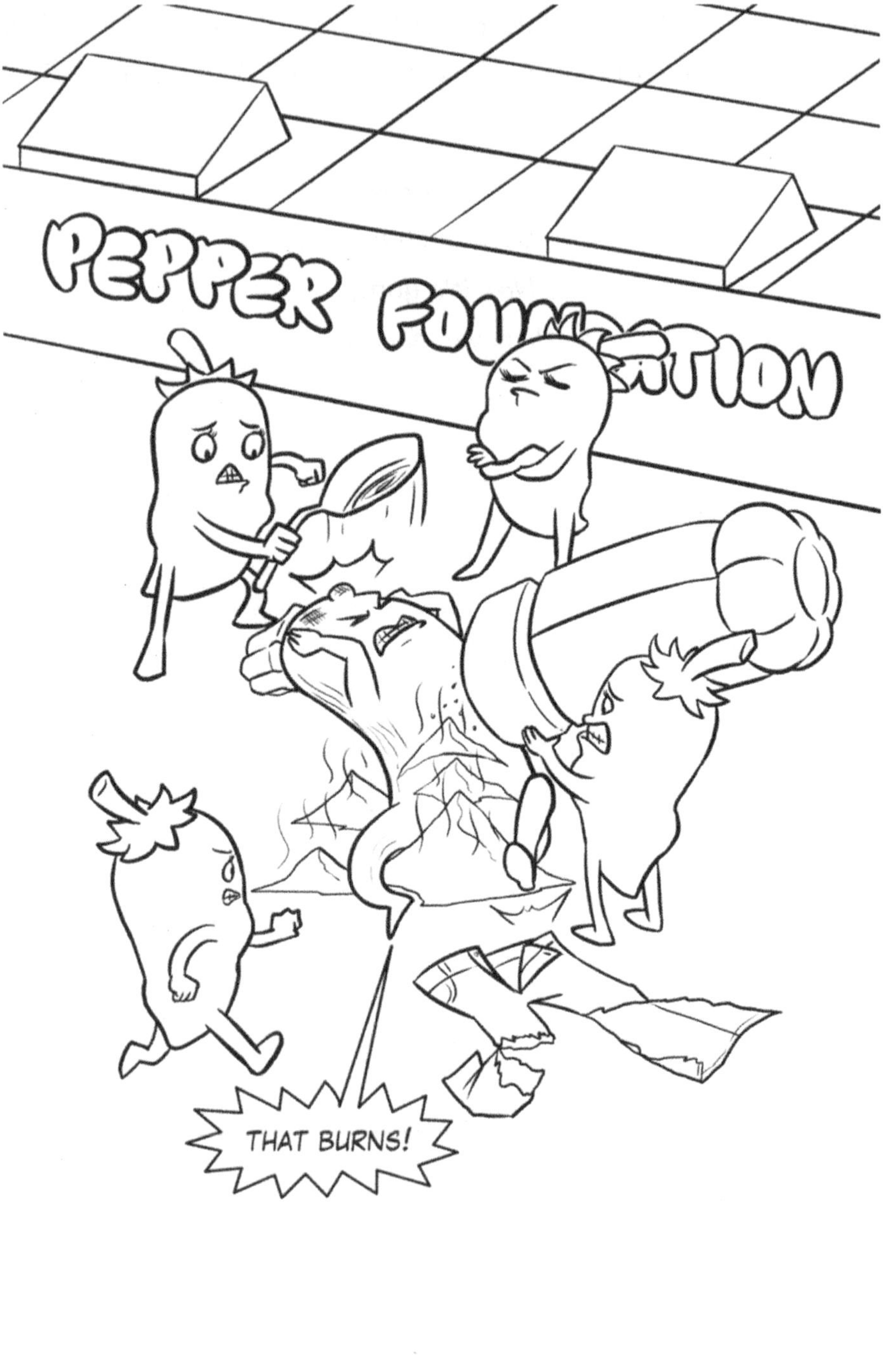
PEPPER FOUNDATION
THAT BURNS!

Determination & Desire II

Now you see how determination and desire are so important in your quest to become fit. Just as Zarkoff overcame challenges of enormous proportions, you too can accomplish something remarkable. You can have it if you really want it. Nothing can stop you.

Weight has long been an issue for many of you. Some of you could stand to lose a lot of it. Guess what? The larger you are right now, the more amazing you're going to be when you lose it *and keep it off*. That's the way you have to look at it. Your friends and family will view you in an entirely different light.

This runs much deeper than the actual weight loss. The weight is just the tip of the iceberg, for the root of it is *you*. Your determination and desire made it happen. Your newfound confidence will spread into other areas of your life. You will realize that you can do *anything*. All you have to do is set your mind to it.

Getting physically fit is a foundation you can build upon. Build the castle of your dreams and be the queen. Life is short, so just go for it. Apply yourself and be the king of your domain. It's as much your world as anyone else's. No one has the right to push you around. Show those doubters what you're capable of doing.

Get physically fit and let that spark light the wildfire. Anything and everything are possible when you have that fire in your eyes. Burn down those barriers and blast through the fence that cages you. Come out swinging and get what you want. It's your right to claim what's been yours for a long time. Your prize has been lying dormant and unopened just waiting for you to come get it. It was yours at birth and you didn't even know it. Now you understand that you count!

You're just as important as that perky little neighbor of yours who prances around thinking she's the hottest, smartest, thinnest, sexiest, richest, most sophisticated girl in the world. Well, she's not a bit better than you. Her world may be an illusion that could crash at any moment.

Regardless of what others are, or appear to be, possess or don't possess, or say and do, they're not any better than you. The point is we never know what's going on behind closed doors of what appears to be a perfect castle. It could be a pleasant dream or a living nightmare.

People who generally put on the biggest airs, pretend they're the greatest show on earth, and brag about this and that, are really sort of pathetic. They're so insecure that they cocoon themselves into an illusionary world that makes them feel good about who and what they really are.

Never feel like *anyone* is better than you. So what if you're currently overweight? As I stated earlier, it's only going to make your feat more incredible. We're all created by a higher power and no human can tell you what you can and can't do. Never let anyone intimidate you because you've got them placed on an unobtainable pedestal.

Climb up there and take a look around for yourself. You have as much right as anyone to mark your territory amongst the termagants (no need to look it up, synonym for bitch) that populate Perkyville. Claw your way to the top and see for yourself. Kick up a little dust and show Perkyville who's the new mayor.

Send that perky shrew running to her shrink as her hierarchical world crumbles with a little dose of reality. "How dare that fat girl lose all that weight and invade my world!" she'll cry to her shrink. He'll nod his head in agreement as her check clears his bank account and he daydreams about his mistress. Prickly little prancer termagant will find out she's not the ruler of your world. *You and you alone* rule that domain.

Be the rising star! It's never too late, so make a stand. Accomplish a fantastic feat and kick those termagants' butts out of Perkyville. Claim your crown and sit upon the throne that was created for you. It certainly doesn't belong to the pretentious termagant whose world was shattered last week when she broke a nail. Show them who's the new tough girl, the girl with the newly thin body, the happy-from-the-inside girl, the girl with so much confidence it radiates outward like a shining star. Rule Perkyville.

When you lose that weight, and do so in a way that you keep it off, you're going to be unstoppable. Your confidence will be built on a rock-solid foundation, unlike those prefab, all-style-and-no-substance Perkyville residences. Unleash yourself from the chains that bind, free up those desires, and let nothing stand in your way. Be determined and get what you want, for you deserve it.

I lost weight,
Fit as can be.
Get outta my way,
You can't stop me!

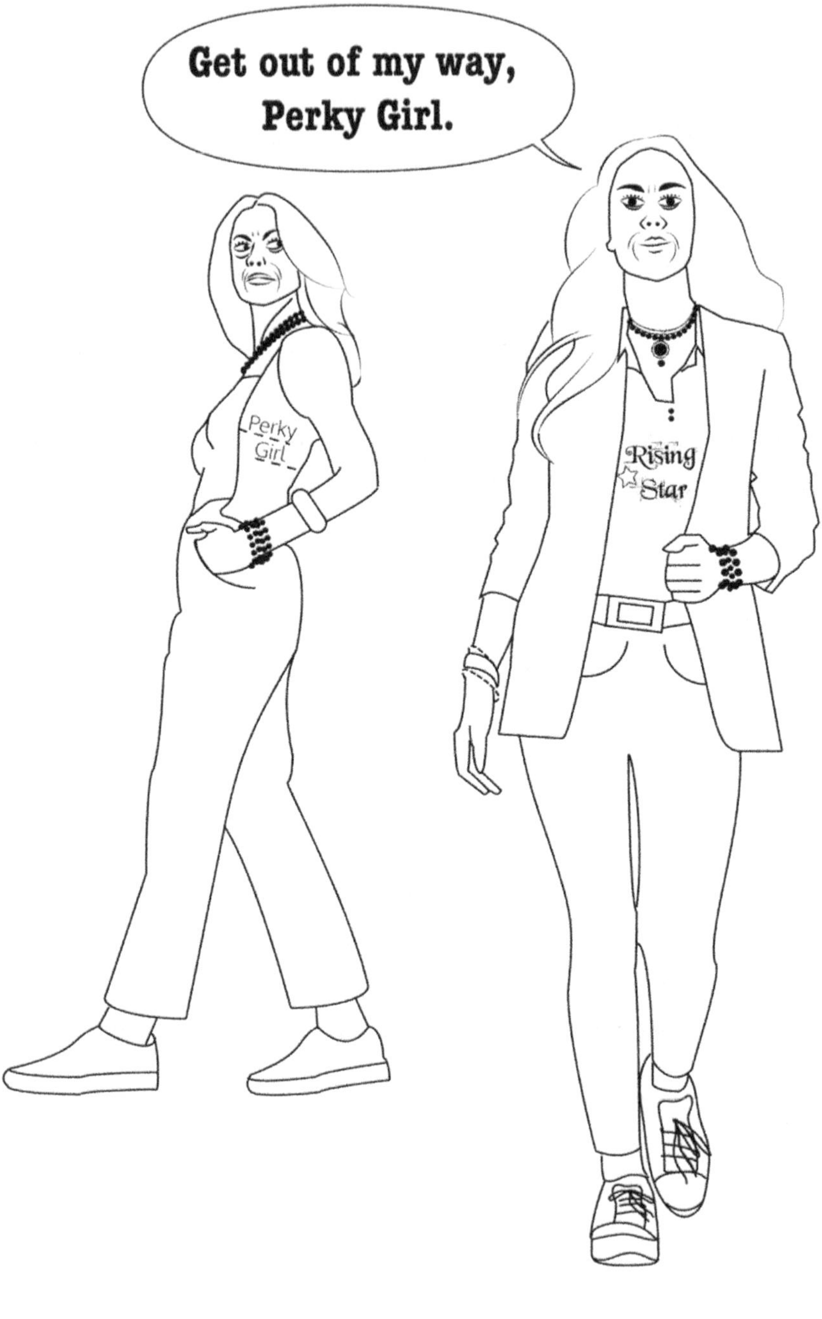
Get out of my way, Perky Girl.
Perky Girl
Rising Star

Finish Your Journey in Style

We're senior citizens. Our lives have been defined by who we are, what we've done, the decisions we've made, and our personal set of ethics. We all have a reputation at this point in our lives. The people who know us best have likely accepted us the way we are until they chunk us into the grave or the furnace. After that, I have no idea what happens. It's probably out of our control at that point, but who really knows, not me.

What we can control is the remainder of our life here in this reality. It may be just a playground that exists before we enter a more important realm, or maybe this is everything. Like I said, I simply don't know. We've got a decade of good living at the most before our mechanics gradually begin to fail. It's the nature of living and dying. Let's make the best of it.

Most of you have children, grandchildren, or other loved ones who have become the most important treasures in your lives. Money certainly takes a back seat to pure love, especially as we age and acquire wisdom. Money is just a lubricant that may or may not make life a little easier, but the people you care about are what really counts.

Maybe you see yourself passing on at a certain time, in a certain way, and that's the way you know it will be. You can still go out with a bang. The journey isn't over until the guy in the white suit throws that blanket over your cold body. If you're reading this, then you're still warm and breathing.

It ain't over til it's over, as they say at the ballgame. And that's what this whole existence feels like sometimes, a game and nothing more. When you step back and look at the big picture, so much of what we humans do means absolutely nothing. Much of it is just a bunch of superficial nothingness that fills the time between birth and death. All that material stuff and mindless so-called entertainment are just limited hangouts that prevent us from attaining full awareness.

There's probably a good reason why those monks and other religious figures live in a silent world, meditate, and avoid all the distractions that surround humanity. It allows them to bypass the unimportant and focus on the important. It lets them view eternity as it relates to our little several-decades experience in these physical bodies.

Our bodies are a shell that encases the real us, and we're stuck with our bodies until they finally fade away. I would call that shell a fairly important item, as it seems to provide shelter for our existential self. Whatever the heck that's inside our shell is important and should be sheltered with care. Major religions even emphasize the importance of the physical body. It is the house where the important stuff resides and should be treated with respect.

That brings us full circle to the importance of being healthy and fit. We're all old enough to have minor aches and pains, if not major ones. We've possibly experienced major medical procedures. Arthritis is something that many of us have to deal with on a daily basis. Our eyesight, hearing, and teeth aren't what they used to be, at least for most of us.

Even the simple stuff doesn't come easy. Bending down to pick something up isn't quite as automatic as it once was.

Once you get down there you may ask yourself, "What else can I do while I'm down here?" And last, but definitely not least, are our minds and mental capabilities. Consider yourself lucky if you escape a slow mental decline as we creep into our seventh, eighth, and ninth decades.

It's the nature of aging and apparently the way life is designed. We're born with this energetic body that knows nothing. We gain knowledge and wisdom as our bodies head in the other direction. Experience and physical decline meet in the middle somewhere around the age of forty. They wave and say hello as the body slowly heads south, while experience, knowledge and wisdom continue rising upwards.

Most of us are way past forty, so we're well aware of that general physical decline. We're reminded every day as we tackle something and realize it's not quite as easy as it used to be. The point here is we have to accept the fact that we're going to experience aging and its consequences. However, we don't have to speed up the process by engaging in bad habits. Eating right and exercising alone can stall the process.

As a matter of fact, until a hundred years ago, eating right and exercising were the norms. Society wasn't yet bombarded with processed foods. Humans had to move their bodies on a daily basis just to survive. Obesity wasn't even an issue except in rare cases. We were like wild animals in a natural habitat.

If you'll take notice, you don't see a lot of fat animals roaming around in the wild. Do you know why? It's because it's a lean, mean, dangerous game of survival out there and fat slows you down. Slow down for just a moment and a natural predator already has its sights set on tonight's dinner. If that doesn't happen, then maybe you'll find yourself left behind the pack because you can't keep up.

In nature, that's sometimes a death sentence as there is safety in numbers. A hungry wolf can corner only one animal at a time, usually the weakest, as the others run away to safety. The bottom line here is that the lean and fit, of any species, is better suited for survival. Not only that, but the strong and quick are more likely to experience *quality* time. Every minute of life has the potential to be a pleasure instead of a burden. You just *live better* when you're lean, strong and fit.

This principle is especially applied to humans. Until recent history, our species was similar to those surviving the wild. Life was difficult and physical tasks were the norm. That kept our bodies moving constantly, for if we stopped, we wouldn't survive the year. Nature and the elements or hunger would do us in. Laziness wasn't an option if you wanted to survive.

It was only when we became overweight that many of our problems began. As technology took over, we regressed and forgot who and what we are. We're machines that need to be used and maintained properly. Compare a machine that's efficiently pumping out its product verses a machine that's sitting by the wayside all rusty and broken.

The one that's working and producing is the equivalent of a human body eating right and exercising. It's moving and being plied with a high-quality fuel, oil, and everything else it needs. The rusty, broken-down version is the sofa-sitter who doesn't move and stuffs him or herself with a dirty human version of low-quality fuel. Too much of that and before long the body is broken down, rusty, and ready for the human junkyard.

Folks, we're stuck with what we were born with and what we've done with it since. Whatever shape your body is in, it's never too late to make a change. It's just a matter of making the effort. What's to lose? So what if you miss a couple of episodes of a staged reality show. Is that the end of your world?

Get out there and show somebody something. Make a name for yourself as you exit this particular existence and head towards the next one. Make it fun and enjoy it. You'll really enjoy it as you see real progress. There are no excuses. The reasons not to do it are just mental blocks that can be knocked down, little barriers that can be squashed in a moment. Show somebody what you're capable of doing. Do what it takes to become lean, strong and healthy. Show them what a motivated geezer is capable of accomplishing. You can do it!

Yes, we're old,
But we ain't done.
We're gonna get fit,
And have some FUN!

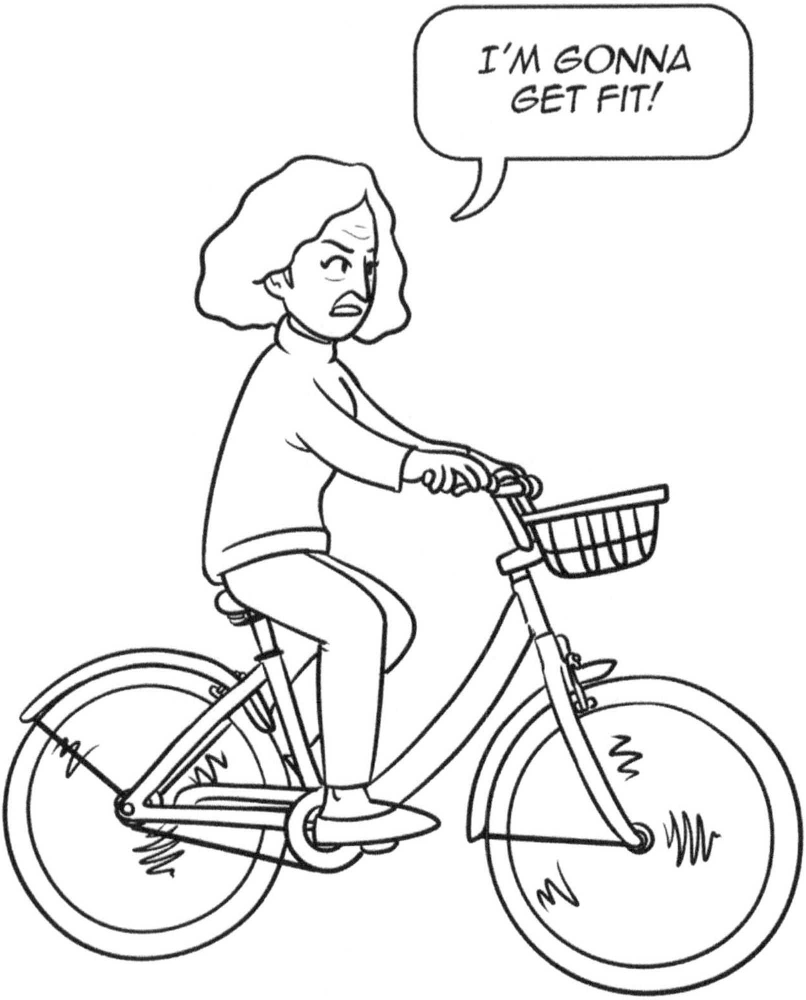
I'M GONNA GET FIT!

CHAPTER 12

Survival Recipes

"Progress is nothing but complicated simplicity."
A. T. Needham

Be Realistic

Extravagant and fancy recipes can be fun and wonderful. There are bunches of them out there that are extremely healthy. If you like them and have time, then schedule one for every meal. If you do this, however, beware of a self-laid trap. It's a psychological thing.

I think many people, especially when they're starting their fitness and nutrition program, have an "all or nothing" attitude. The problem with this black-or-white-only approach is it turns into "nothing' more often than "all." They set the bar too high and when they finally realize it, they're psychologically defeated.

It's a lot better to take the slower, steadier approach and methodically plow through your exercise tasks and nutritional goals. I know I've been preaching this throughout the book as it applies to nearly every aspect of the program. It doesn't stop with the meal planning segment either. You have to be realistic and take into consideration your lifestyle, time constraints, and your true day-to-day activities.

For example, it sounds ambitious to plan a perfect, healthy, multi-course dinner every evening, and possibly even one or more additional meals daily. I commend you for setting such goals in order to attain success. The meals are mile markers in your overall journey towards becoming fit and healthy. Many of you have the time to pull this off. Many of you, however, will find that you set unrealistic goals for yourself. Then you'll crash and burn and feel like a loser.

If you don't think that you can manage those time-consuming healthy meals on a regular basis, then leave yourself a psychological "out." By this, I mean a Plan B, or even a Plan C. Have a strategy to fall back on when it becomes crunch time and the pressure is on. Come through in the clutch and escape with a quicker version of Plan A that still holds true, or at least stays close, to your nutrition values.

It may not be the prettiest meal around and land you on a television cooking show, but it will allow you to survive, to stay in the game, to still be lingering around with a chance to win. A psychological defeat is the worst possible outcome and you want to avoid this at all costs. Sneak through the maze of obstacles and come out the other side. You may be slightly battered, but you'll be alive and still in the race.

It all revolves around a split-second decision that is affected by many factors. Time and exhaustion are the two main barriers. No matter how well you plan your schedule, there's always something that creeps in and chews up a piece of your valuable time. This has to be accounted for in some manner, and too often it manifests itself as a quick, convenient, unhealthy meal. You simply don't have time to cook the magnificent, aesthetic dish you so desired.

Pure exhaustion is an incredible modifier of your lofty expectations. You may come home after a particularly trying day and plop yourself down on the sofa. Then you look over at that menu that you so ambitiously planned for the evening. It's going to require thirty minutes of preparation and cooking and you can't forget the dreaded cleanup. Another glance spots a bag of potato chips, a box of cookies, or some other processed snack that requires no effort to prepare and consume. This is the split-second that will determine failure or success.

The trap here is the fact that you've allowed yourself only two options. You're totally exhausted, and we've all been there, and you simply don't have the energy to cook a full meal. The only other option is that processed, high-fat, salty, sweet quick-fix that's going to wreck your nutritional program. You've neglected to prepare and there's no grey area within which to operate. You've left yourself with no out, no escape, no back-door exit.

This brings me back around to my primary point. Keep things simple and they're easier to manage. Be armed with a collection of middle-ground nutritional weapons that can be prepared relatively quickly. Be prepared for those days, and you know they're coming, that stab you in the back when you're riding high. Time and exhaustion are two tough opponents, but with some proper planning and preparation, you can knock them off their high horse.

As I mentioned earlier, you may not win in a pretty manner, but you will win. You'll wake up in the morning feeling good about yourself. You'll be proud you survived and didn't cave in to the temptations of the quick and easy way out. Every time you survive an attack from these powerful forces, you become stronger from the inside. Soon you'll be so powerful that nothing can overtake you. They may reach in and bite you, but they're not going to drag you into the darkness below and chew you up. You're too strong.

I want to remind you of something before I delve into our recipe specifics. *Always clean your food.* I'm mainly speaking about our unprocessed selections. It's likely that your fruits and veggies have been poisoned at some point with pesticides. Wash that stuff off immediately. Do you really think anything that kills insects is harmless? Insects are tough survivors and they don't go down easily. Any poison that kills them is going to do you harm. That's simple common sense. I'm constantly amazed at how many people won't take time to clean their food. Don't be a dummy.

How about washing your meat before cooking it? I've read by the "experts" that we shouldn't do it, so I'm not going to give advice. I do, however, wonder about certain things. You never really know the history behind that particular cut of meat. How many hands has it been through on its journey from butcher to consumer?

I sometimes picture this scenario in my mind. Your nice ribeye steak is in its final stage of packaging. Paul the packer accidently drops it on the floor just before he gets ready to seal it in the package. He looks around and notes that no one witnessed it. Instead of washing it, he places the dirty meat into the package and seals it. Off it goes until it lands on your broiling pan.

"Umm good!" you say as you gobble down your delicious steak seasoned with an array of various germs, floor dirt and decayed crawling insects. "Umm, that broiled dog doo that fell off Paul's shoes is so delicious!" Once again, I'm not telling you to wash your meat before cooking it. No, no, no, I would never do that.

Okay, let's get back to our subject at hand. I prefer organic food over non-organic, but I'm always on guard. Even if it claims to be organic, I still assume it has been contaminated. You've been around long enough to know that lying is a natural human trait. We've been lied to many times and maybe told a few ourselves. Corporations are made up of humans and therefore are capable of stretching the truth. We can't always depend on them to act in our best interest, especially when there's big money as motivation. Therefore, I wash my organic food to be safe.

The following recipes are broken down into three categories. Many of these I hesitate to call recipes, for they are nothing more than survival outlets. They're relatively quick and easy, and in reality, simply an alternative to a prepared meal. Some of them are even microwave options. I'm no fan of this, but it's much better than reaching for the processed stuff that can destroy your program.

One other note along these lines, purchase a small toaster oven. It's an efficient tool which speeds up the emergency survival operation. Stay away from the ones that require an engineering degree or help from your grandkid to operate. That's right, you ole geezer.

I'm not going to list very many of these "recipes," for there are literally countless options out there that are healthy. Just take some of these extremely simple ideas and run with them. Create your own versions, modify mine, or simply start from scratch and innovate with some fresh ideas. If you've read this book, you now know what to eat, how to prepare it, and what to leave off that contaminates it. Get out there and design a plan that will work for your personal lifestyle. You're old and geezed-up, but you're as wise as they come.

No time, a little time, and lots of time are your meal options. It will vary on a personal level as to what you want and what is realistic. Be armed and loaded with your weapons so you don't fall in defeat. Have a few "no time" and "little time" fallback options always at your fingertips to engage the time and exhaustion opponents. Treat this as if it were a military operation with situational alternative strategies dependent on the enemies' particular tactical aggressions. It's war!

Just remember this. If you wake in the morning feeling terrible because you slipped up and ate the wrong foods, there's no one or nothing to blame but yourself. Don't even try to shift the blame elsewhere. Likewise, when you wake up feeling proud of yourself for staying true to your basic nutritional plan, you're not going to get big kudos from anyone. You have to pat yourself on the back and move on. There's a whole other day and night just waiting to pounce on you and destroy your well-laid plans. Be a warrior and survive.

The following ideas I'll present *will* satisfy your hunger. They can substitute for real meals. Some of them you may combine, but you had better go about it in a sane manner. Go crazy and you'll be paying a big price in the form of weight gain and major disappointment. After reading this book you know what to do, so don't kid yourself. Be careful and be responsible.

I could tell you to grab some fruit or veggies instead of these concoctions, but I would be taking the easy way out. I know as well as anyone that there are certain times when your body needs a feeling of satisfaction, something of substance in that belly. I promise you these will do the trick. They're quick and easy and are incredible weapons in your fitness battle. I call them crisis foods, as it seems a crisis lurks around every corner in this never-ending war against processed foods.

Here's a little starter fluid, in the form of recipes, if you can call them that. They're really just a little kick in the butt to get that mind of yours rolling in the right direction. I'm only listing a few, but it's enough to stir your geezer creativity. They are the simplest of the simple, but that's the mentality that wins in the end. Add natural spices to any or all of these. You don't need to be told again which ones to use. Mix them up and experiment. They substitute for the fatty flavor options.

Any four-year-old can decipher these most basic recipes. They are in no particular order. It's simply a matter of putting them together and making them work. As I said earlier, if you have time and enjoy it, prepare a fine healthy meal. There are countless great recipes floating around out there. I tend to prefer those myself. Just remember that real life is a tough opponent. These outrageously simplistic survival meals can keep you in the game. Don't laugh at them because you may find yourself depending on them. I trust that you'll design a plan that works for *you*.

One last thing, there's a rumor floating around that unless you make a genuine attempt at becoming fit, you will go to Hell. I heard it from my drunk Uncle Homer just before he passed out one night. Damn, that's a harsh penalty!

I seriously doubt what my juicehead uncle muttered is true, as he was also smoking funny cigarettes that night. Uncle Homer was known for telling some whopper lies. Anyway, let's not take any chances. Let's all start shaping up. These recipes should help. Forever is a long time.

Eat good stuff,
And you'll survive.
Eat good stuff,
To stay alive!

No Time (3 minutes)

HEALTHY LEFTOVERS: Did you prepare a healthy dish earlier in the day, or maybe yesterday? As I mentioned earlier, I'm no fan of microwaving, but it's a much better option than opening yourself up to a cookie/potato chip attack. It's even better if you have the time to reheat it in your toaster oven. Try to get into the habit of never letting anything sit around for more than 24 hours. We're into freshness here. You got that, you old geezer?

CHEESE & STUFF ON CRACKERS: I know this goes beyond simple and seems like it needs no explanation. The problem is it's a potential disaster if approached the wrong way. Here's the proper way to go about preparing this survival recipe.

Make sure your crackers are as healthy as can be. The less salt, the healthier, as you well know. I've found that the heartier crackers seem to have less fat proportionally than the little wussy ones that fall apart when you touch them. Spend that extra money and keep some quality crackers handy and ready to go. If you're a natural tight-ass with money, then it's time for you to see the light and shape up. It's your life at stake.

As far as the cheese goes, it's the same mentality. Don't be afraid to spend a little extra money and get some good stuff. You're all about quality over quantity when it comes to this dangerous item. Go on a cheese binge and you're not going to like what you see in the mirror. Experiment and find some favorites. Do not overdo the cheese! In case you missed it, *do not overdo the cheese!*

Now it's time for the good stuff. Make these cracker-topping items the star of the show. They are the centerpiece of this survival weaponry arsenal. Olives, sliced hot peppers or tomatoes are all quick and easy selections. Any and every veggie you can think of will send you in the right direction. There's no limit to the creativity here. Fruits, *lean* meats, lentils, any of these are options and so many more.

At this point dot each cracker with a bit of sauce if you like. Salsa, steak sauce, a little barbeque sauce, mustard and many more are viable options. You've read this book so you know what they are. One thing they're *not* is fat. Get your geezer magnifying glass and read the fat content statistic. Throw that dangerous bottle into the garbage if it's fatty.

It's only crackers and toppings. You can go in two different directions here. Do the right thing. Use that geezed-up, wise ole medulla and make the right choice. Don't be a dummy Zarkoff and screw this up. A hundred tiny decisions equal success!

NUTS: Here's another one that would seem like it needs no explanation. Yes, you can replace a full meal with nuts alone. Surround yourself with a variety of nuts. Keep them at home, at work, in your car, everywhere! Yes, they do contain a higher proportion of fat than our other survival dishes, but it's the good fat. Please trust me on this. There's no need to call cousin Doc Bernie for verification. Isn't he a touch overweight anyway?

These delightful creatures are the ultimate survival meal. By that I mean the convenience factor is off the charts. Pour some into your hand and eat. It's that simple. I'd bet that a human could survive an extraordinary length of time on nuts alone. Even pudgy Doc Bernie would probably agree with that.

The preceding paragraphs mean NOTHING if the nuts have been ruined by humans. Salt, oils, bad fats, gimmicky flavoring, and stuff much worse than those are the norm when it comes to grocery store nut shopping. All that crap negates every healthy aspect of what we just discussed. I know you're used to a lifetime of being conditioned by those nut-polluters. That's okay, it's not too late to change.

Here's what you do. You find a healthy store that has lots of options in the nut department. Many sell nuts by bulk, as little or as much as you want. You open up your tight-ass wallet and prepare to spend some money, lots of it. You purchase a wide variety of nuts. Most have a relatively long shelf life. They are *all* unsalted. They are *all* either raw or dry roasted. There is *nothing* added to them at all. Do you understand? If not, please reread this paragraph.

Okay, so you're all shriveled and puckered up because you actually parted with a sizable amount of money to purchase nuts. And they're not even the tasty kind you like! Well, now your heirs have less to argue about when you slide away into geezer afterlife. I would guess that's a good thing.

There's an incredible variety of nuts out there in this world. Brazil nuts, walnuts, almonds, cashews, chestnuts, these are just a few of them. There's always the dependable peanut. Macadamia nuts, pistachio nuts and pine nuts are excellent inheritance reducers. Search them out and find them.

If you want a little more taste, use that geezer-acquired wisdom and unleash your creativity. A droplet of hot sauce should do the trick. Nuts are an incredible weapon in your battle to become lean and strong. They leave you feeling full and energized. I don't care what cousin Bernie says.

SANDWICH: You've been eating sandwiches since dear ole Aunt Blanche made your first one. You remember Aunt Blanche. She was the aunt that claimed your family was of royal heritage and other assorted fabricated falsehoods. God bless her embellishing soul.

Sandwiches are a valuable resource in the real-world struggle to get and remain fit. When prepared properly they are one of the healthiest survival meals in your arsenal. They're balanced with a perfect mix of veggies, protein and complex carbohydrates. They're 24-hour soldiers that can be utilized at any time.

Here's how you make a sandwich, and it's not Aunt Blanche's way. I'm so sorry that she led you astray at such an early age. Aunt Blanche told you that sandwiches had to be loaded up with gobs of mayonnaise. You should have known you couldn't trust her when you discovered that your "Came-over-on-the-Mayflower" family was completely bogus. Maybe it was the vodka talking.

A healthy sandwich starts with the bread. Make sure it's a healthy, whole, natural-as-can-be choice. If it's whiter than snow you're off to a bad start. Feed that stuff to the animals, although they're probably too smart to eat it. Fresh and natural are what you're looking for in bread.

The next step is critical. Old habits creep in and people automatically slather their bread with gooey globs of mayonnaise. At this point you might as well go shopping for some larger clothes, because you're now on a weight-gaining program. If you don't believe me, break out that magnifying glass again and read the horrific fat and calorie content on the label. Mustard is a *much* better choice. If you don't like mustard then go dry. Mayonnaise is for sumo wrestlers.

Now it's time for the meat. Lean chicken or turkey is always a winner. Some sort of veggie burger is an option. You're looking for two things here and the concept is really simple. Lean and fresh, that's all you need to know. Don't go trying to fool yourself and pile a big chunk of fatty meat on your sandwich. I've seen some people add bacon to their sandwiches. Keep doing that and the clothes you have on will be on the Goodwill shelf pretty soon. Kiss that pretty dress goodbye because a bacon diet is going to puff you up like that marshmallow cartoon character. He loves bacon.

It's cheese time. Either go cheese-less or go easy. Make sure it's a quality cheese, not the plastic sliced stuff that pretends to be cheese. Don't turn this thing into a multi-layered cheese sandwich, regardless of the quality. Keep it balanced. You may fool yourself and think you're not overdoing it, but you won't be fooling your body. It will be Goodwill donation time again if you become a cheese-head.

Now it's time to load that baby up with veggies. Any and all veggies will work. Hopefully you've been responsible with moderate portions of meat and cheese. This leaves lots of room to pile on the veggies. Pile it high and squash it down. Now you have a nutritious, low-calorie meal. Eat it now or place it in a cooler for later in the day. Congratulations on surviving another day in the jungle.

CHIPS & SALSA: You're probably asking, "Is Spyder going to complicate this one also? How hard is it to eat salsa?" Well, this one is relatively simple. The main issue here is the chips. Once again, I've found that some of the more expensive ones are by far a better quality than the cheapos.

If you're one of those penny-pincher types, then cringe up and part with a couple of extra dollars. If your spouse or mate is one of those types, chain him or her up in the basement Zarkoff-style until he or she sees the light. Steal his or her wallet and count out the money in front of them. Torture them as they watch their precious money changing hands. Come back later and offer them a delicious chip.

The salsa itself is also an important decision. Just use your gut and your instincts on this one. The less salt, the more natural, these are the type of things you're looking for. If it happens to cost a little more, then just steal money from your mate. Or maybe cancel your cable TV subscription and use that fortune to finance your salsa and chip bill. Geezers don't need to be worrying about an extra dollar or two. We've already got the afterlife breathing down our necks, just waiting to punish us for all the fun we had in the 70's.

Do you want some protein to leave you with that satisfied feeling? More often than not, I take a high quality can of beans and mix it with the salsa. Once again, it's going to cost a few extra cents for the good stuff, so go raid your spouse's retirement fund to fund it. He or she is chained up in the basement, so they'll never know.

Drain the beans, rinse thoroughly so as to clean them of all salt and preservatives, and quickly heat them in a small pot. Mix the hot beans into the salsa and now you have a relatively healthy meal that is balanced. It could be more natural, but it will suffice.

Here's one last note regarding the salsa. If you have time, make your own. That way you control the ingredients and the sodium content. Be creative here. You're a survivor and you do what it takes. Don't forget to feed the prisoner downstairs.

CANNED PROTEIN: Canned meats make for a quick protein fix. I sometimes eat them for dinner, but their pure convenience makes them an excellent lunch-on-the-go selection. If you don't mind looking a little weird and silly, just eat it right out of the can like I do. If you prefer the less animalistic approach, properly place it in some sort of bowl or plate.

Restrictions apply here as usual. You know nothing's easy when you're old and geezed-up. We're all a bunch of has-beens who have decided we're not done yet. We're going to get fit and stay fit until it's completely out of our control. We're going to make one last big splash before we blast off into eternity. Eternity is a long time.

I can just see the Great Decider reviewing your case when your soul goes before judgement. "Susie girl, I was going to send you down below for your bad behavior during your college days, but since you turned your life around and started eating unsalted tuna and other boring foods, I'm going to give you a break and send you to the pearly gates upstairs. Congratulations on becoming fit at such an advanced age."

There you have it. To avoid eternal difficulties, you're going to have to eat canned meats in a boring manner. That absolutely means no mayonnaise with your tuna. It has to be packed in water, no oils. You will make extreme efforts to find versions with no salt or very little salt. Turkey, chicken, or other types of fish are allowed. A few healthy crackers are allowed. You can also top them with an approved topping. You've read this book and know what they are. Beef, pork, and any other fatties that may tempt you are off the table.

Another form of canned protein is beans. There are so many varieties, so mix them up regularly. They're the perfect survivalist food. If you come home from work and you're exhausted, pull out a can of unsalted or lightly salted beans. Drain and rinse them. God forbid there's a grain of salt or a molecule of preservative lurking in there somewhere. Heat in a pot on high and in two minutes you have a meal. A little hot sauce or another approved topping can really add some flavor. Ole toked-up Uncle Homer would not approve of any bad toppings.

I'm sure there are other forms of canned protein that I've missed. Keep your eyes open while shopping and you'll find them. Make sure to put on those thick geezer eyeglasses and read the fine print before purchasing.

CEREAL: Good cereals can energize and push you through the day. Of course, there are certain restrictions that apply. Sugar Sweeties and Sugar Boogars won't make the cut. As a matter of fact, very few processed cereals will. Most of these kiddie-marketed products contain enough sugar to make you want to climb the walls of the Empire State Building and jump off. I won't even mention the loads of discredited artificial flavorings and colorings that exist in certain ones.

If you need a survivalist cereal fix, your choices are limited. Shredded wheat is an excellent choice. Trickery has been known to exist even with this wonderful cereal, so break out those geezer glasses again for the fine print. Oatmeal is always a good choice. A touch of honey on it does wonders. You can even use the one-minute variety here if you desire. We're in survival territory here.

Of course, I still recommend the steel-cut unprocessed version if you have the time. It's more nutrient dense and healthier in my opinion. I'm sure my cousin Doc Bernie would love to debate me on that one all night long. I don't have time for bickering, so I'll just agree with him and send him on his merry way. He's not going to change me though, although he does make me consume more alcohol.

Do you like milk on your cereal? Try to stay away from the whole milk, or at least go very light with it. It's a calorie and fat monster and needs to be treated as such. The low-fat option is a better choice in my opinion. You don't really need milk anyway. You're just doing it because cocktail-juiced Aunt Blanche put it on your cereal decades ago. As a matter of fact, I always eat my cereal dry.

So, so tired,
Such a long day.
A quick recipe,
I'll be okay!

A Little Time (10 minutes)

STEAMED VEGGIES: Steamed veggies are about as good as it gets. They're cooked the right way. They're packed with nutrition, low in calories, and natural as can be. The trick is to keep them that way. Don't go ruining them with salt, butter, margarine or another geezer-life-shortening substance. We're dancing around our graves already so we don't need a push.

Mix up your selections and you can't go wrong. Eat as much as you want because uncontaminated steamed veggies are fillers that leave you feeling totally satisfied, yet never stuffed. If you ever feel the need to overeat, this is where you do it. This meal everyday will definitely send you to the clothes rack for the right reason. Losing weight!

There's no need for expansion on this wonderful dish. Wash your veggies and steam them as long as you want. Anywhere from raw to well-done will do the trick. Make them your way and gobble them down.

Those fatblobs that have pestering you for years will melt away if you continue this good behavior. Steamed veggies, some lean protein, a long daily walk around the neighborhood, and you're racing towards the fitness finish line. Girls, you'll be looking so good you won't know what to do with yourselves. Keep up the good work and watch out for those Zarkoff types. They'll be hunting you down.

RICE & BEANS: This combo will definitely leave you satisfied and energized. Yes, they contain some calories, but they're the good carb kind and not the fatty kind. This would be another contentious subject for ole cousin Doc Bernie. He is Mister Carb Hater. Judging from cuz Bernie and his ample paunch he needs to stop preaching and start learning. Maybe he's not eating carbs, but something's making that stomach expand. Maybe he needs to go back to college.

I won't spend a lot of time on the bean part of this. You know what to do, drain, rinse and cook. Regarding the rice, go for a healthy version. The white, bleachy stuff has been depleted of certain nutrients. Some genius years ago decided it was a good idea. He probably got his education from the same higher-learning institution as cuz Bernie.

I like brown rice because you can easily find it. There are also black and red varieties if you want to search for them. Good ole brown rice does the trick for me. I like the totally unprocessed version of any rice, but for survivalist reasons the quick-cooking varieties will suffice. We are in a war here and we have to win any way we can.

It's very easy. Start cooking the rice. Pour in the rinsed canned beans and give it a couple of minutes. Add a veggie if you like. Chopped onions are a nice choice. Drain the water and pour in into your dish. Add a little hot sauce or salsa. Sit back and enjoy as cuz Bernie spouts off about how you shouldn't consume carbs.

BOILED CORN: I just love corn-on-the-cob. Those Central Americans are really on to something. They have these little stands that serve nothing but delicious, huge ears of grilled corn. They'll try to salt it for you, but decline that one. Do take them up on their offer of a liberal squeeze of lime juice. That's so tasty and healthy.

Boiling the corn is a quick survivalist method of preparing this incredible food. Once again, it's classified by cuz Bernie as a dreaded carb, but pay no attention to ole doughnut butt. You can also bake your corn. It's a little drier than the boiled option, but the lime juice takes care of that issue.

As far as other toppings, we don't have to go through all that again. Be creative with some hot sauce, Worcestershire sauce, low-sodium soy sauce, or something that doesn't create the Watusi-wobble. Don't ruin a good thing with butter or margarine. Please!

QUICK SALAD: Keep your salad quick and simple, especially if you're in total exhaustion survival territory. You could even have it pre-prepared. That's the smart way. Quick doesn't necessarily mean small. Pile those veggies as high as you like, for they're going to fill you up, blast you off with nutrition, and burn away like rocket smoke. They're the perfect foods for losing weight. And guess what, they're basically all carbs with a splash of protein. Carbs! How do you like that, cuz?

Do you need a little protein addition? Add some tuna, lean chicken or turkey, tofu, or some sort of lentil. Do remember that the veggies are the main attraction here. Keep any cheese at a bare minimum. Add some spoon-size shredded wheat for a little crunch and texture if you like. And *please* don't go pouring some creamy, fatty dressing on this otherwise perfect dish. Do you really have to be told again? Of course not, you geezed ole wise coot.

I need food,
Time is tight.
I'll eat healthy,
I'll eat right!

Lots of Time (30 minutes)

VEGGIE SOUP: Do you want to lose weight? Replace one fatty meal with this super healthy dish and you're well on your way. The great thing about this particular dish is you can eat all you want. Satisfy your tummy because everything in it is absolutely good for you. We're not using stock as our base. Instead, it's low-sodium vegetable juice. V8 is a popular brand.

Experiment with the amounts because you'll want to make this fresh every day. After you've made a couple of batches, you'll get a feel for it. Eat it all up and make a fresh one the next day. Some like it thick and super-heavy on the vegetables, while others like their soup a little less dense.

You may find yourself interchanging between the two or an in-between version. A lighter, less-hearty version is a great first course if you follow it with something healthy. You may prefer the heartier version if it's a stand-alone meal. You'll have to play around with the water/juice amounts to figure out what works for you.

Always remember that *nothing* is going to melt those excess pounds off overnight, but this particular dish is as good as it gets. Your geezed-up metabolism isn't as fine-tuned as those youngsters, so don't place yourself in fantasyland and expect overnight miracles. That being said, I can't say enough good things about this incredible dish. Take those daily walks or some other cardio exercise, eat this every day, and you'll be a superstar weight-loser in several months.

The real secret behind this masterpiece is the unlimited variety it presents. Mix and match any and every vegetable in the world, and the amounts of each. Infinite combinations are available when you look at it like this. For example, a lot of onion and a bit of celery could be a version. A lot of carrots, a lot of bell peppers, and a touch of another veggie could be one. A little squash and a little of something else will work. Just one veggie can make a dish. Now you're getting the picture. Use what you have and don't worry about it.

If you've read this far into this book, you know you *always* keep a few fresh veggies nearby ready for action. Simply grab one or two or ten of them and make your soup. This is no Einstein project. There's only one thing you need to remember and that is don't throw any bad crap in there. Keep it simple and you can't go wrong. Come on, geezer, you can do it.

Let's discuss adding some protein to your veggie soup. If you're getting your protein elsewhere, there's no need to add any. I've gone through different phases of this, sometimes all veggies and no added protein, sometimes a little added protein, and sometimes heavier on the protein. I'll remind you again, this isn't a big deal either way as long as you keep your protein lean and mean.

Tiny lentils are a mainstay in my soup at the moment. Throw them into the concoction early and let them simmer away. They cook much quicker than the bigger beans. Tofu is a great protein choice. Leftover chicken, turkey or fish will also work. *Lean is the key here.* Don't you dare start messing around with fatty meats or you'll turn into a fatty meat yourself. You'll have no one to blame but your geezy self.

Don't be scared of spices. Go overboard with spices in all your dishes, but especially this one. Don't be afraid to throw in some of those exotic flavors. They're virtually calorie-free and healthy as can be. I personally look upon them as nature's medicine. You get that free flavor without all those calories. That kind of stuff keeps a geezer's body running smoothly.

Do you like hot and spicy? Throw in a jalapeno or even a fierier pepper if you really like the heat. You know what's allowed and what's not allowed. Keep your soup interesting and you'll never get tired of it. Make this soup your trustworthy friend and you won't regret it. I promise that.

The following recipe makes approximately 2-3 hearty servings. I'm time-efficiency obsessed, so I'm still chopping as the soup starts souping. After all, these recipes are all about minimum effort and time to obtain maximum benefit. Here's how you do it. Don't fall asleep on me, geezer. I know it's your nap time now.

It's time to start cooking. Pick a cooking pot that's not too big or too small for the job. Keep this pot handy and ready to go at all times. Imagine you're dead tired and all you want to do is eat and relax. You won't have time or energy to go around searching for your magic pot. That critical minute may dissuade you from making the effort. This may sound like overkill, but I'm warning you. It's your weakest moment and you're exhausted. That's when those potato chips and cookies start looking like a viable option. Don't let that happen!

Add a cup or two of water in your magic pot and start heating it. I like to go with high heat and get the train rolling quickly. Start chopping the slower cooking veggies and place them into the magic pot first. Carrots would be an example of this. Next come any other slower cooking ingredients, such as lentils, rice, quinoa, or similar items.

Is your soup heating? Now is the time to add 20 ounces of low-sodium V8 juice, or another similar brand. Always feel free to use *less* of the juice. The less juice, the less calories. You can make up the difference by adding more water.

Keep chopping on one, two, three, or ten veggies, throwing them into the mix as you finish. Tofu cooks relatively quick, so toss that into the soup if you like. Do you need more vegetable juice or water? Feel free to pour some more in there.

Now it's spice time. Once again, have them handy and ready to go. Too much effort and you'll sadly neglect these healthy, flavorful additions. You're a tired ole decrepit geezer. Liberally pour one, two, five, or ten of them into the mix. Mix and match these differently with every new batch. Don't laugh, because this is the flavor that's replacing all that fatty taste that you used to crave.

At this point decide if you want a thick and hearty version, or something lighter. It all depends on your mood at the moment. Whatever the case, don't make the mistake of making a serving that's too small. That may leave you unsatisfied and vulnerable to a cookie/chip attack afterwards. Any overeating should begin and end with the soup. Make that belly happy with the good stuff.

We're all about being time-optimal with this dish, so get it right to the boiling point and then turn it down very low. Cover the pot with the magic cover and go sit down. Enjoy a glass of wine and relax. Daydream about the pool guy. Let it simmer for twenty minutes or two hours, or however long you desire. Get up occasionally to stir the soup. Add some vegetable juice or water if necessary.

It's time to eat! All those veggies and their compatible buddies have blended together and smell so good. Umm, that first taste is so delicious. Enjoy your big bowl of soup and congratulate yourself on making it through another day. Tomorrow is coming soon and you're going to have to do it all over again. You're a winner.

SMALL-BUTT NACHOS: Many of us love the flavor and spice of Mexican food. Like any other cuisine, you can go lean and healthy, or you can opt for the fat-butt style. It's all about making the right decisions at crunch time. Start with a healthy selection and make sure you don't contaminate it with a fat-butt substance. It's those little choices that make the difference in butt size.

Big-butters like big meals laced with numerous butt-growing ingredients. Small-butters usually pay attention to what goes into their mouths and tend to order from the small-butt menu. The following nacho dish has some calories, no doubt about it. However, I've removed most of the butt-growing ingredients, drastically lowering the calorie count. Once again, it's a collection of numerous tiny decisions that make all the difference.

I lived in Texas for several years. Their excellent nachos spoiled me for life. Have you ever received your restaurant nachos and the chips underneath are cold? That's because they put no soul into their cooking. Following will be a small-butt version of nachos that are cooked properly and taste so good that even big-butters will love them.

Start with a high-quality bag of chips. As we've discussed in the past, they're a bit more costly, so quit puckering up and getting red in the face every time you spend a dollar and start living. I like those blue chips lately as they just seem healthy. Organic is always the better option whatever chip you choose.

If you have a little more time, here is an excellent idea to cut back on calories. Pucker up and get red-faced again and buy some high-quality tortillas. The big difference here is the fact they haven't been fried. That means less grease makes its way into your body. For all you girls, that's good news. This means you're well on your way to being classified as a small-butter, but that doesn't mean your current medium-butt or even your big-butt isn't pretty. I'm sure every one of your butts is beautiful.

If you choose the butt-reduction option, and I really like this option, prepare your tortillas this way. Tear them into large chip sizes and place them on your baking tray. Bake them on high heat for a few minutes. Keep a close eye on them or your fire alarm will start making a super-annoying noise. This is an extra step and requires a bit of time, but those nachos are going to be super healthy. Remove them when you see a little browning and crispness.

Now let's assume we're back to the bagged chips. You'll do the same thing. Spread your chips on your baking tray and bake them for a few minutes at a fairly high temperature. Then take your dog for a walk and accidently forget about the nachos and set your house on fire. Just kidding.

Get the chips nice and hot and remove them. Your next items you've previously prepared and now they're placed upon the chips. If you don't like one or more of these items, make up for it with more of another ingredient. They're all classified as small to medium-butt items, so pile them high.

The small-butt selections are sliced jalapeno peppers and olives. You are not limited to these, for with a little creativity you can come up with a vast array of small-butt selections. Chopped poblano peppers, bell peppers and corn are good examples. Fresh cilantro is always tasty in this dish. There is no limit to what can be done here. Use that geezed brain and innovate.

This next butt-reducing ingredient is critical if you like a little protein in your nachos. The under-appreciated bean is an excellent small-butt ingredient, for utilized properly it is nearly a perfect food. Take your drained and rinsed low-sodium beans and spread them upon the chips. Make sure the beans are dry so they don't soak water into your chips. You can't be messing with that crispness that we all love.

You can always use some lean chicken or turkey breast meat instead of beans if you prefer, or you could do a bean/meat combo. I've even heard of canned tuna being used, but don't tell anyone from Texas that you've committed such a heinous crime. Whatever you do, don't ever forget that the veggies are the star of this show. Your goal should be filling yourself with as many veggies as possible. We're looking for that satisfied feeling without advancing to the super-big-butt category.

Now place your dish back into the oven. Keep a close eye on it and when it's a few minutes from perfection remove it again and cover it with cheese. You know the dangers of cheese, so go sparingly in this department. The cheese will melt quickly. When it looks good, remove it from the oven and go to the next step.

The following items you have already prepared. You actually could have placed them upon the nachos earlier if you prefer. It's really a matter of personal preference. These items are chopped tomatoes and onions, and a sliced avocado. Cabbage or lettuce might also be a nice addition. Have a jar of quality salsa available. Place these items on the nachos and there you have it. Small-butt nachos are a long-time favorite of mine. Enjoy!

BAKED POTATO: The potato has been pushed around too long. It's always been a bit undervalued and disrespected. If I were a potato, I would be on the streets marching and protesting the fact that I've been proclaimed a side dish. A baked potato is a complete meal once you doctor it up with some healthy toppings and spices. The sweet potato should be considered veggie royalty with all its nutrients.

Most of you know how to bake a potato. It's the doctoring-up part of it that goes horribly wrong for many people. So many delicious, healthy toppings can be added to this delicacy, yet people seem automatically programmed to scoop up the heart-clogger stuff and pile it on. You know what they are, butter, margarine, sour cream, bacon and all their other villainous cousins.

Vodka-swilling Aunt Blanche introduced these unfortunates to potato destruction via bad toppings, and they made it a lifelong habit. Then these same people have the nerve to declare that a potato is the reason they're an overweight wobble machine. They're wobble machines because of all the crap they put on the potato. The potato alone has never once created a wobble machine. Dummy, dummy, watch what you put in your tummy, tummy.

Guess what pure fat does when it enters your body. I can tell you this, it doesn't turn into lean muscle. No, it stays just what it is, pure unadulterated fat. That gooey glob of fat simply relocates from the refrigerator to your buttocks. Once the butter fat settles in the right buttock, sour cream is invited to be its neighbor in the left buttock. "Don't worry, there's room for everyone here," the happy settlers proclaim. "These warm, floppy, bouncy, geezer buttocks are a much better home than that cold ole refrigerator."

Bacon is quickly invited to the party and the buttocks expand even more. More fatty items move into their geezy, saggy buttock accommodations. Soon the geezer's buttocks are overrun with fat population and the metropolitan area has surpassed Los Angeles in size. The geezer has grown a bouncy butt and then has the nerve to blame it on a baked potato.

Really? Was it really that wonderful, nutrition dense, nearly perfect potato that spread out and homesteaded your butt? Could it possibly have been due to all that fatty crap that you loaded onto it? Eat all the fatty stuff you want, but don't go around blaming the potato for your bouncy butt. The potato is simply a fall guy for some illogical decisions on the part of the bouncy-butt geezer. The potato is innocent of all charges.

There you have it. A baked potato is a survivalist dreamfood. It fills you up, stays with you, and does *not* make you fat. I've harped enough on what toppings should adorn your potato. Worcestershire sauce, low-sodium soy sauce, steak sauce, salsa, and countless other creative concoctions are good choices. A touch of cheese is okay if you don't go overboard. Just stay away from tipsy Aunt Blanche's fat-maker toppings unless you truly desire a bouncy butt.

BAKED POTATO CHIPS: Since we're discussing the horribly mistreated potato, this dish needs to be mentioned. Baked potato chips can satisfy you more than the bagged, processed, nutrition-less grease monsters you find on the grocery shelves. They can be a stand-alone meal in your never-ending quest for survival.

Here's how to make them. Get the oven going to a high temperature. You'll have to experiment as to what temperature works for you. Sometimes I'll start a little on the low side and crank it up at the end for exceptional crispness.

Cut a large potato or two into slices of varying thickness. You'll never know how thick you want them until you've experimented somewhat. I like the super-thin ones along with the thicker ones. Place the chips on a slightly oiled pan and into the oven. Go upstairs and call cousin Daisy. Listen to her moan about her miserable marriage and forget about the chips until the fire department knocks on your door.

Once you move into your new home because the other one burned to the ground, try making these again. Pull them out of the oven at the perfect moment. That last surge of high heat can really make them tasty. Now, what are you going to top them with?

Do we really have to get into this again? Don't ruin your chips with butt-growing substances! Ketchup is okay if you're sane about the amount. Mustard is an excellent choice, especially if you purchase the quality stuff. Penny-pinchers, let loose of some of that green and start living with some decent mustard. Come on, you're nearly dead at this stage of life, and you're still worried about a couple of dollars!

I won't bother you with what toppings are allowed and what are not allowed. If you don't know by now, then it's time to hang up your hat and give up. I know you're not going to do that. You're a winner. Make your chips tasty and flavorful by using the right toppings. You can do it, you old geezer!

FROZEN STUFF: Survival is accomplished by whatever methods available. That freezer of yours needs to be filled with good stuff only. Take a few moments and ruthlessly throw all your garbage-fatty food into the dumpster. Maybe some hungry raccoon will eat it. Do you see that little carton of sausages hidden in the back of the freezer that you bought in the early 70's? It's time to finally kiss it goodbye. Now go out and buy some healthy stuff and have it handy and ready to go.

In a time-pinch the frozen goodies can bail you out and you can stay on track. Keep some wise choices available. Frozen fish, scallops, shrimp, and the pre-discussed veggie burgers are a good start. There are also some great, healthy, frozen veggie pizzas in the marketplace now. Buy the stuff that either thaws quickly or it's made to go right into the oven. Remember, this is emergency food that keeps you away from the cookies and cream.

When you're totally wiped out and exhausted, you're not thinking straight. You can't allow those old cravings to grab hold. Make the right decision and make it quick. Chase those dastardly, big-butt-loving demons out of your kitchen before they sink their claws into you. Tell them to go see your friend Bessie down the block. She loves fatty stuff.

One last note about the frozen pizza option. I don't have to remind you to stay away from meaty pizzas, do I? Meaty pizza equates to meaty girl. You're so pretty, so don't mess yourself up by becoming meaty. Load your pizza ridiculously high with extra fresh veggies before you place it into the oven. Spice it up if you like. You've just converted it into a satisfying, yet incredibly healthy meal. I've eaten hundreds of these over the decades.

That's it for the staying-in-the-game recipes. Create some of your own. Use these valuable weapons. You'll wake up in the morning and be so proud that you're still standing tall and strong. You can do it. You know you can. Survive, baby!

I'm getting hungry,
Got lots of time.
I'm cooking healthy,
I'm gonna be fine!

My Personal Summation and Thanks

If you're reading this there's a good chance you've read my book. I thank you from the bottom of my heart. Writing a book is such a personal experience. It means so much when others choose to spend their precious time on my creation. There are a million other ways you could have spent your time, yet you chose my book. I am so grateful.

We're at an age of reflection. We're at a stage of life where certain things begin to take on value and others fall by the wayside. The old saying "You can't take it with you when you die," starts to make sense. There's more in our rearview mirror than is ahead of us.

We've all dealt with hardships. Death, divorce, sickness, deception, lies, greed, the list goes on and on. We've seen loved ones pass, experienced physical and emotional pain, and we've been hurt so bad that we wanted to die. We fight our own individual battles and we win some and lose some. It's been quite the journey, this thing we call life. All we can do is hang on as the world spins and hope we're not thrown off into the cosmos. I think no one has it completely figured out.

I wish all of you the best. I wish you joy and happiness, for they are so hard to find. I wish you peace and serenity, loving relations with your family and friends, and financial security.

You have become a piece of me by reading my book. I truly mean it. I hope it entertained you in some way as I know I drifted into pure silliness at times. I hope you use my information to become healthy and fit. I'm very confident in what I'm promoting. It will work if you will work.

So, that's it. Carry on with your lives as I will do the same. I don't expect any great changes in the way the world operates. It would be nice if someone or something took it by the reins and transformed it into a planet of pure love, joy and happiness. But it hasn't happened yet and I don't see it happening in our lifetime.

What we can do is try to make the world better by doing good things and showing compassion to every living creature. If all of us take this small step, maybe we can make a difference. To love others, you have to love yourself. I hope my book has grabbed a few of you and you're on your way to getting fit. You'll love yourself more and you can spread the love. Zarkoff Zucchini would be proud. Thank you and goodbye until next time, Spyder.

Thank you, readers,
It's been great.
You can do it,
Get in shape!